Micromanipulation in Assisted Conception

This practical handbook provides an extremely comprehensive, highly illustrated and up-to-date guide to micromanipulation techniques in assisted conception in a clinical setting. It includes detailed, illustrated descriptions of all the common micromanipulation systems currently in use in in vitro fertilization (IVF) laboratories around the world and explains clearly how to optimize their successful use. The volume covers state-of-the-art techniques, including intracytoplasmic sperm injection (ICSI), and procedures such as assisted hatching and blastomere biopsy (for pre-implantation genetic diagnosis). Valuable information on troubleshooting the potential mechanical and technical difficulties that can arise is provided to help all practitioners of these techniques, including trainee embryologists and consultant obstetricians, and technicians and scientists involved in animal transgenesis and cloning. It will undoubtedly be of immense value to all doctors and scientists working with assisted reproductive technologies.

Steven D. Fleming is currently a senior lecturer in reproductive medicine in the Department of Obstetrics and Gynaecology, University of Sydney (based at Westmead Hospital) and Scientific Director of Westmead Fertility Centre. After completing his PhD in 1987, he undertook postdoctoral research in the Human Reproduction Unit of the Department of Obstetrics and Gynaecology at the Royal North Shore Hospital in Sydney. From 1993 to 1997 he was appointed Lecturer in Obstetrics and Gynaecology at the University of Nottingham, UK, where he established the world's first master's degree in assisted reproduction technology with Simon Fishel as well as a summer school with Lars Hamberger at the University of Gothenburg in Sweden. He has also been invited to lecture on courses at the Bourn Hall Clinic in Cambridge and at University College London, UK, and he has acted as a consultant to assisted reproduction centres in Egypt, Greece, Jordan, Israel, Malaysia and Thailand. Since returning to Sydney in 1998, he has been elected on to the committee and appointed Chairman of the Education Sub-Committee of Scientists in Reproductive Technology, the scientific arm of the Fertility Society of Australia. He is the recipient of a National Health and Medical Research Council grant, and his extensive research activities have resulted in numerous publications in various books and peer-reviewed journals, as well as invitations to speak at and chair sessions at national and international conferences.

Robert S. King received his BSc in biological science from the University of Sussex in 1988 and his MSc in zoology from Cambridge University in 1992, investigating the role of birth date in neuronal identity. Since then, he has held various sales and marketing positions with Merck Sharp and Dohme, Narishige Europe Limited and Eppendorf Scientific. He is currently a product manager for Gene Transfer Instrumentation with Bio-Rad Laboratories in the San Francisco Bay area. In 1996, he was invited to lecture on microinjection at the annual meeting of the Middle East Fertility Society in Alexandria, Egypt. Over the last seven years, he has installed Narishige and Eppendorf microinjection systems in laboratories in the Middle East, Europe, Japan and North America, and trained researchers and embryologists in various microinjection techniques, including ICSI.

Micromanipulation in Assisted Conception

A Users' Manual and Troubleshooting Guide

Steven D. Fleming
and Robert S. King

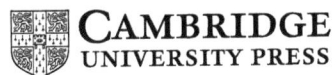

CAMBRIDGE
UNIVERSITY PRESS

CAMBRIDGE UNIVERSITY PRESS
Cambridge, New York, Melbourne, Madrid, Cape Town,
Singapore, São Paulo, Delhi, Mexico City

Cambridge University Press
The Edinburgh Building, Cambridge CB2 8RU, UK

Published in the United States of America by Cambridge University Press, New York

www.cambridge.org
Information on this title: www.cambridge.org/9781107406940

First published 2003
First paperback edition 2012

A catalogue record for this publication is available from the British Library

Library of Congress Cataloguing in Publication Data
Fleming, Steven D.
Micromanipulation in assisted conception: a users' manual and troubleshooting guide /
Steven D. Fleming & Robert S. King.
    p. cm.
Includes bibliographical references and index.
ISBN 0 521 64847 5
1. Fertilization in vitro, Human – Handbooks, manuals, etc. 2. Human reproductive
technology – Handbooks, manuals, etc. 3. Conception – Technological
innovations – Handbooks, manuals, etc. 4. Microsurgery – Handbooks, manuals, etc.
I. King, Robert S. II. Title.
RG135.F54 2003
618.1′78059–dc21   2003041954

ISBN 978-0-521-64847-9 Hardback
ISBN 978-1-107-40694-0 Paperback

Contents

Foreword

This is no ordinary book. It is a detailed description, such as has never been compiled before, of the current status of micromanipulation procedures. It describes in detail the various pieces of equipment and supplies necessary to set up the sophisticated procedures used in the treatment of male infertility, in characterizing early-stage embryos, and in performing procedures of mouse transgenesis. It is gratifying to see that this work is grounded in the belief that the key to micromanipulation is understanding the instruments, selecting the appropriate equipment, and picking the ideal consumables.

Since the first success of in vitro fertilization (IVF) in 1978, the field has been transformed by a steady stream of discovery and technological progress that has led to the expansion of the indications, such as the treatment of severe male infertility by intracytoplasmic sperm injection (ICSI) and the identification of genetic disorders by pre-implantation genetic diagnosis (PGD). These discoveries and techniques are grouped under the term 'assisted reproduction techniques'. For the first time, this book describes in a clear and concise manner the hows, whys and therefores of such procedures. It has been written to be readable and usable by research fellows, embryologists and technicians who need some insight into the technical developments, and who wish to know the A to Z of micromanipulation as seen and performed by the two authors.

It is always exciting to browse through a new book, particularly a manual, but as we go along we often notice that the information is too polished, presented from an ideal standpoint, and dealing with theoretical situations. Such material makes a good book, but from a practical point of view often may not prove to be very useful. During the preparation of this manual, the authors could have been trapped by the irresistible drive to be comprehensive and make a large book that would have lost practical usefulness and contact with the reality of micromanipulation.

Instead, Steven Fleming and Robert King have produced a work that stays on track. The authors deliver a quick, practical troubleshooting manual for the laboratory. This work will help scientists, embryologists and technicians feel secure in setting up their systems and dealing with the daily difficulties of micromanipulation. The manual integrates current successful procedures and some newer ones, such as nuclear transplantation and genetic engineering.

In short, the work is dynamic. There is an authoritative exposition of the different steps of micromanipulation, ranging from the routine of well-established procedures to the generation of new experimental animals. This manual represents a milestone in the literature of reproductive medicine and will benefit all who read it.

Gianpiero D. Palermo, M.D.
Director of Andrology and Assisted Fertilization,
Center for Reproductive Medicine and Infertility
Associate Professor of Reproductive Medicine,
Weill Medical College of Cornell University

Preface

A number of good books have been published on the scientific and technical aspects of micromanipulation. However, they are usually aimed at the experienced practitioner with limited benefit to those working in an environment that is often largely devoid of expert technical support. In contrast, the primary objective of this book is to provide an easy-to-follow, step-by-step guide to micromanipulation techniques, with an emphasis on troubleshooting the myriad difficulties inevitably encountered. Indeed, the original idea for this book arose from a chance meeting between the authors. We realized that we shared a common experience despite our diverse backgrounds. Having introduced students to the equipment and techniques involved in micromanipulation, much of our time was then spent acting on a long-distance consultancy basis once these students found themselves back in the 'real world' of a clinical assisted reproduction centre. In this respect, the authors have also recognized that many of these challenges are most likely common to those working within the related fields of human assisted reproduction, livestock production, endangered species preservation, and transgenic research. Therefore, an attempt has been made to direct the material at a broad readership wherever relevant.

It is important to appreciate that this is fundamentally a technical manual. Hence, the chapters are designed to be read not in any particular order but as required. Related information within the same chapter as well as within different chapters is cross-referenced wherever necessary. Abbreviations litter this field of work and, therefore, a list of abbreviations that relate specifically to the information in this book has been provided. Likewise, a glossary of terms has been provided to explain much of the terminology used within this book. Finally, full contact details for all the suppliers of equipment and consumables listed in this book have been provided; this list is by no means exhaustive, and neither is it intended to recommend one distributor over another.

While every effort has been made to ensure the technical information contained in this book is as up to date as possible, it should be noted that manufacturers reserve the right to change product specifications, to discontinue old product lines, and to introduce new instruments without prior notice. New products will invariably be introduced in the future, and it is hoped that these instruments can be covered in future editions.

The authors welcome feedback and further discussion regarding content.

Acknowledgements

The authors would like to thank the following individuals for their assistance in the preparation of this book: Eisuke Arinobe (Olympus Optical Company Limited) for providing one of the figures in Chapter 3; Bill Brown (Research Instruments Limited) for providing most of the information and figures for Chapter 5; Simon Cooke (IVF Australia at CityWest) for providing most of the information and figures for the section on visualization of the meiotic spindle for ICSI in Chapter 12; Chris Hall and David Hutchinson (Narishige Europe Limited) for information in Chapter 3; Joyce Harper (University College, London) for reviewing Chapter 9; Usanee Jetsawangsri (Jetanin Institute for Assisted Reproduction, Bangkok) for providing most of the figures in Chapter 9; Josephine Joya (Children's Medical Research Institute, Sydney) and Frances Lemckert (Children's Hospital at Westmead, Sydney) for providing most of the information and figures for Chapter 11; David Mortimer (Oozoa Biomedical Incorporated) for reviewing Chapters 2 and 7; Adair Oesterle and Dale Fleming (Sutter Instrument Company) for providing some of the information in Chapter 10; Norbert Rottmann (Eppendorf AG) for providing some of the information and figures for Chapter 4; and Aki Wakamiya (Nikon Corporation) for providing some of the figures in Chapter 3.

Glossary

Agglutination: The sticking together of large numbers of motile spermatozoa due to the presence of anti-sperm antibodies.

Aneuploidy: A condition where there is a loss or gain of chromosomes resulting in an alteration to the normal complement within a cell.

Assisted hatching: The partial or complete removal of the zona pellucida by zona drilling or by enzymatic means, the rationale being that this will enhance the ability of the blastocyst to escape from the zona pellucida and implant into the uterus.

Asthenozoospermia: Lower than normal percentage of progressively motile spermatozoa in the ejaculate.

Azoospermia: The total absence of spermatozoa within the ejaculate.

Blastomere: A cell of a pre-implantation embryo, from the two-cell stage to the blastocyst.

Blastomere biopsy: Removal of one or more blastomeres from an embryo for pre-implantation genetic diagnosis.

Calcium ionophore: A drug, such as A23187, that opens calcium channels in the plasmalemma, allowing calcium to enter the cell.

Cleavage: Series of mitotic cell divisions by which a zygote is transformed into a blastocyst.

Congenital bilateral absence of the vas deferens: Abnormality, often associated with the cystic fibrosis mutation, in which the vas deferens fails to develop on both sides, resulting in obstructive azoospermia.

Corona radiata: The layer of granulosa cells immediately surrounding the oocyte and in contact with the zona pellucida. Also termed the zona radiata.

Cryptozoospermia: An ejaculate that appears azoospermic until concentrated down by centrifugation, after which a few spermatozoa can be identified.

Cumulus oophorus: The cloud-like layer of granulosa cells that surrounds the oocyte and connects it to the granulosa.

Epididymis: A long, narrow, coiled tube lying on the anterodorsal aspect of the testis. The epididymis connects the rete testis to the vas deferens and is the site where spermatozoa undergo further maturation.

Fragile oocyte syndrome: A condition where oocytes that appear morphologically normal usually degenerate following injection. These oocytes are typically very easy to inject, their oolemma offering little resistance.

Globozoospermia: A condition in which spermatozoa lack an acrosome due to impaired spermiogenesis.

Headstage: The moving section of a manipulator (as opposed to the controller), usually mounted on the illumination support limb of a microscope.

Hypo-osmotic swelling test: The immersion of spermatozoa within hypo-osmotic media to determine the integrity of their plasmalemma. Intact cells take up water from the surrounding media by osmosis and swell to accommodate their increase in volume.

Hypospermatogenesis: A lower-than-normal level of spermatogenesis.

Immotile cilia syndrome: A lack of motility or aberrant motility of the cilium or flagellum of the spermatozoon, due to abnormal development or function of the axoneme. One typical example of this syndrome is Kartagener's Syndrome, in which the dynein arms of the axoneme are either too short or absent.

Manipulator: Any device that allows a probe or micropipette to be positioned in one or more dimensions (*see also Micromanipulator*).

Manipulator, coarse: Distinct from a micromanipulator, this device allows only approximate positioning in one or more dimensions, i.e. it has a lower resolution than a micromanipulator.

Micro-epididymal sperm aspiration: The collection of spermatozoa from the epididymis by passing a hypodermic needle into the surgically exposed epididymis under local or general anaesthesia, and then applying gentle suction.

Microinjection sperm transfer: The transfer of one or more spermatozoa into the perivitelline space using an injection pipette, and subsequently termed subzonal insemination.

Micromanipulator: A device for positioning a probe or micropipette extremely precisely in three dimensions, often to resolutions of less than 1 μm. Usually used in conjunction with a *coarse manipulator*.

Monopronucleate: Having a single pronucleus.

Multipronucleate: Having more than two pronuclei.

Non-obstructive azoospermia: Azoospermia due to failed or impaired spermatogenesis.

Normozoospermia: Normal density of spermatozoa within the ejaculate with a normal percentage of progressive motility and normal morphology.

Obstructive azoospermia: Azoospermia due to a blockage in the reproductive tract.

Oligozoospermia: Lower-than-normal density of spermatozoa in the ejaculate.

Oocyte: A diploid (primary) or haploid (secondary) germ cell that gives rise to an ovum via meiosis.

Oocyte activation: The stimulation of the oocyte by the fertilizing spermatozoon that results in the completion of fertilization and initiation of cleavage.

Oogenesis: Production and growth of ova that occurs within the ovary.

Oogonium: A premeiotic diploid germ cell that gives rise to oocytes via mitosis.

Oolemma: Another term for the vitelline membrane, the membrane surrounding and secreted by an oocyte.

Ooplasm: The cytoplasm of an oocyte.

Oscillin: The original term used to describe the putative factor released from the spermatozoon at fertilization, responsible for causing the oscillations in intracellular calcium that bring about egg activation.

Ovum: Mature, haploid female gamete.

Partial zona dissection: Another term for *zona drilling* and originally devised to enhance the passage of spermatozoa into the perivitelline space during in vitro fertilization.

Percutaneous epididymal sperm aspiration: The collection of spermatozoa from the epididymis by passing a hypodermic needle through the skin and into the epididymis under local or general anaesthesia, and then applying gentle suction.

Perivitelline space: The space surrounding the oocyte, lying between the oolemma and zona pellucida.

Phosphodiesterase inhibitors: Drugs such as pentoxifylline and caffeine that inhibit the breakdown of cyclic adenosine monophosphate (cAMP) by phosphodiesterase. The consequent elevation in cAMP causes enhancement of sperm motility.

Plasmalemma: The cell membrane.

Polygyny: Polyploidy as a result of a failure of the fertilized oocyte to extrude the second polar body.

Polyploidy: A condition in which there is a gain of one or more sets of chromosomes, resulting in an increase in the normal complement within a cell.

Polyspermy: Entry of more than one spermatozoon into an oocyte during fertilization, resulting in polyploidy.

Pre-implantation genetic diagnosis: The use of molecular biological techniques, such as fluorescent in situ hybridization and the polymerase chain reaction, to determine the chromosomal and genetic constitution of an embryo prior to its transfer to the uterus.

Pronucleus: The nucleus of a gamete that appears within a zygote at fertilization, just prior to *syngamy*.

Rescue intracytoplasmic sperm injection (ICSI): ICSI performed upon an oocyte that has failed to fertilize following in vitro fertilization.

Retrograde ejaculation: Ejaculation into the bladder instead of through the urethra, due to failure of the sphincter muscle at the neck of the bladder.

Seminiferous tubules: The long coiled tubules within the testis where spermatogenesis occurs.

Sertoli cell: A large cell within the testis responsible for the sustenance of spermatogonia, spermatocytes and spermatids.

Sertoli cell-only syndrome: A condition in which spermatogonia are largely or totally absent within the seminiferous tubules.

Spermatid: Immature, haploid spermatozoon.

Spermatocyte: A diploid (primary) or haploid (secondary) germ cell that gives rise to spermatids via meiosis.

Spermatogenesis: Production and growth of spermatozoa that occurs within the testis.

Spermatogenic arrest: A condition in which spermatogenesis fails to continue beyond a certain stage of germ cell development for genetic or other reasons.

Spermatogonium: A premeiotic diploid germ cell that gives rise to spermatocytes via mitosis.

Spermatozoon: Mature, haploid male gamete.

Spermiogenesis: Maturation of spermatids into spermatozoa.

Split ejaculate: An ejaculate that has been collected into two separate receptacles, one containing the initial part and the other containing the remainder.

Strict criteria: Highly specific morphological criteria that spermatozoa must meet in order to be considered normal. Also termed Tygerberg strict criteria and Kruger strict criteria.

Subzonal insemination: Another, more commonly used term for *microinjection sperm transfer*.

Suction-mediated aspiration of the rete testis: The collection of spermatozoa from the rete testis by passing a hypodermic needle through the skin and into the rete testis under local or general anaesthesia, and then applying gentle suction.

Syngamy: The fusion of the male and female pronuclei.

Teratozoospermia: Lower-than-normal percentage of morphologically normal spermatozoa in the ejaculate.

Testicular sperm aspiration: The collection of spermatozoa from the testis by passing a hypodermic needle through the skin and into the testis under local or general anaesthesia, and then applying gentle suction.

Testicular sperm extraction: The collection of spermatozoa from the testis by excising part of the surgically exposed testis under local or general anaesthesia.

Tripronucleate: Having three pronuclei.

Vital dyes: Dyes that have a molecular size too large to cross an intact cell plasmalemma, used to determine cell viability.

***x*-axis:** The horizontally oriented axis aligned from left to right, with respect to the microscope.

***y*-axis:** The horizontally oriented axis aligned from front to back, with respect to the microscope.

***z*-axis:** The vertically oriented (up-and-down) axis.

Zona drilling: The making of a passage through the *zona pellucida* by mechanical or chemical means, or with the use of a laser.

Zona pellucida: Acellular, striated glycoprotein membrane normally surrounding the oocyte.

Zona radiata: Another term for the corona radiata.

Zygote: The fertilized ovum, prior to cleavage.

Abbreviations

AH	assisted hatching
cAMP	cyclic adenosine monophosphate
CBAVD	congenital bilateral absence of the vas deferens
COC	cumulus–oocyte complex
DIC	differential interference contrast
DMEM	Dulbecco's modified Eagle's medium
EBSS	Earle's balanced salt solution
EDTA	ethylene diamine tetra-acetic acid
EKRB	enriched Krebs–Ringer bicarbonate
ELSI	elongated spermatid injection
EMEM	Eagle's modified minimal essential medium with Earle's Salts
ESC	embryonic stem cell
ET	embryo transfer
FACS	fluorescence-activated cell sorting
FBS	fetal bovine serum
FCS	fetal calf serum
FISH	fluorescent in situ hybridization
FSH	follicle-stimulating hormone
GIFT	gamete intrafalloplan transfer
GV	germinal vesicle
GVBD	germinal vesicle breakdown
hCG	human chorionic gonadotrophin
HIC	high insemination concentration
HMEM	Hepes-buffered minimal essential medium
hMG	human menopausal gonadotrophin
HOST	hypo-osmotic swelling test
HSA	human serum albumin
HTF	human tubal fluid
ICM	inner cell mass

ICSI	intracytoplasmic sperm injection
IUI	intrauterine insemination
IVF	in vitro fertilization
IVM	in vitro maturation
LASU	laser setting-up device
LH	luteinizing hormone
LIF	leukaemia inhibitory factor
MEM	minimal essential medium
MESA	micro-epididymal sperm aspiration
MHC	major histocompatibility complex
MI	metaphase 1
MII	metaphase 2
MIST	microinjection sperm transfer
OHSS	ovarian hyperstimulation syndrome
PB	polar body
PB1	first polar body
PB2	second polar body
PBS	phosphate-buffered saline
PCOD	polycystic ovarian disease
PCR	polymerase chain reaction
PESA	percutaneous epididymal sperm aspiration
PGD	pre-implantation genetic diagnosis
PMSG	pregnant mare's serum gonadotrophin
PN	pronucleus
PVP	polyvinylpyrrolidone
PVS	perivitelline space
PZD	partial zona dissection
ROSI	round spermatid injection
ROSNI	round spermatid nucleus injection
SAS	screw-actuated syringe
SCNT	somatic cell nuclear transfer
SESI	secondary spermatocyte injection
SMART	suction-mediated aspiration of the rete testis
SSR	surgical sperm recovery
SUZI	subzonal insemination
TAE	Tris-acetate/ethylene diamine tetra-acetic acid
TCM	tissue culture medium
TESA	testicular sperm aspiration
TESE	testicular sperm extraction
TMC	total motile count

TNF   tumour necrosis factor
VSUG   velocity sedimentation under unit gravity
WHO   World Health Organization
ZD   zona drilling
ZIFT   zygote intrafallopian transfer
ZP   zona pellucida

1 Micromanipulation in human assisted conception: an overview

1.1 A SHORT HISTORY AND BACKGROUND TO IN VITRO FERTILIZATION, INTRACYTOPLASMIC SPERM INJECTION AND ASSOCIATED TECHNIQUES

On 25 July in 1978, Louise Joy Brown, the world's first baby to be born as a result of in vitro fertilization (IVF), heralded a breakthrough in the alleviation of infertility. Over a million babies have now been born as a result of IVF. However, this relatively simple technique of placing eggs into medium containing thousands of sperm is of benefit only to those patients with the ability to produce large numbers of highly motile, normally shaped spermatozoa. Cases involving sperm disorders, however, are less likely to possess an adequate number of functional spermatozoa, with normal cleavage of any fertilized eggs also being less likely to occur.

Initially, most patients with male-factor infertility were treated empirically (e.g. using anti-oestrogens, gonadotrophins, androgens and antibiotics) in an attempt to optimize their semen profile, but without any great proven success. Modifications in preparation (e.g. discontinuous density gradient centrifugation purification and metabolic stimulation with phosphodiesterase inhibitors) and insemination procedures (e.g. high insemination concentration and short-duration inseminations) improve the fertilizing potential of spermatozoa but only in those amenable to such treatment (e.g. those with more than 500 000 progressively motile sperm). Hence, those with severe male-factor infertility have had to wait until the last decade of the twentieth century, during which time the application of micromanipulation technology and surgical sperm-recovery techniques have allowed us to offer hope to these patients.

It was not until almost a decade after the birth of Louise Brown that micromanipulation techniques were first applied successfully to the treatment of male-factor infertility (see Table 1.1). Following the initial development of a zona drilling (ZD) technique in a mouse model (Gordon and

Table 1.1 *Chronological evolution of micromanipulation techniques*

Year	Technique	Pioneers in the field
1987	MIST[a]	Laws-King *et al.*
1988	MIST[a]	Ng *et al.*
1988	ZD	Gordon *et al.*
1988	PZD	Cohen *et al.*
1988	ICSI	Lanzendorf *et al.*
1990	AH	Cohen *et al.*
1990	PGD[b]	Handyside *et al.*
1992	ICSI	Palermo *et al.*
1995	ELSI	Fishel *et al.*
1995	ROSI	Tesarik *et al.*
1998	SESI	Sofikitis *et al.*

[a] MIST later became termed SUZI. [b] PGD relies upon the techniques of ZD and blastomere biopsy.

ELSI, elongated spermatid injection; ROSI, round spermatid injection; SESI, secondary spermatocyte injection.

Talansky, 1986), various methods were rapidly adapted for use in the alleviation of male-factor infertility. Partial zona dissection (PZD) was introduced in an attempt to improve the chances of fertilization by sperm failing to overcome the zona pellucida (ZP), the oocyte's first and major barrier (Cohen *et al.*, 1988; Gordon *et al.*, 1988). Unfortunately, this never proved to be a reliably effective remedy (especially in terms of normal fertilization, which was less than 25%), presumably due to the varied aetiology of male infertility. At around the same time, the technique of microinjection sperm transfer (MIST) was pioneered (Laws-King *et al.*, 1987; Ng *et al.*, 1988). This comprised the injection of 5–20 sperm into the perivitelline space (PVS) between the ZP and oolemma, and was later termed subzonal insemination (SUZI). It was used successfully with both freshly ejaculated and frozen sperm, and pregnancies were achieved following embryo transfer (ET) and zygote intrafallopian transfer (ZIFT). Incredibly, this technique was reported to have been used to achieve fertilization even in an individual with immotile cilia syndrome (Bongso *et al.*, 1989). However, monospermic fertilization rates were generally less than 25%; consequently, less than 70% of patients progressed to ET, resulting in pregnancy rates of less than 10%. Also, SUZI was unable to overcome infertility resulting from an inability of spermatozoa to undergo the acrosome reaction (Sathananthan *et al.*, 1989). Centres in the USA and Singapore then began to push the SUZI technique one step further, so pioneering intracytoplasmic sperm injection (ICSI) in humans (Lanzendorf *et al.*, 1988; Ng *et al.*, 1991). However, it was not until 1992 that the first pregnancies in humans were reported, with implantation rates of about 20% per embryo replaced (Palermo *et al.*, 1992). The efficacy of ICSI rapidly became apparent as other centres around the world confirmed the initial data of Palermo and colleagues. Meanwhile, ZD techniques were being applied to embryos as a putative means of assisted hatching (AH) (Cohen *et al.*, 1990), and this development also facilitated blastomere biopsy methods for pre-implantation genetic diagnosis (PGD).

Surgical sperm recovery can be used in conjunction with ICSI for patients with obstructive or non-obstructive azoospermia, making fertilization a possibility even for very severe cases, such as hypospermatogenesis, Sertoli cell-only syndrome and spermatogenic arrest, where pockets of spermatogenic activity not identified by previous biopsy may persist. Sperm may be recovered from the epididymis by percutaneous epididymal sperm aspiration (PESA) or micro-epididymal sperm aspiration (MESA), or from the testis by suction-mediated aspiration of the rete testis (SMART), testicular sperm aspiration (TESA) or testicular sperm extraction (TESE), the least invasive technique necessary being the preferred approach. Sperm recovered surgically are usually motile when aspirated or following a short period of in vitro culture. Even if the sperm should prove totally and permanently immotile, they may nevertheless be viable and can be identified as such using vital dyes (e.g. trypan blue; see section 2.1.4) and selected for ICSI using the hypo-osmotic swelling test (HOST; see section 2.1.4), which is non-toxic. For patients with obstructive azoospermia, such as failed vasectomy reversals and those with congenital bilateral absence of the vas deferens (CBAVD), pregnancy rates of more than 30% arc possible. Those with non-obstructive azoospermia tend to have lower pregnancy rates, those with more severe aetiologies, such as immotile cilia syndrome and globozoospermia (spermatozoa devoid of their acrosomal cap), having very limited success.

Allied to various techniques of surgical sperm recovery, ICSI has become a powerful means of overcoming infertility in azoospermic patients. Indeed, freshly collected and frozen-thawed sperm from the ejaculate, epididymis or testis have all been found to be equally suitable for ICSI (Nagy *et al.*, 1995c). Even patients with globozoospermia were found to be capable of achieving pregnancy with the aid of ICSI (Lundin *et al.*, 1994). However, it is important to appreciate that ICSI is not the panacea for all forms of infertility.

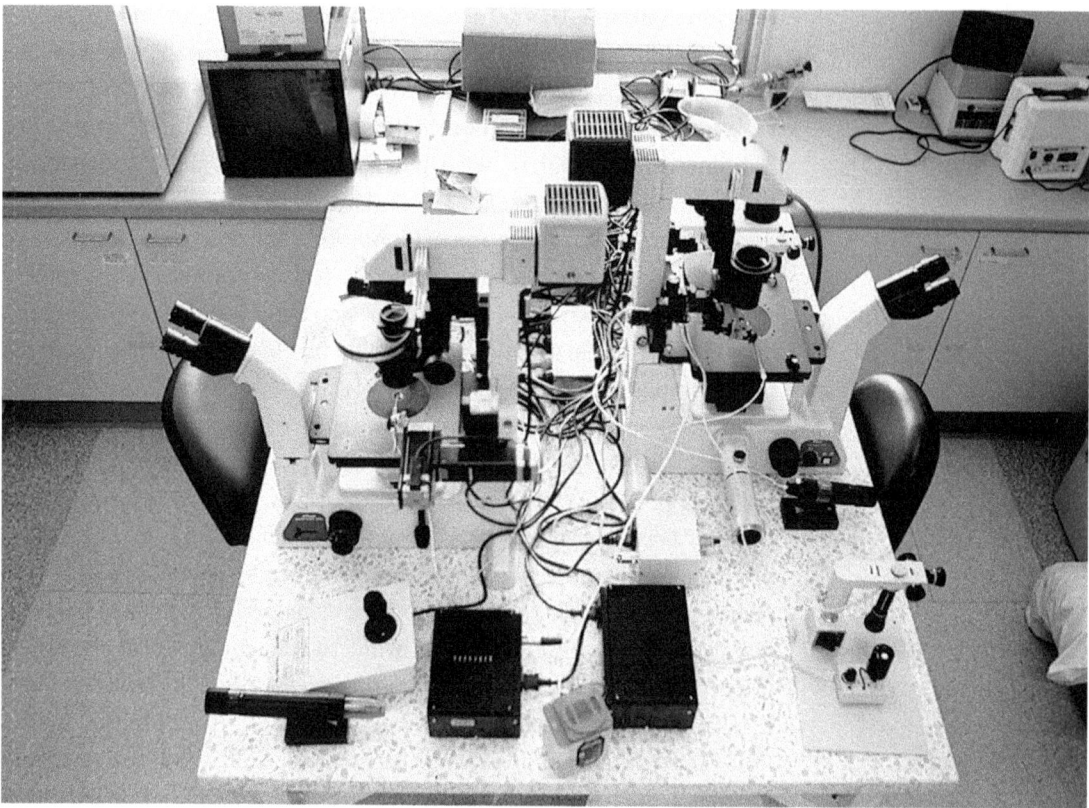

Figure 1.1 This micromanipulation workstation is comprised of two inverted microscopes supported by a solid table made from terrazzo concrete. Micromanipulators are mounted on to the microscope pillars and bear microtool holders that are connected to microinjectors. Hoffman modulation contrast is employed to optimize optics using plastic Petri dishes, and the microscope stages are heated to help maintain cell viability. Video cameras are fitted to the microscopes for the purpose of viewing and recording procedures using the TV monitor and video recorder.

As a result of the development of ICSI, the modern infertility laboratory is now typified by the presence of inverted microscopes bearing micromanipulation equipment employing microtools (see Figure 1.1). ICSI mimics the later stages of fertilization, ensuring delivery of the requirements of the oocyte for fertilization to proceed with subsequent embryogenesis. The essential factors provided by the sperm are:

- paternal DNA for the embryonic genome;
- the proximal centriole from the neck of the sperm, which helps form the mitotic spindle for cell division;
- an egg-activating sperm cytosolic factor, originally termed 'oscillin' due to its ability to stimulate transient elevations of intracellular calcium within the oocyte.

Employing specific steps designed to convey these factors to the oocyte, ICSI results in fertilization, cleavage, pregnancy, implantation and live birth rates comparable to those achieved with standard, routine IVF.

Unfortunately, in some individuals mature sperm cannot be found despite extensive regional testicular biopsy. Usually, such patients have

Figure 1.2 Spermatogenesis occurs within the seminiferous tubules of the testis, where all stages of sperm cell are nurtured by Sertoli cells. As spermatogenesis proceeds, the sperm cells migrate from the basal lamina to the lumen of the seminiferous tubule. Diploid spermatogonia proliferate mitotically to give rise to primary spermatocytes, and these divide meiotically to yield haploid secondary spermatocytes. The secondary spermatocytes undergo a further meiotic division and, hence, each primary spermatocyte gives rise to four round spermatids, each of which is destined to differentiate into a functional mature spermatozoon.

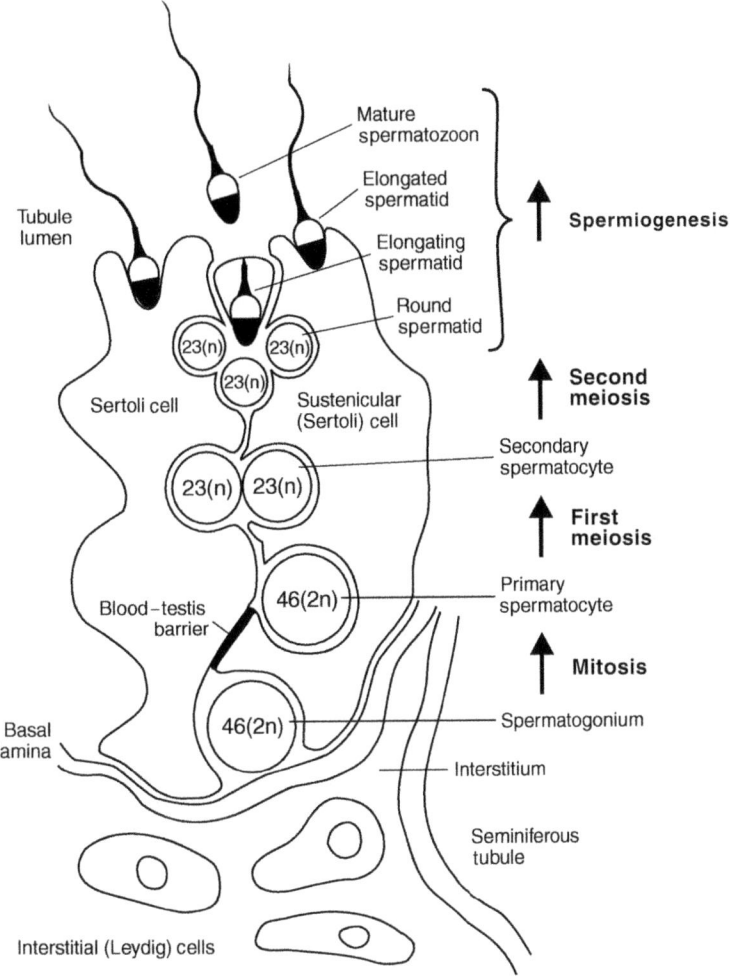

suffered either early or late spermatogenic arrest. Depending on the stage of maturation arrest, it may be possible to identify spermatogonia, spermatocytes and spermatids. Secondary spermatocytes and spermatids, like spermatozoa, are haploid gametes that have yet to undergo spermiogenesis (see Figure 1.2), a process of differentiation designed largely for sperm transport. During spermiogenesis, a round spermatid becomes elongated to form a spermatozoon. Nevertheless, all three components required by the oocyte for fertilization and embryogenesis would appear to be present in these immature haploid gametes. In practice, elongated spermatids have been injected using the ICSI technique (Fishel *et al.*, 1995a), and round spermatids and secondary spermatocytes have been incorporated into the egg using either electrofusion or ICSI (Sofikitis *et al.*, 1998; Tesarik *et al.*, 1995).

Compared with the use of spermatozoa, fertilization rates when using immature sperm are far lower, and pregnancy rates are lower with round spermatids than with elongated spermatids. The first live birth from a spermatid pregnancy was reported from the UK in 1995 (Fishel *et al.*, 1995a), this from elongated spermatid ICSI (ELSI). Pregnancies using round spermatid ICSI (ROSI) were reported in the same year (Tesarik *et al.*, 1995). More recently, a pregnancy following assisted fertilization using a secondary spermatocyte has been reported (Sofikitis *et al.*, 1998). Naturally, the data available in this area are somewhat limited. Nevertheless, a study conducted by Bob Schoysman's group in Belgium has provided some useful information (Vanderzwalmen *et al.*, 1997). By comparing spermatid ICSI with and without using the calcium ionophore A23187, their work suggests a requirement of the oocyte for exogenous activation by extracellular calcium under these circumstances. Indeed, it has been suggested that the oocyte-activating pattern of spermatids is inappropriate for development (Yazawa *et al.*, 2000). Hence, it may be that the ICSI technique for spermatids requires further modification or that round spermatids contain insufficient oscillin, if any at all. Alternatively, in vitro maturation (IVM) of immature sperm may prove to be the way forward in the treatment of such individuals (Aslam and Fishel, 1998; Tesarik *et al.*, 1998; Tesarik *et al.*, 1999). Indeed, elongated spermatids derived from the IVM of round spermatids have been shown to be capable of supporting fertilization and embryogenesis (Cremades *et al.*, 2001).

1.2 THE LEARNING CURVE AND ICSI TRAINING

ICSI is now considered a routine technique and, consequently, experienced embryologists are usually expected to be proficient in it. However, it remains one of the most demanding techniques to master, due partly to its inherent technical difficulty and partly to the heterogeneity of the cases encountered for treatment. Hence, the learning curve is invariably a long one, and it is not unusual to experience a dip in performance at an early stage following the acquisition of apparent proficiency in the technique. Therefore, it is important to establish training criteria and performance thresholds that should be met in order to attain the experience necessary to treat patients independently. Equally, it is desirable that appropriate quality control measures be implemented in order to ensure that such performance thresholds, once achieved, are maintained.

The first requirement should be that the trainee is fully conversant with the setting up and operation of the micromanipulation equipment. This may seem like an obvious statement; however, eagerness to perform ICSI sometimes enables trainees to convince themselves and others that they know how to use the equipment properly when in fact they do not. In this respect, it is most important that the trainee be encouraged to develop a routine of adjusting the equipment to a preset zero point and of following a step-by-step procedure from coarse through to fine control.

Once the trainee has become familiar with the micromanipulation controls, they can then proceed to setting up and acquiring a feel for the sensitivity and control of the injectors. The most suitable approach for this is to concentrate on one injector at a time, ideally using similar material to that which will be used in practice. For example, the trainee can begin by practising with aspirating one or more of the following:

- an immature oocyte;
- an oocyte that has failed to fertilize;
- a polyploid zygote.

Control of the holding pipette has to be practised until the trainee is able to efficiently place the oocyte with its polar body (if it has one) in the appropriate position without undue distortion of the oolemma. This can be followed by practice on the other injector, using spermatozoa that are not required for patient treatment. This involves simply aspirating spermatozoa into and out of an injecting pipette, assessing the control required to bring them to a point just short of the pipette opening, and holding them in that position.

Familiarity with the micromanipulators and injectors allows the trainee to progress to using them concurrently so that they may effectively manipulate the gametes in a way that mimics a treatment scenario. A good initial exercise is to practise permanently damaging the flagellum of spermatozoa before aspirating them into an injection pipette and stabilizing them at a given point within the pipette. Next, mock injections (without spermatozoa) can be practised on the type of oocytes described above, to learn how to effectively penetrate the ZP and oolemma. Only once these techniques have been perfected should the trainee proceed to attempting to inject a spermatozoon into an oocyte (it is important to be aware that national or state regulations may have to come into consideration at this point).

Generally accepted criteria for competence in ICSI include an oocyte degeneration rate of less than 15% (ideally, less than 10%) and a fertilization rate of more than 50% (ideally, more than 60%). However, it is neither in the interest of the patients nor fair to the trainee to allow them to initially put their training into practice in an unrestricted manner. Therefore, it is good policy for certain milestones to be reached whilst the trainee attains greater independence. For example, a trainee can be restricted to injecting just three oocytes in cases where there are at least 12 mature oocytes for ICSI. Once the trainee has demonstrated an ability to achieve fertilization in one or two of the three oocytes injected (without damaging more than one of them) on three consecutive occasions, they may be considered ready to progress to dealing with half of the oocytes in a given case. Again, though, there should be at least 12 mature oocytes available for ICSI. Similar performance thresholds can then be applied before allowing the trainee to progress to handling an entire case independently. Nevertheless, no trainee should be pressured into accepting increased responsibility before they feel ready, and there should always be provision for stepping back to the security of having to handle only half case-loads for both trainee and ICSI-trained embryologist alike. This is a valid point when one considers the fact that there is often a dip in performance at some stage during the apprenticeship of an embryologist aiming to become competent at ICSI. Once trained, annual returns on the percentage of oocytes damaged, fertilized, cleaved and resulting in good-quality embryos provide a good form of quality assurance. Naturally, pregnancies resulting from embryos derived through ICSI provide further quality assurance, but they are also subject to variables other than injection technique.

1.3   PATIENT GROUPS AMENABLE TO TREATMENT WITH ICSI

It could be argued that all patient groups should be treated with ICSI. However, this argument is neither valid nor proven, and it should be remembered that ICSI is labour-intensive and is a more invasive technique than standard IVF. Therefore, especially while there remain concerns over the long-term safety of ICSI, it should be viewed as an insemination option only for specific aetiologies of infertility. The groups most amenable to treatment with ICSI are predominantly male-factor patients, although there are also some female-factor patients that fall into this category (see Table 1.2).

1.3.1   Oligo-, astheno- and teratozoospermia

In the absence of any prior treatment information, varying degrees of oligo-, astheno- and teratozoospermia constitute the typical parameters that can be used to determine the most appropriate form of treatment for patients. Clearly, those patients with severe oligozoospermia (including those with cryptozoospermia and azoospermia) or severe asthenozoospermia (including cryopreserved sperm presenting upon thawing with poor motility, and those patients with immotile cilia syndrome) readily fall into the category of patients amenable to treatment with ICSI (see Table 1.2). The degree of teratozoospermia that renders a patient suitable

Table 1.2 *Patient groups typically amenable to treatment with ICSI*

Asthenozoospermia
Azoospermia
Cryptozoospermia
Ejaculatory dysfunction
Globozoospermia
Oligozoospermia
Repeated fertilization failure with standard IVF
Teratozoospermia

for treatment with ICSI is less easy to define. This is partly because of the different staining techniques and criteria for normal morphology employed, and partly because of the large coefficient of variation that is known to exist with the assessment of sperm morphology. Also, in view of the variation in normal morphology that is known to exist even between sequential ejaculates, it is preferable that analysis of sperm morphology be carried out on the sample to be used on the day. Nevertheless, patients with teratozoospermia due to globozoospermia clearly fall into the ICSI category of treatment. Furthermore, apart from those patients with globozoospermia, the degree of oligoasthenoteratozoospermia does not appear to influence ICSI outcome (Fishel *et al.*, 1995b; Nagy *et al.*, 1995a; Svalander *et al.*, 1996).

Where such impairments of sperm quality are less severe, in the majority of cases there is good evidence that high insemination concentration (HIC) IVF will result in successful fertilization (Fishel *et al.*, 1995b; Hall *et al.*, 1995a). This is presumably due to the effective number of fertile sperm that this technique makes available to the oocyte. Furthermore, the separation of spermatozoa from semen using density gradient separation is known to enhance the percentage of morphologically normal, motile spermatozoa in the insemination preparation (Fleming *et al.*, 1994; Hall *et al.*, 1995b; Vanderzwalmen *et al.*, 1991). However, the efficacy and consistency of density gradient separation is believed to be impaired in samples from oligozoospermic and asthenozoospermic individuals. Indeed, this also appears to hold true for patients with very severe teratozoospermia (less than 5% normal morphology, using Kruger strict criteria; Kruger *et al.*, 1987). In this category, density gradient separation results in no improvement, whereas it enhances sperm morphology in those with less severe teratozoospermia (5–14% normal morphology, using strict criteria) and normozoospermia (greater than 14% normal morphology, using strict criteria; Fleming *et al.*, 1994; Hall *et al.*, 1995b).

Table 1.3 *Semen analysis parameters and recommended modes of insemination*

Category	Parameters	Mode of insemination
ICSI only	TMC < 5 million or Normal morphology < 1% or A + B motility < 25%	ICSI
Split treatment	TMC ≥ 10 million and A + B motility ≥ 25% 0% grade A motility or Normal morphology <5%	ICSI/HIC-IVF
IVF only	TMC ≥ 10 million and A + B motility ≥ 25% 1–9% grade A motility or Normal morphology 5–14% ≥ 10% grade A motility	HIC-IVF/IVF
	and Normal morphology ≥ 15%	IVF

Where a split mode of insemination is indicated, the first line of treatment is listed before the second line of treatment, the latter being employed only if there are at least ten eggs available (at least six mature eggs should be available for ICSI in ICSI/HIC splits). Morphological analysis and motility are based upon WHO criteria (World Health Organization, 1999).
TMC, total motile count.

Hence, with a view to choosing the most appropriate choice of treatment, various factors must be taken into consideration when analysing the raw ejaculate (see Table 1.3). These factors include the total motile count, the quality of sperm progression (rather than the percentage of motile spermatozoa), and the percentage of morphologically normal spermatozoa present, before and after preparation.

1.3.2 Anti-sperm antibodies

Certain groups of men, with a high titre of anti-sperm antibodies, may be treated more effectively with ICSI. In this respect, the presence of anti-sperm antibodies within seminal fluid, as a result of disruption of the blood–testis barrier by inflammation, gonadal trauma or vasectomy, leads to greater impairment of fertility than their presence within serum. The presence of anti-sperm antibodies is often revealed by patchy or linear

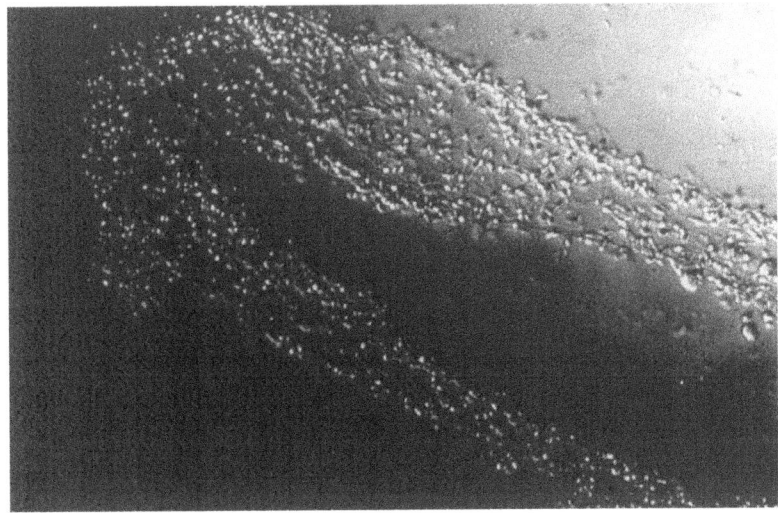

Figure 1.3 Semen that contains antibodies may present as either patchy or linear agglutination of motile spermatozoa. In this example, linear agglutination is apparent, the spermatozoa having been immobilized into long swathes.

agglutination of spermatozoa (see Figure 1.3). Again, the titre or isotype of antibody present does not appear to influence ICSI outcome.

1.3.3   Non-ejaculated spermatozoa

Patients from whom spermatozoa are recovered following retrograde ejaculation or surgical sperm recovery are also amenable to treatment with ICSI. The reason for this is that sperm motility and viability may be affected adversely by exposure to acidic conditions during retrograde ejaculation, and standard IVF using epididymal or testicular sperm results in poor fertilization rates, regardless of the concentration and motility of sperm recovered (Silber *et al.*, 1994). In this respect, it is known that spermatozoa recovered from the epididymis exhibit markedly impaired motility, progression and morphology compared with those from the ejaculate (Ord *et al.*, 1992).

1.3.4   Poor or failed fertilization

A cycle of standard IVF may result in poor or failed fertilization due to a sperm factor, an oocyte factor or, occasionally, a combination of both. However, it is well known that the majority of cases will succeed with a successive cycle of IVF (Lipitz *et al.*, 1994). Therefore, it is important to ascertain, if possible, the cause of the poor result, and, if appropriate, to attempt a further cycle of IVF (preferably HIC-IVF) before proceeding to ICSI. Also, it is possible to perform rescue ICSI on the morning that a failed fertilization is discovered (Nagy *et al.*, 1993b; Tsirigotis *et al.*, 1994; Sjogren *et al.*, 1995; Lundin *et al.*, 1996). However, there may be national regulations preventing this practice (e.g. as laid down by the Human Fertilisation and Embryology Authority in the UK) due to the perceived increased risk of resultant polyspermia or chromosomal aberration within aged oocytes. Also, it should be appreciated that the success rate of this technique, even with the use of a freshly prepared sperm sample, is very low (Kuczynski *et al.*, 2002; Lundin *et al.*, 1996).

If the cause of fertilization failure can be traced to total failure of spermatozoa to bind to the ZP, presumably due to some morphological or biochemical impairment, then ICSI is warranted in any future cycle of treatment. Ideally, the ability of donor sperm to bind to the unfertilized oocytes should be tested as a positive control. Likewise, ICSI would be the future treatment of choice in the event that binding is good but the spermatozoa have failed to fuse with the oolemma due to an unusual thickness (greater than 15 μm) of the ZP, this feature being observed more often in oocytes aspirated from perimenopausal women. However, if poor fertilization has resulted simply because few of the oocytes prove to be mature, or due to an unusually poor semen sample on the day of treatment, then the indications are that a further cycle of IVF may well succeed. In this instance, a split treatment of ICSI/HIC-IVF is optimal as this resolves the issue while guarding against a successive fertilization failure.

1.3.5 Pre-implantation genetic diagnosis

Patients who opt for PGD of their embryos before transfer, e.g. to avoid the transmission of sex-linked disease for which one or both parents are known to be carriers, are particularly suitable for treatment by ICSI. This is because of the increased likelihood of a misdiagnosis of blastomeres biopsied from embryos resulting from standard IVF, due to the possibility of there being additional spermatozoa embedded in the ZP or even free within the PVS. The techniques of fluorescent in situ hybridization (FISH) and polymerase chain reaction (PCR) used in PGD are certainly sensitive enough to pick up a stray X- or Y-bearing spermatozoon leading to an erroneous result.

1.3.6 Other indications

In some patient subgroups, poor-quality embryos are believed to be the result of overexposure of oocytes to excessive levels of reactive oxygen species generated by spermatozoa during standard IVF and especially during HIC-IVF. There is evidence that this effect may be abrogated by reducing the duration of insemination to as little as one hour (Gianaroli *et al.*, 1996a; Gianaroli *et al.*, 1996b; Hall and Fleming, 2001). Clearly, the use of ICSI in such situations avoids this potential problem altogether.

Occasionally, standard IVF may result in a repeated high incidence of polyspermy, leading to embryos that are not suitable for transfer. One option in such instances is to reduce the insemination concentration to below usual levels, but with this practice there is always the risk of a failed fertilization. Reducing the duration of exposure of the gametes to one hour is another option, but this is not guaranteed to solve the problem. An alternative option is to employ ICSI, so ensuring that only a single spermatozoon enters each oocyte.

1.4 PATIENT GROUPS NOT AMENABLE TO TREATMENT WITH ICSI

Since ICSI is a powerful, invasive technique able to short-circuit most barriers to fertilization, it should be used responsibly and with care. As such, there do exist patient subgroups that clearly should not be encouraged to have treatment by ICSI. For example, a very small number of men are known to produce spermatozoa that are all aneuploid, those that are diploid or polyploid usually being identified easily by virtue of their large head size, making it impossible to aspirate them into an ICSI pipette of standard dimensions.

Another subgroup of patients that do not respond well to treatment with ICSI include those that consistently produce very poor-quality oocytes, characterized by a centrally located dark area of ooplasm, typical of degenerating oocytes. These oocytes often fail to fertilize, fertilize abnormally (i.e. monopronucleate or tripronucleate zygotes result), or degenerate following injection. Yet another patient subgroup appears to produce fragile oocytes, their oocytes appearing normal in appearance but usually degenerating following injection. Ironically, such oocytes are usually easy to inject as a result of their poor membrane integrity, but this is often an ominous indication for a poor prognosis. Therefore, it may be prudent to employ IVF in patients presenting with this fragile oocyte syndrome, even if the fertilization rates prove to be low, rather than subject them to ICSI with resultant degeneration of all the oocytes.

Finally, it has to be accepted that current success rates with ICSI from patients in whom only immature spermatozoa can be retrieved are currently extremely disappointing. There are probably several reasons for this, including the difficulty in identifying viable, round spermatids and secondary spermatocytes in unstained specimens at the level of the light microscope. Therefore, patient groups in which only immature spermatozoa can be recovered are consequently not particularly amenable to treatment with ICSI, at least until better methods are developed that result in higher fertilization and pregnancy rates.

2 Media and other consumables for micromanipulation

This intention of this chapter is not to provide a fully comprehensive listing of all consumables, and suppliers thereof, that may be used for micromanipulation. Rather, the emphasis is on the requirement for specific types of materials to perform different aspects of micromanipulation technique. In most instances, a given type of consumable is often provided by a number of different suppliers, the choice usually being determined by personal preference. In this respect, most of the suppliers listed are either internationally well established or those with which the authors have dealt with in the past. Therefore, although these may not be the very best available, in most instances they have at least been tried and have been proven suitable for the purpose for which they are intended.

2.1 MATERIALS REQUIRED FOR THE PREPARATION OF SPERMATOZOA

It must be appreciated that spermatozoa are living cells and, therefore, should be handled gently during preparation. This point is particularly pertinent to samples with reduced viability, such as those sometimes recovered from surgical aspiration of the epididymis or testis. Also, occasionally samples with an intrinsically short lifespan are encountered. Therefore, handling should be minimized to that sufficient to provide spermatozoa in a condition free of debris, suitable for micromanipulation. In this respect, parameters such as the buffer employed in the medium to maintain physiological pH and the temperature at which the medium is maintained are less critical, as human spermatozoa are particularly susceptible only to acidic conditions and do not exhibit 'cold-shock'. Hence, they may be prepared at room temperature using bicarbonate-buffered medium without any detrimental effect. Indeed, it may be deleterious to samples with compromised viability to store them in an incubator set at 37 °C.

Figure 2.1 To be suitable for semen collection, specimen jars must be non-toxic and sterile, such as the urine collection containers available from LIP and Sarstedt.

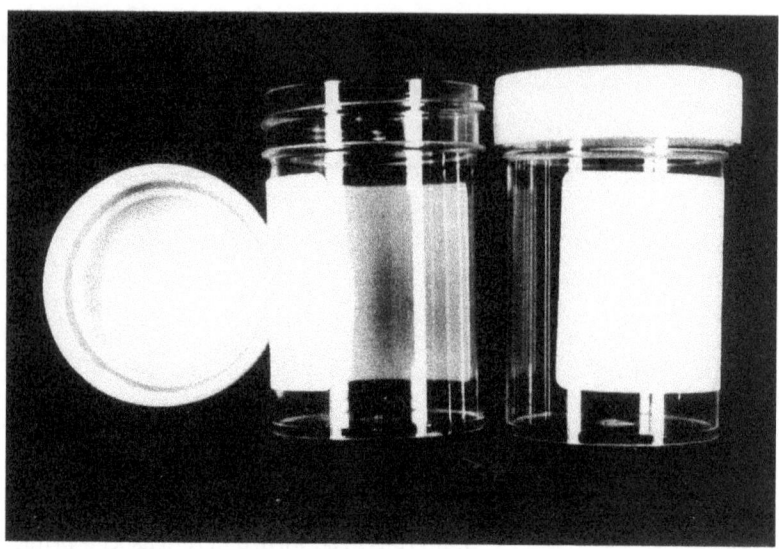

2.1.1 Plasticware and glass consumables

Semen may be produced as a combined or split ejaculate, and can be collected directly into sterile specimen jars (see Figure 2.1). Split ejaculates are particularly beneficial where low numbers of spermatozoa are present within a large volume of seminal plasma. This is because preparation of the initial, spermatozoa-rich part of the semen sample may be performed more efficiently due to the reduced volume of ejaculate, resulting in a better yield.

Handling of the ejaculate and surgically recovered aspirate or biopsy can be achieved with either sterile, tissue-culture-grade plastic (such as that available from Falcon) or glass Pasteur pipettes (such as those available from Sigma). However, if using glass pipettes, it is important to use those manufactured from borosilicate glass, as those manufactured from soda-lime release sodium ions into the medium, and these are detrimental to embryogenesis. Also, it is necessary to flame the opening of glass Pasteur pipettes in order to create a bevel, so avoiding the scratching of any plasticware that could release potentially toxic shards of plastic into the medium. Of course, if glass Pasteur pipettes have been bevelled or flame-sterilized, then it is essential that they are allowed to cool before handling any semen or suspension of spermatozoa within medium. In the case of plastic pipettes, it is good practice to assess their suitability for the handling of spermatozoa by first conducting a sperm survival test, as a means of quality control.

Density gradients for the separation of spermatozoa from seminal plasma can be prepared in sterile, tissue-culture-grade plastic, conical,

15-ml centrifuge tubes (such as those available from Falcon). Similarly, all washing of spermatozoa may be carried out in these tubes. Any microfuging of spermatozoa, useful when very low numbers of spermatozoa have to be concentrated into a minimal volume of media, can be performed using sterile 1.5-ml microtubes (such as those available from Eppendorf). Epididymal and testicular aspirates and biopsies may be collected into small, sterile, tissue-culture-grade plastic Petri dishes (such as those available from Falcon). Sterile hypodermic needles and scalpel blades or mini tissue homogenizers can be used for the disaggregation of biopsies. Epididymal and testicular aspirates and macerates are often maintained as pools of media under prewashed light mineral oil (such as that available from Sigma). Washing of the oil by mixing and equilibration with culture medium (3 : 1, v/v) at room temperature for at least two days is strongly advised. The purpose of this is to remove any water-soluble endotoxins that may be present and would otherwise leach into any culture medium that is to be overlaid with the oil.

2.1.2 Culture media

Essentially, culture medium is a buffered solution of physiological salts, amino acids and vitamins able to satisfy the nutritive requirements of cells and tissues. The different types of media that may be employed for the preparation of spermatozoa are wide-ranging, and there are several chemically defined media that are commercially available (see Table 2.1).

Different suppliers often supply similar media. However, one should be aware that there might be subtle differences between the same media from different suppliers (e.g. minimal essential medium (MEM) from Gibco BRL contains adenosine and guanosine, which are not present in MEM supplied by Sigma; although these purines may not affect spermatozoa adversely, they are known to contribute to the meiotic arrest of oocytes).

The standard simple salt solutions are generally cheaper and can be prepared in-house or obtained commercially. However, they may require the addition of exogenous protein such as human serum albumin (HSA; e.g. from Sigma), antibiotics such as penicillin (e.g. from GlaxoSmithKline) and streptomycin (e.g. from Sigma), and an energy source such as sodium pyruvate (e.g. from Sigma). The addition of protein is primarily for the coating of any pipettes, centrifuge tubes, Petri dishes and culture plates that the spermatozoa may come into contact with. Albumin has a secondary benefit in that it acts as an additional buffer. Antibiotics are necessary as the culture media and conditions used to incubate gametes and embryos are also ideal for the growth and proliferation of any bacteria that may be present. Cell culture purists may argue against the non-physiological

Table 2.1 *Commercially available media used in sperm preparation*

Medium	Supplier	Product no.
EBSS	Sigma	E7883
Gamete™-20/-100	Vitrolife Fertility Systems	10006/7
HMEM	Sigma	M7278
HTF Medium	Irvine Scientific	9962
IVF™-20/-100	Vitrolife Fertility Systems	10008/9
Modified HTF Medium	Irvine Scientific	9963
Quinn's Advantage Medium with Hepes	SAGE BioPharma	ART-1024
SpermRinse™-20/-100	Vitrolife Fertility Systems	10011/0
Sperm Preparation Medium	Medicult Imperial Laboratories	1070
Sperm Washing Medium	Irvine Scientific	9983
Universal IVF Medium	Medicult Imperial Laboratories	1031

This list is by no means exhaustive but is provided to give an indication of the variety of media that may be used successfully for the preparation of spermatozoa. Both bicarbonate- and Hepes-buffered media are listed, as both are suitable for this purpose.

EBSS, Earle's balanced salt solution; HMEM, Hepes–buffered minimal essential medium; HTF, human tubal fluid.

use of antibiotics, as these can influence the behaviour of cells in culture, and may argue for reliance on good aseptic technique alone. However, this is of limited value if bacteria are present in the material at source, as can be the case, and it is debatable whether a limited supply of precious human material should be subjected to the risks inherent in antibiotic-free culture. An example of a typical complete medium, based upon a bicarbonate-buffered simple salt solution, which can be prepared easily for the preparation of spermatozoa is EBSS (see Table 2.2).

Naturally, good aseptic technique should be applied during preparation of medium. Any non-sterile constituents should be diluted in an aliquot of the culture medium and filter-sterilized through a 0.22–μm filter (such as that available from Millipore) (any filter, especially those sterilized with ethylene oxide, should be prewashed with 5–10 ml diluent to remove any potentially toxic coating). Homologous serum is usually prepared by centrifugation of freshly collected whole blood at 800 g for 10 min to separate the plasma from the red blood cells. The plasma can then be transferred into a glass inactivation tube and allowed to clot, leaving a serum exudate. The serum should then be heat-inactivated for at least 30 min at 56 °C to inactivate complement and destroy any viruses that may be present. However, some practitioners leave out the heat-inactivation procedure as they believe this to be unnecessary, providing no benefit to gamete function

Table 2.2 *Constituents necessary for the preparation of complete EBSS*

Constituent	Supplier	Product no.
EBSS	Sigma	E7883
0.00104% (w/v) Sodium pyruvate	Sigma	P4562
0.00604% (w/v) Benzyl penicillin	Glaxo	1088
4.5% HSA	Sigma	A8763

Synthetic serum substitutes (such as that available from Irvine Scientific) are an alternative source of protein, but they are still comprised predominantly of HSA. However, in some countries (e.g. Australia), it should be noted that there is tight restriction on the import of media containing a source of protein, especially that of human origin. In such circumstances, 10% patient's own (homologous) serum may be used in place of HSA.

and embryogenesis. On the other hand, the use of serum from patients who are known to have endometriosis or high levels of anti-sperm antibodies should be avoided as this is known to be detrimental. Obviously, serum from patients who have tested positive for human immunodeficiency virus (HIV) I and II or hepatitis B or C must not be used. Once pyruvate has been added to the medium, it may be stored refrigerated for up to two weeks and aliquots removed for use as required. The limiting factor for the storage of the medium is the pyruvate, since it becomes denatured after a relatively short period of time.

Pharmaceutical-grade media such as those available from Vitrolife are usually complete media (requiring no exogenous additives) and are prepared more rigorously. Even so, it is good practice to check the osmolarity (this should be 285–290 mosmol/kg), to record the expiry dates and batch numbers of all media used, and to test new batches before use, for the purpose of quality control. Human sperm survival and mouse embryogenesis tests may be employed for this purpose.

2.1.3 Density gradient centrifugation media

The ability of cervical mucus to differentially select viable from non-viable spermatozoa is bypassed during assisted conception. Consequently, different methods have been developed to separate normal spermatozoa from seminal plasma, dead and immature sperm, leucocytes and bacteria. These include swim-up, self-migration sedimentation, glass wool filtration, and 'entrapment' using Ficoll, Nycodenz or Percoll discontinuous gradient centrifugation. Separation by density gradient centrifugation is dependent mainly upon differences in density, spermatozoa with

Table 2.3 *Commercially available density gradient centrifugation media*

Medium	Supplier	Product no.
Isolate	Irvine Scientific	99264
IxaPrep	Medicult Imperial Laboratories	1020
PureCeption	SAGE BioPharma	ART-2100
PureSperm	NidaCon International AB	AB PS-0100
SpermGrad™-100	Vitrolife Fertility Systems	10022
SupraSperm	Medicult Imperial Laboratories	1021/2

morphologically normal heads being collected in more concentrated fractions of the gradient since they possess a dense and homogeneous nucleus. Hence, this tends to be the preferred method.

The density gradient medium Percoll (Pharmacia Corporation) is a colloidal suspension of silica particles that are coated with polyvinyl pyrrolidone. (N.B. Pharmacia has stated that this is not licensed for human use. Part of the rationale for this is that Percoll commonly has endotoxin levels of between 25 and 50 EU/ml. Ironically, Percoll has been used successfully for this purpose for many years in the past, with no known adverse effects.) It was the most commonly used density gradient centrifugation medium for sperm preparation, but it has now been superseded by similar preparations (see Table 2.3), such as Isolate (Irvine Scientific), IxaPrep (Medicult Imperial Laboratories) and PureSperm (NidaCon International AB). Isolate and PureSperm are iso-osmotic colloidal suspensions of silica particles coated with reactive silane. IxaPrep is based upon sucrose rather than silica. One benefit of the colloidal particles within these media is that they provide buoyant density that helps cushion spermatozoa during centrifugation, thereby minimizing any disruptive effects on the sperm nuclear chromatin arrangement. Preparation with density gradient media also enhances the percentage of spermatozoa with a normal morphology, providing the ejaculate contains 5% or more normal forms (Fleming *et al.*, 1994; Hall *et al.*, 1995b). Isolate, IxaPrep and PureSperm are supplied ready to use, whereas media such as Percoll require preparation at different concentrations, depending on the discontinuous gradient to be employed. For convenience, gradients may be prepared and refrigerated before use.

2.1.4 Media for stimulating motility and assessing sperm viability

Phosphodiesterase inhibitors such as pentoxifylline stimulate the flagellar movements of spermatozoa by virtue of their ability to elevate intracellular levels of the cyclic nucleotide, cyclic adenosine monophosphate (cAMP).

Table 2.4 *Commercially available vital dyes*

Vital dye	Supplier	Product no.
Bisbenzimide	Hoechst	H258
Propidium iodide	Sigma	P4170
Trypan blue	Sigma	T-8154

Table 2.5 *Formulations for the preparation of hypo-osmotic media*

Jeyendran *et al.* (1984)	Verheyen *et al.* (1997)
0.735% Sodium citrate	50% EBSS
1.351% Fructose	0.48% Hepes
	1% HSA

All hypo-osmotic media are prepared using distilled, deionized (e.g. milli-Q) water.

Hence, incubation in medium containing pentoxifylline has proven useful in the past for improving the motility of asthenozoospermic samples prior to SUZI (Yovich *et al.*, 1990). However, the same technique can also be used to improve the motility of spermatozoa so that those that are viable but barely moving may be identified more easily. Pentoxifylline is available commercially (e.g. from Sigma) and is readily soluble in culture medium, but it should be filter-sterilized before addition. Typically, it is used in the concentration range 0.36–3.60 mM, lower concentrations being used for longer exposures so as to avoid a burn-out effect (Mahajan *et al.*, 1994; Moohan *et al.*, 1993).

Some samples of spermatozoa are irreversibly immotile but viable. The percentage of viable cells present can be assessed using vital dyes that are excluded by those spermatozoa whose plasmalemma remains intact, dead or dying cells exhibiting leaky cell membranes. For example, an aliquot of prepared spermatozoa within culture medium can be mixed with 0.4% trypan blue (1 : 1, v/v) for this purpose. These dyes are available commercially (see Table 2.4).

However, these dyes are potentially toxic to viable spermatozoa. Therefore, the preferred method for the identification of viable sperm before use for ICSI is HOST. Hypo-osmotic medium for this purpose can be prepared in various ways (see Table 2.5).

The preparation and use of hypo-osmotic medium for the purpose of assessing sperm viability was originally reported by Jeyendran *et al.* (1984).

However, it has recently been proposed that a 50% solution of culture medium in distilled water does not compromise the viability of the spermatozoa under investigation to the same extent, and allows a more accurate evaluation of viability (Verheyen et al., 1997). Hypo-osmotic medium, already prepared for use, is also available from commercial sources (e.g. HYPO™-10 from Vitrolife Fertility Systems).

2.2 MATERIALS REQUIRED FOR THE PREPARATION OF OOCYTES

Unlike spermatozoa, mature oocytes are particularly susceptible to deviations in pH and temperature outside of the physiological range. Therefore, the type of buffer employed in the medium to maintain physiological pH and the temperature at which the medium is maintained are extremely important. Exposure of oocytes to unfavourable conditions may not necessarily be reflected by lower fertilization rates but will certainly result in lower pregnancy rates, often as a direct result of low cleavage rates and poor embryo quality.

2.2.1 Plasticware and glass consumables

Oocytes are best handled using sterile glass Pasteur pipettes (such as those available from Sigma), pulled over a flame source to an appropriate diameter. The point made earlier regarding the need to use pipettes manufactured from borosilicate glass is particularly pertinent to the handling of oocytes, as embryogenesis begins in oogenesis. However, it is only necessary to flame the opening of glass Pasteur pipettes to be used for the handling of the cumulus–oocyte complex (COC). The removal of the cumulus oophorus and handling of denuded oocytes is achieved with the aid of pulled pipettes, which cannot be flame-bevelled. Handheld pipettors with pulled pipettes of a diameter approximating that required for denudation are also available commercially (see Table 2.6), but these do not always meet the dimensions required for oocytes, which can vary from the expected size. In this respect, it is extremely important that the oocyte does not become distorted through an attempt to squeeze it into a pipette that is too narrow, otherwise damage to the cytoskeleton may occur, resulting in either failed cleavage or poor embryo quality. Conversely, if the diameter of the pipette is too great, then it will take an inordinate amount of time to denude the oocytes, leading to their prolonged exposure to adverse conditions that exist outside the incubator. The use of hand-pulled glass Pasteur pipettes can meet the requirements for denudation of oocytes, whatever their dimensions.

At oocyte retrieval, the follicular aspirate is usually collected into sterile embryo culture tubes (such as those available from Falcon). The COC

Table 2.6 *Commercially available micropipettes for denuding human oocytes*

Supplier	Product no	Internal diameter (μm)
COOK IVF	K-FPIP-1130	130
	K-FPIP-1140	140
	K-FPIP-1170	170
	K-FPIP-1600	600
Humagen Fertility Diagnostics Inc.	10-MDP-120	120
	10-MDP-150	150
	10-MDP-190	190
MidAtlantic Diagnostics Inc.	MXL3-125	125
	MXL3-150	150
	MXL3-175	175

is identified most easily after the aspirate has been tipped into a large, sterile, tissue-culture-grade plastic Petri dish (such as those available from Falcon). Those COCs so identified may then be washed and stored in small, sterile, tissue-culture-grade plastic Petri dishes, organ culture dishes, or four-well embryo culture plates (such as those available from Falcon). They may be maintained either in a closed culture system of drops or pools of media under prewashed light mineral oil (such as that available from Sigma) or in an open culture system. Prewashing of the oil that is used for the closed culture of oocytes is particularly important, as explained earlier (see section 2.1.1).

2.2.2 Culture media

Media for the flushing of follicles and aspiration of oocytes may be buffered with bicarbonate and/or Hepes (see Table 2.7). Antibiotics and heparin (2–10 IU/ml) may be added to prevent contamination of the COC and clotting of the aspirate, respectively. However, some of the commercially available media developed for this purpose also include antibiotic- and heparin-free preparations. The rationale for this is that some patients are allergic to penicillin and some practitioners believe the heparin to be toxic to the COC.

Some of the media (those that are bicarbonate-buffered) listed earlier in this chapter (see Table 2.1) that may be employed for the preparation of spermatozoa may also be used in the preparation of oocytes. However, these tend to be more appropriate for the washing and holding of oocytes within a CO_2 incubator before micromanipulation. In addition, media

Table 2.7 *Commercially available media used in oocyte aspiration*

Medium	Supplier	Product no.
ASP™-100	Vitrolife Fertility Systems	10001
Flushing Medium	Medicult Imperial Laboratories	1083
Hartman's Solution	Baxter Healthcare Corporation	B2324
IVF™-20/-100	Vitrolife Fertility Systems	10008
Quinn's Advantage Medium with Hepes	SAGE BioPharma	ART-1024
Modified HTF Medium	Irvine Scientific	9963
SynVitro Flush	Medicult Imperial Laboratories	1076

Media that are buffered using Hepes are also appropriate for oocyte denudation and micromanipulation procedures.

Table 2.8 *Commercially available media used in oocyte preparation*

Medium	Supplier	Product no.
EBSS	Sigma	E7883
HTF Medium	Irvine Scientific	9962
IVF™-20/-100	Vitrolife Fertility Systems	10008
Quinn's Fertilisation Medium	SAGE BioPharma	ART-1020
Universal IVF Medium	Medicult Imperial Laboratories	1031

formulated especially for this purpose are available commercially (see Table 2.8).

In addition, the denudation of the COC requires the use of a medium containing hyaluronidase, an enzyme that aids the removal of the oocyte (surrounded by its corona radiata) from its surrounding cumulus oophorus by degrading the extracellular matrix that holds together the cumulus cells. Since this procedure must be carried out quickly to avoid prolonged exposure of the oocyte to hyaluronidase, the medium employed may be buffered with either bicarbonate or Hepes. For example, a Hepes-buffered medium for the denudation of oocytes can be prepared easily using MEM (see Table 2.9).

Again, good aseptic technique should be applied during constitution of this medium, which may be stored refrigerated for up to two weeks and aliquots removed for use as required. In some places, concerns over the clinical use of animal extracts, such as hyaluronidase, have led to the investigation of alternative plant extracts. One such plant extract, coronase, has been tested in its use for the denudation of human oocytes and has been found to be a suitable alternative (Parinaud *et al.*, 1998).

Table 2.9 *Formulation for the preparation of denudation medium*

Constituent	Supplier	Product no.
HMEM	Sigma	M7278
0.00104% (w/v) Sodium pyruvate	Sigma	P4562
0.00604% (w/v) Benzyl penicillin	GlaxoSmithKline	1088
4.5% HSA	Sigma	A8763
80 IU/ml Hyaluronidase	Sigma	H3506

2.3 MATERIALS REQUIRED FOR MICROMANIPULATION PROCEDURES

Micromanipulation procedures are usually performed outside of an incubator over the objective lens of an inverted microscope, there often being a limited working distance between the lens and the condenser. Therefore, the materials used during these procedures tend to be specific to the demands imposed by these conditions. However, a variety of methods using different materials have been utilized. This section will concentrate on those materials used most commonly.

2.3.1 Plasticware and glass consumables

Gametes or embryos are usually placed into drops of media overlaid with light mineral oil (such as that available from Sigma). The purpose of this closed culture system is to isolate a maximal number of cells within a single vessel, whilst buffering against non-physiological ambient temperatures and limiting the risk of microbial contamination should the procedure be performed outside of a laminar flow hood. Although the period of time that the gametes will be maintained under oil during various procedures should be limited, prewashing of the oil is still highly recommended (see section 2.1.1). Typically, the drops of media and oil are placed into shallow, sterile, tissue-culture-grade plastic Petri dishes (such as those available from Falcon) or prewashed and heat-sterilized glass slides bearing one or two centrally placed concave wells (such as those available from BDH). Slides may be washed with detergent (e.g. 1% Liquinox), rinsed thoroughly with distilled water, and heat-sterilized for 40 min at 180 °C in an oven. However, even the shallow lid of an ordinary sterile, tissue-culture-grade plastic Petri dish will suffice.

Direct manipulation of gametes and embryos is achieved through the use of microtools constructed from borosilicate glass capillary tubes (0.975–1.025 mm o.d., 0.6 mm i.d., 100 mm long). These may be forged into pipettes for holding oocytes and embryos, aspirating and injecting spermatozoa, AH and blastomere biopsy, the diameter and opening of the

Table 2.10 *Suppliers of micropipettes for micromanipulation*

COOK IVF
Eppendorf
Humagen
Research Instruments
SAGE BioPharma
The Pipette Company

pipette being manufactured according to use (see Chapter 10). They can be forged straight, but they often possess one or more bends so that they may be inserted into a micromanipulation vessel without the tool holders having to be in the same plane. They may be manufactured in-house, but they are also available commercially from a number of sources (see Table 2.10).

2.3.2 Culture media

The same types of media that may be employed for the preparation of spermatozoa and oocytes (see Tables 2.1, 2.7 and 2.8) may also be used during micromanipulation procedures. However, a Hepes-buffered medium such as HMEM (see Table 2.9) supplemented with penicillin, pyruvate and HSA is recommended for any prolonged procedure performed outside of an incubator, Hepes being an excellent buffer that is not dependent upon an atmosphere containing 5% CO_2 in order to maintain physiological pH. This is particularly relevant to the novice, who invariably takes longer to perform any given procedure. More experienced practitioners may wish to avoid the potentially toxic effects of Hepes altogether by employing a bicarbonate-buffered medium instead. There still remains some debate over the relative merits of these different buffering systems for the purpose of micromanipulation, and therefore personal preference tends to prevail.

Spermatozoa may be manipulated in standard culture medium, but this practice is suitable only for the experienced practitioner, as the spermatozoa are more mobile and greater control is required during their aspiration and injection under such conditions. Therefore, it is recommended that they be placed into a 10% solution of polyvinylpyrrolidone (PVP), which is a relatively inert viscous solution that hampers sperm progression, making them easier to manipulate and inject. PVP may be prepared in-house, but it is also available commercially (see Table 2.11).

Ideally, any source of PVP should be tested for toxicity, especially if prepared in-house, as it has been reported that different types differentially affect the cleavage rate and morphology of mouse embryos (Bras *et al.*, 1994).

Table 2.11 *Suppliers of PVP*

Preparation	Supplier	Product no.
ICSI™-100	Vitrolife Fertility Systems	10016
PVP (lyophilized powder)	Irvine Scientific	99219
PVP 10% Solution	SAGE BioPharma	ART-4005
PVP Clinical Grade	Medicult Imperial Laboratories	1090
PVP Medium	Medicult Imperial Laboratories	1089
PVP Solution	Irvine Scientific	99311

Table 2.12 *Formulation for the preparation of hypertonic medium*

Constituent	Supplier	Product no.
80% EBSS	Sigma	E7883
20% Sucrose (0.5 M in PBS)	Sigma	(D5780)

The sucrose solution is prepared using Dulbecco's phosphate buffered saline (PBS) containing 10% homologous serum. Once prepared, this medium can then be filter-sterilized and stored in a refrigerator.

Table 2.13 *Commercial sources of acidified Tyrode's used for ZD*

Medium	Supplier	Product no.
Acidified Hepes HTF	SAGE BioPharma	ART-4013
Acidified Tyrode's solution	Medicult Imperial Laboratories	1060
Tyrode's solution – acidified	Irvine Scientific	9962
ZD™-10	Vitrolife Fertility Systems	10002

Blastomere biopsy is facilitated by the use of Ca^{2+}/Mg^{2+}-free medium (Dumoulin *et al.*, 1998). Again, this is also available from commercial sources (e.g. EB™-10 from Vitrolife Fertility Systems).

Techniques such as PZD and SUZI are often performed in a hypertonic medium containing sucrose, which causes shrinkage of the oocyte resulting in an enlarged PVS, so minimizing the risk of any damage to the oocyte during the procedure (see Table 2.12).

AH and blastomere biopsy techniques are increasingly reliant on the use of laser technology for breaching the ZP. However, this is still typically achieved using an acidified (pH 2.3–2.5) Tyrode's solution that can be prepared 'in-house' or obtained from a commercial supplier (see Table 2.13).

3 Narishige micromanipulation workstation systems

Eiichi Narishige established the Narishige Scientific Instrument Laboratory in Tokyo in 1953. Quickly becoming renowned throughout Japan for producing high-quality mechanical micromanipulators and stereotaxic equipment, Narishige concentrated on selling to physiology and neuroscience research facilities in Japan and, later, the West. The first hydraulic micromanipulator, a single-axis device designed to place microelectrodes into the brains of experimental animals, followed in 1969, and the first three-axis hydraulic micromanipulator was produced in the early 1980s (Cohen *et al.*, 1992). The advent of three hydraulic axes controlled by a single joystick allowed true microsurgical manipulation in much the same way that the original Leitz and DeFonbrune joystick models had. The main advantage of the Narishige system over the traditional Leitz manipulator was the ability to mount the moving (slave) headstage on to the microscope, but with the joystick controller positioned remotely.

In 1985, Narishige Company Limited was established, also in Tokyo, as a separate entity from Narishige Scientific. Unlike Narishige Scientific, which sold instruments directly to end users, Narishige Company distributed through the big four microscope companies, Leica, Zeiss, Olympus and Nikon. With the power of the big four's sales teams behind it, sales of Narishige equipment began to increase steadily. New markets were identified, including SUZI and animal ICSI around 1987. One of the first establishments to develop this technique, the Dutch-Speaking Free University of Brussels (AZ-VUB), was already a customer of the Nikon Corporation. Nikon, recognizing the potential of this new market, approached Narishige to build a range of three-axis, oil-hydraulic, joystick-controlled micromanipulators. A joint venture was formed between the two companies and the Nikon-Narishige NT-8 micromanipulation workstation was conceived. The NT-8 and its successor, the NT-88, proved to be phenomenally successful, and it was estimated that by the end of 1995 over

Figure 3.1 The Olympus version of the Narishige upright joystick, known as the 'Ergo-Stick', featured a wooden handrest and a lower-profile appearance.

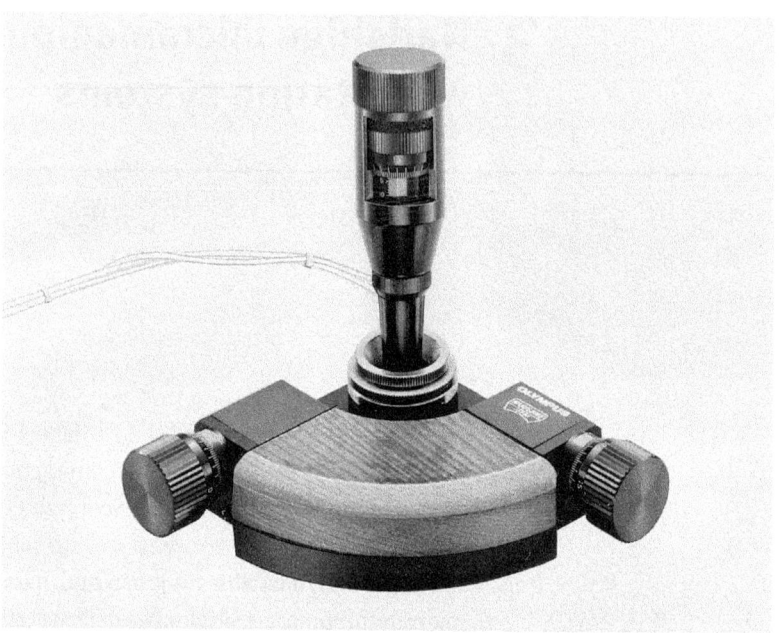

three-quarters of the world's ICSI centres were using Narishige-type micromanipulators.

Around 1994, an Olympus version of the Narishige upright joystick was conceived after a joint meeting of the two companies. The ONO-121 was dubbed the 'Ergo-Stick' and featured a wooden handrest and a lower-profile appearance (see Figure 3.1). It seemed to receive a somewhat cool reception from some users, however, due mainly to the inaccessible z-axis control, and it was discontinued in the autumn of 1997. Throughout this time, Narishige continued to sell its own system directly to end users as well as through its dealer network.

Both the Olympus and the Nikon ranges have undergone recent upgrades. The latest Olympus system (code number ON2–99D; see Figure 3.2) features a hanging joystick, rather than the upright style of the old Ergo-Stick. The latest incarnation of the Nikon system (code number NT-88NE; see Figure 3.3) also features a hanging-style joystick. Although opinions differ as to whether an upright or a hanging joystick is best for microsurgical procedures like ICSI, the fact that both Nikon and Olympus have chosen to market hanging-style joysticks suggests that they are more popular. Indeed, the ratios of Narishige's European sales of hanging to upright joysticks between 1995 and 1998 were estimated to be eight to one (Hall, personal communication 1999). In some cases, it is possible to identify equivalent components from the different companies, as

Figure 3.2 The Olympus 'ON' micromanipulation system.

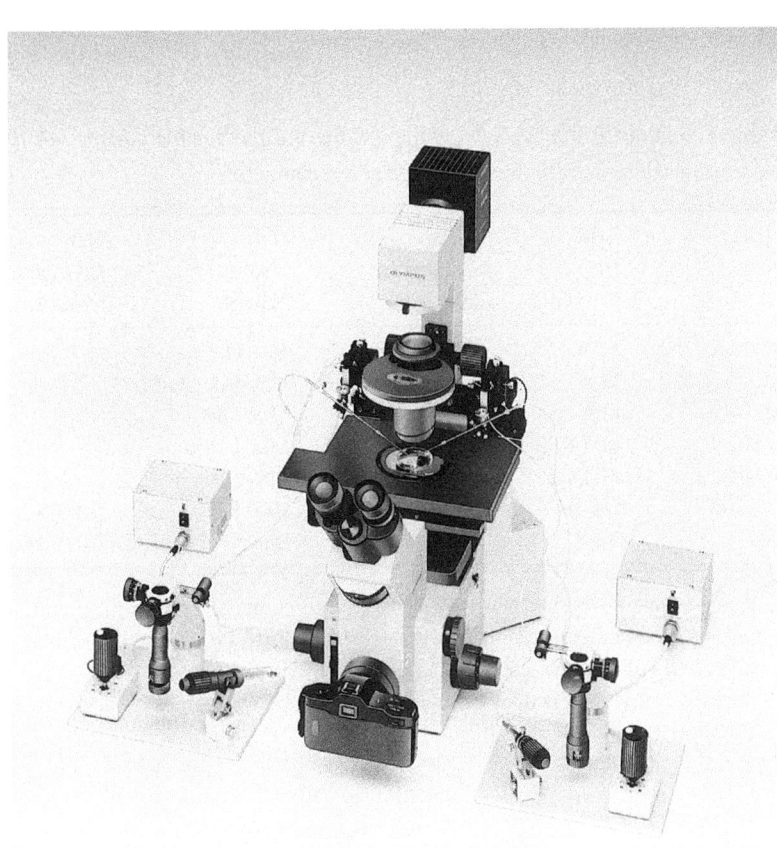

Figure 3.3 The Nikon–Narishige micromanipulation system.

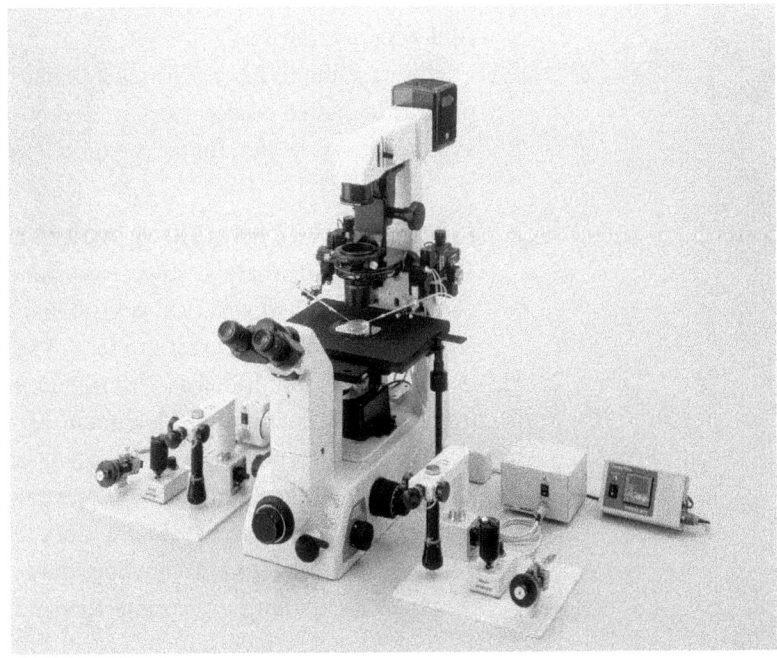

Table 3.1 *Equivalent models found in previous and existing Narishige, Nikon–Narishige and Olympus–Narishige instruments*

New Narishige	Old Narishige	New Nikon NT-88NE	Old Nikon NT-88	New Olympus ON2–99D*	Old Olympus
MMO-202ND	MMO-202D	MO-188NE	MO-188	–	No equivalent**
MMO-202N	MMO-202	No equivalent**	No equivalent**	–	ONO-121
MM-89	MM-88	MM-188NE	MM-188	–	No equivalent**
MM-89	MM-88B	MM-188NE	MM-188B	–	No equivalent**
MMN-1	MMN-1	MN-188NE	MN-188	–	ONM-1
IM-50B	IM-5B	IM-16	IM-188	N-IM-55–2	No equivalent**
IM-16	IM-6	IM-16	IM-6	N-IM-26–2	No equivalent**

* The new Olympus system is supplied in one piece, comprising mounting adaptor and coarse and fine manipulators, making installation considerably simpler (but note that this system can be installed only on Olympus microscopes).

** Where no direct equivalent exists, the microscope companies tend to supply Narishige-original instruments.

illustrated in Table 3.1, and it is even possible to mix components from different manufacturers, although this is not recommended.

Perhaps it should be noted at this point that to this day Narishige offers a bewildering array of instruments for this application, which can be confusing to the first-time buyer and the seasoned practitioner alike. The best way to keep up to date is to stay in touch with the local microscope dealer representative.

The instruments described in this chapter represent most of the current products and their predecessors at the time of going to press, although it is expected that new, but similar, products will come to replace them in time.

3.1 INSTALLING THE NARISHIGE WORKSTATION

The assembly of the Narishige workstation (including the Olympus–Narishige and Nikon–Narishige versions) can be a daunting task. The user is provided with a great number of boxes, nuts and bolts, and a set of instructions that have been translated, sometimes rather too literally, from Japanese. Furthermore, it is not uncommon to find that illustrations in the instruction books are somewhat different from the instrument provided. With a little planning and perseverance, however, assembly is not usually a major difficulty (the trick is not to panic).

Ideally, the distributor from whom they were purchased should set up the micromanipulators, microinjectors and other accessories at the same time as the microscope. In most parts of the world, Narishige equipment may be purchased through any of the big four microscope manufacturers, whose dealers should have the capability to install the complete system. However, the Narishige construction can be as daunting to the microscope company representative as it is to the end user, and, in all fairness, the microscope companies are in business to sell microscopes and cannot be expected to be experts in micromanipulation. Furthermore, since Narishige also sells directly to the end user, the self-assembly scenario is a common one.

The tools required for the construction process are usually supplied with the equipment. However, these tools are cheap Allen (hex) keys, and assembly can be made a lot less painless by using a good-quality set of hexagonal ball-drivers (in metric sizes). The only other tools that may be required are a set of jewellers' flat and cross-headed screwdrivers. Users should not concern themselves with maintenance of the instrument at this stage. The instruments are generally well made and designed to operate for several years before needing a service. Furthermore, it can do more harm than good if complex mechanisms such as hydraulic lines are disassembled by untrained individuals.

The Narishige ICSI workstation is modular in construction. The individual parts are:

- microscope
- mounting adaptor
- coarse manipulators
- micromanipulators, including universal joints
- microinjectors, including tool holders.

The following account details the mounting and configuration of a Narishige-original workstation, comprising mounting adaptor, MMN-1 and MM-89 coarse manipulators, MMO-202 and MMO-202D micromanipulators, and IM-6 and IM-5B microinjectors. These instruments are the range that were sold worldwide by Narishige between 1994 and 1997, a period when the ICSI technique was being adopted most rapidly within Europe. In almost all cases, subsequent models are mounted in a similar fashion. If there is any doubt as to the model number of an instrument, then a small black and silver plate fixed to each instrument will list the model number and the serial number. The first two digits of the serial number refer to the year of manufacture, the rest to the number of that instrument in the production sequence. For example, MM-88 number 95011 was the eleventh MM-88 to be manufactured in 1995.

Figure 3.4 Fitting the mounting adaptor.

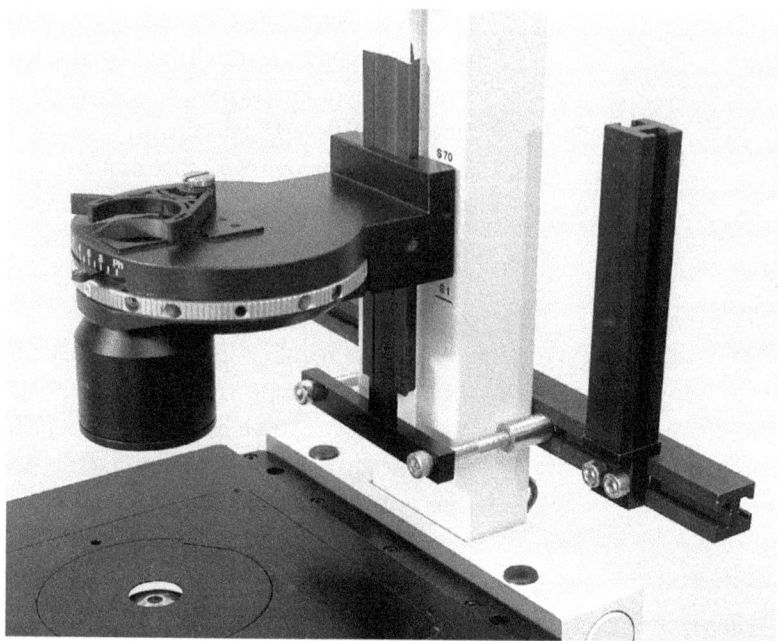

3.1.1 Mounting adaptor – installation

This allows the manipulators to be mounted on to the microscope, usually on to the illumination support pillar (see Figure 3.4). Constructed from black anodized aluminium, with an I-shaped cross-section, the usual configuration is of a horizontal bar, clamped or screwed to the illumination support, with two vertical bars, one on each end (see Figure 3.5). An optional vertical bar with a rotating action, (Narishige code NR) is available; this can be useful for more rapid exchange of pipettes, but it is not essential.

Figures 3.5, 3.6 and 3.7 show alternative ways of mounting the adaptor, depending on the model of microscope. It is easy to see the large number of permutations available for mounting the Narishige manipulators, and it may take some time to find the right one.

If the mounting adaptor is to be used with motorized coarse manipulators, then vertical bars are not required (see Figure 3.7), and the motorized headstages are fitted directly to the horizontal bar (see below).

Mounting adaptors are available for most current makes and models of microscopes (see Table 3.2), and for many microscopes that are no longer available. Adaptors are available with and without vertical bars for mounting mechanical or motorized coarse manipulators, respectively. It is advisable to contact Narishige directly for further information on the

Figure 3.5 Fitting the mounting
adaptor with the vertical bars
set back.

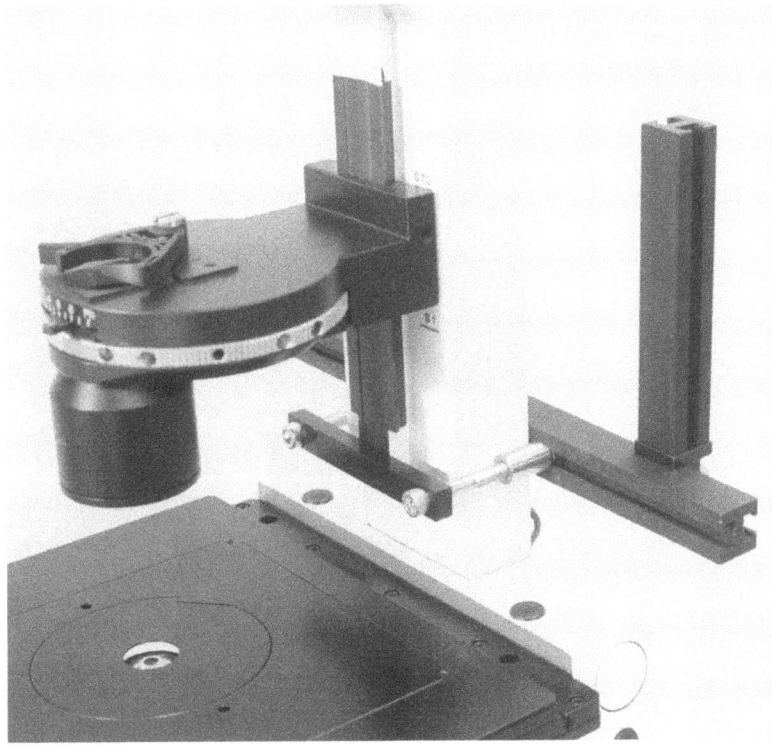

Figure 3.6 Fitting the mounting
adaptor with the vertical bars
hanging down.

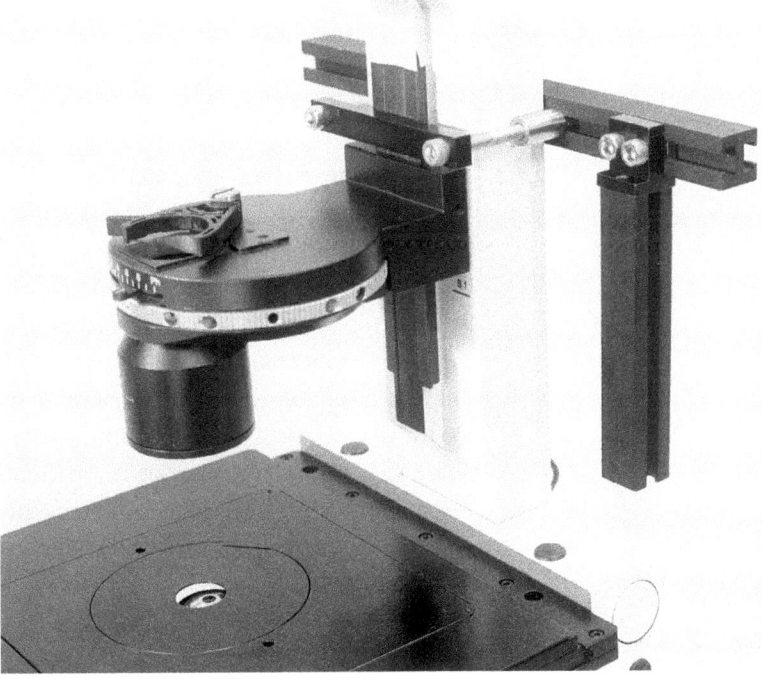

Figure 3.7 Fitting the mounting adaptor to accommodate motorized coarse manipulators.

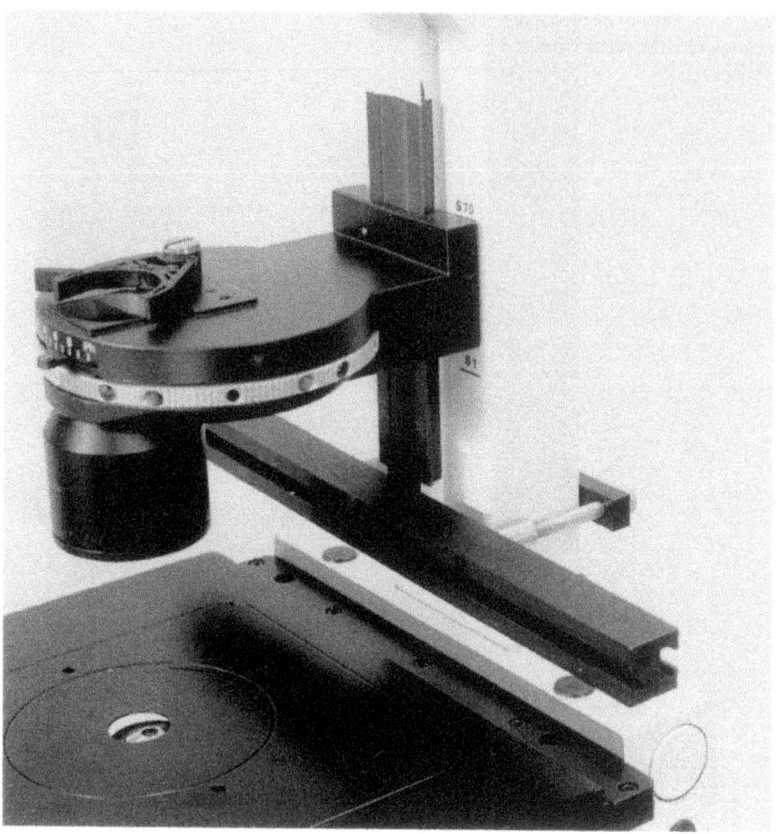

availability and on fitting mounting adaptors to microscopes (see appendix for contact details).

3.1.2 Coarse manipulators – installation

The basic mechanical coarse manipulator, the MMN-1, comprises three mechanical axes set at right angles to each other. Each axis has a total range of 30 mm. Two coarse manipulators are required, one on the left and one on the right of the microscope. They are fitted by means of two large screws into the slot in the vertical pillar of the mounting adaptor. This method of mounting allows the manipulator to be positioned at any point on the vertical portion of the mounting adaptor, which is important since it allows a great amount of variability in the positioning of the manipulators to account for the different construction of different microscopes.

3.1.2.1 Fitting the MMN-1

Assemble the MMN-1 according to the instructions supplied. Using the two large screws and nuts that have been provided, fit the MMN-1 to the

Table 3.2 *Selecting the appropriate mounting adaptor for the microscope*

Microscope	Narishige mounting adaptor code
Leica DM IL	NL-3
Leica DM IRB/E	NL-6
Leica DM IRB/E	NL-6-2 (without vertical bars)
Nikon TMD	NN-B
Nikon Diaphot 200/300	NN-H
Nikon Diaphot 200/300	NN-I (with rotating vertical bars)
Nikon Diaphot 200/300	NN-H-2 (without vertical bars)
Nikon TE 200/300	NN-H
Nikon TE 200/300	NN-I (with rotating vertical bars)
Nikon TE 200/300	NN-H-2 (without vertical bars)
Olympus CK-2	NO-ADK
Olympus IMT-2	NO-ADM
Olympus IX-50, -70	NO-PIX
Olympus IX-50, -70	NO-PIX-2 (without vertical bars)
Zeiss Axiovert 10, 100, 135	NZ-6
Zeiss Axiovert 10, 100, 135	NZ-17 (without vertical bars)
Axiovert 200	NZ-19 (without vertical bars)
Rotating vertical bar	NR

These are Narishige's code numbers. When ordering through the microscope companies directly, they may have their own, different codes.

All adaptors come with fixed vertical bars (as shown in Figure 3.5), unless stated otherwise.

vertical bar of the mounting adaptor, approximately halfway up. The manipulator can be mounted with the z-axis control knob pointing upwards or downwards, as illustrated in Narishige's instruction manual. Either method is acceptable, and will depend on the type of microscope used. At this point, ensure that the fixing screws are about halfway along their slots on the fixing plate of the MMN-1. Tighten the screws enough to prevent any movement (i.e. finger tight), but do not lock them down fully at this stage. These last two points also apply to the assembly of the MMN-1 in general, since minor adjustments may have to be made at a later stage to ensure the pipettes are oriented correctly in relation to the microscope stage (see section 3.5.5).

Narishige offers an electrical coarse manipulator with joystick control, MM-89, as an alternative to the MMN-1. Like the manual version, the headstage of the MM-89 is fitted to the mounting adaptor, but it is attached to the horizontal portion of the bar (the vertical bars are discarded, as in

Figure 3.8 Fitting the motorized coarse manipulators to the mounting adaptor.

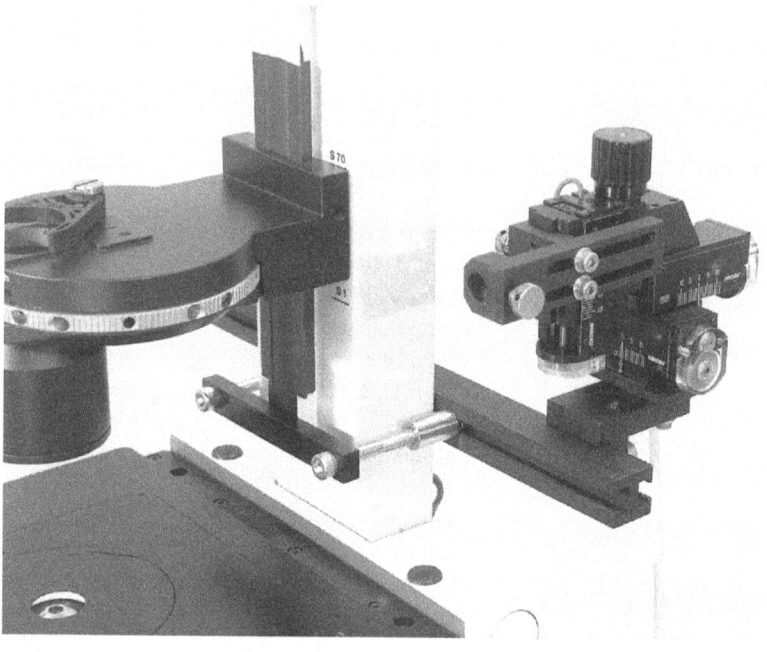

Figure 3.7). Again, two units are required, one for the left and one for the right-hand side.

The MM-89 is fitted with a mechanical z-axis on the headstage, which allows the user to raise and lower the pipette without using the electrical controls.

3.1.2.2 Fitting the MM-89

Using the two large screws provided, fit the MM-89 to the rear of the horizontal portion of the mounting adaptor (see Figure 3.8). Slide it about 4 cm from the outer end of the mounting adaptor bar and tighten the screws finger tight. On the right-hand side (looking from the front) of the main body of the MM-89 headstage is a flat plate with two long slots. Loosen the two screws there and slide the plate so that the screws are approximately in the centre of their slots. Tighten the screws finger tight. Connect the headstage and controller cables to the power supply, and connect the power supply to an outlet. Before switching on the power, check that the correct voltage setting is selected (the selector is found on the back of the power supply box). Use the joystick to adjust the three headstage axes so that they are in the centre of their tracks (there is a scale on the side of each axis to facilitate this). The MM-89 is now ready to accept the hydraulic headstage unit.

3.1.3   **Micromanipulators – installation**

The Narishige micromanipulators are controlled remotely via a hydraulic system. Briefly, a master cylinder with a rolling rubber diaphragm is connected via a 1-m length of tubing to a slave cylinder of equal size. The system is oil-filled and closed to the outside. At the master cylinder end, movements of the hand controller (in this case, a joystick) push a short rod into the diaphragm, which displaces the hydraulic oil and moves out the diaphragm at the slave cylinder by an equal amount. The displacement of the slave diaphragm thus pushes a rod attached to a slide on the headstage. It is this action that moves the pipette holder. There are three axes, which allow the pipette holder to be displaced in any spatial co-ordinate within the micromanipulator's range. The capacity of the master and slave cylinders dictates the maximum range of the headstage sliders, and in fact the Narishige has a larger range of movement (10 mm) than the Nikon (5 mm). In practice, however, this is relatively unimportant since the maximum displacement required is never more than the field of view of the microscope (roughly half a millimetre at $40\times$ magnification). The basic design of the Narishige hydraulic joystick micromanipulator system is essentially the same, whether branded with Narishige, Nikon or Olympus. The only real difference between the current Narishige and Nikon hanging joystick micromanipulators is in the appearance of the joystick controller.

Probably because of the success of the Nikon–Narishige NT-88 system, which featured hydraulic micromanipulators with hanging joystick controls, the MMO-202D has proved to be the most popular variant of the original Narishige range. The MMO-202D's hanging joystick is slightly easier to control and comes with a metal base plate to which the joystick is mounted magnetically. With the MMO-202, the upright joystick is not supplied with a metal base plate, which, since the injectors and joystick controls of the MM-89 coarse electrical manipulators are also mounted magnetically, means that the user must supply their own plate. If the user selects the upright joystick, the MM-89 joystick and the injectors can be left free-standing, but since their footprints are smaller than their predecessors, the MM-88 and IM-6, they are prone to slipping about or even falling over. All these considerations tend to make the hanging joystick variant the preferred choice.

3.1.3.1   *Hydraulic manipulators: a brief history*

- *Mid-1996:* The MMO-202D z-axis is changed so that it works in the same direction as the then current Nikon MO-188 (see section 3.1.3.2).

- *1997:* The Olympus ONO-121 is discontinued.
- *June–December 1997:* The last few MMO-202 and MMO-202D micromanipulators have headstages with fixing rods that screw in rather than slide in.
- *December 1997:* The MMO-202 and MMO-202D are discontinued and replaced with the MMO-202N and MMO-202ND, respectively. Superficially, these instruments are the same as their predecessors. However, the hydraulic headstages of both instruments now have screw-in rather than slide-in fixing rods, and have a rotating mechanism for switching from right-hand to left-hand use. The MMO-202N now comes with a magnetic mount and a metal base plate, which can also be used to mount the control box of the MM-89 and the injector.

3.1.3.2 The z-axis confusion

While the instrument was available, the fine *z*-axis control of a Nikon–Narishige MO-188 would result in the pipette tip moving downwards if the control was twisted clockwise (looking at it from above). As mentioned previously, the Nikon–Narishige instruments were some of the best selling and spearheaded the drive towards ICSI as a routine procedure. Many people learned to perform ICSI with this instrument. It was a source of surprise and annoyance for them, then, to find that the Narishige-original MMO-202D possessed a *z*-axis that worked in the opposite direction. Users who had bought an MO-188 from Nikon, and who then went on to buy an MMO-202D from Narishige as a second system, found themselves having to relearn tricky techniques, such as sperm immobilization and capture. They would instinctively twist the MMO-202D's joystick clockwise to bring the pipette down on the tail of the sperm, and it would instead rise. Some users returned their instruments to Narishige, asking for modifications to be made. Narishige was able to do this, and as a result of so many comments revised the MMO-202D to incorporate a *z*-axis that went the same way as that of the MO-188. This happened in mid-1996. Since that time, every *z*-axis (including that of the upright joystick, the MMO-202) has operated as the original MO-188 did.

3.1.3.3 Installing the MMO-202D

The MMO-202D headstage is fitted to the coarse manipulator with a 10-mm-diameter rod, which fits into a hole on the coarse manipulator (see Figure 3.9). The MMO-202D is supplied as a right-handed version, but it is capable of being mounted on either side of the microscope. Examination of the headstage reveals the letters 'L' and 'R' on adjacent faces. If the headstage is mounted on the right-hand side of the microscope, then the

Figure 3.9 Fitting the hydraulic headstage to the coarse manipulator. The headstage bears the letters 'L' and 'R' on adjacent faces. If the headstage is mounted on the right-hand side of the microscope, then the 'R' should be facing forward. If the headstage is mounted on the left, then the 'L' should be facing forward.

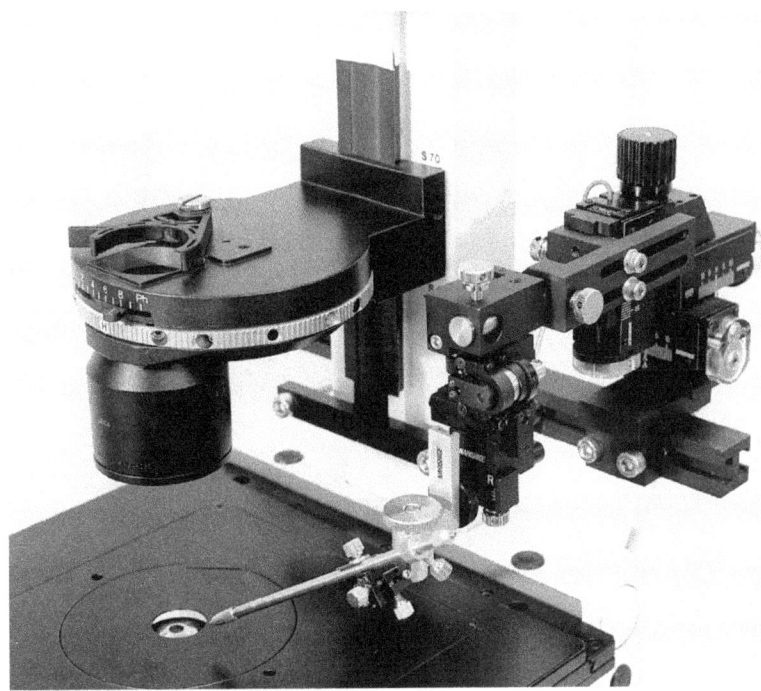

'R' should be facing forward; if the headstage is mounted on the left, then the fixing rod should be inserted into the headstage at 90 degrees, with the 'L' facing forward.

3.1.3.4 Installing the MMO-202

Fitting the MMO-202 is exactly as described above, with the exception that the joystick is free-standing rather than mounted magnetically, as shown in Figure 3.10, which also shows the MMN-1 coarse manipulator in place of the electrical model.

Once the headstage of the micromanipulator is in place, the universal joint can be fitted and the tool holder of the microinjector inserted (see Figure 3.11).

3.1.4 Universal joints

The original universal joint, a ball-and-socket affair (part number B8-C), allowed the tool holder to be positioned in almost any orientation, but it suffered greatly from the fact that it was notoriously difficult to make fine adjustments. Furthermore, should the locknut be overtightened, irreparable damage to the ball-and-socket arrangement would result. In

Figure 3.10 Mounting the upright joystick micro-manipulator (MMO-202).

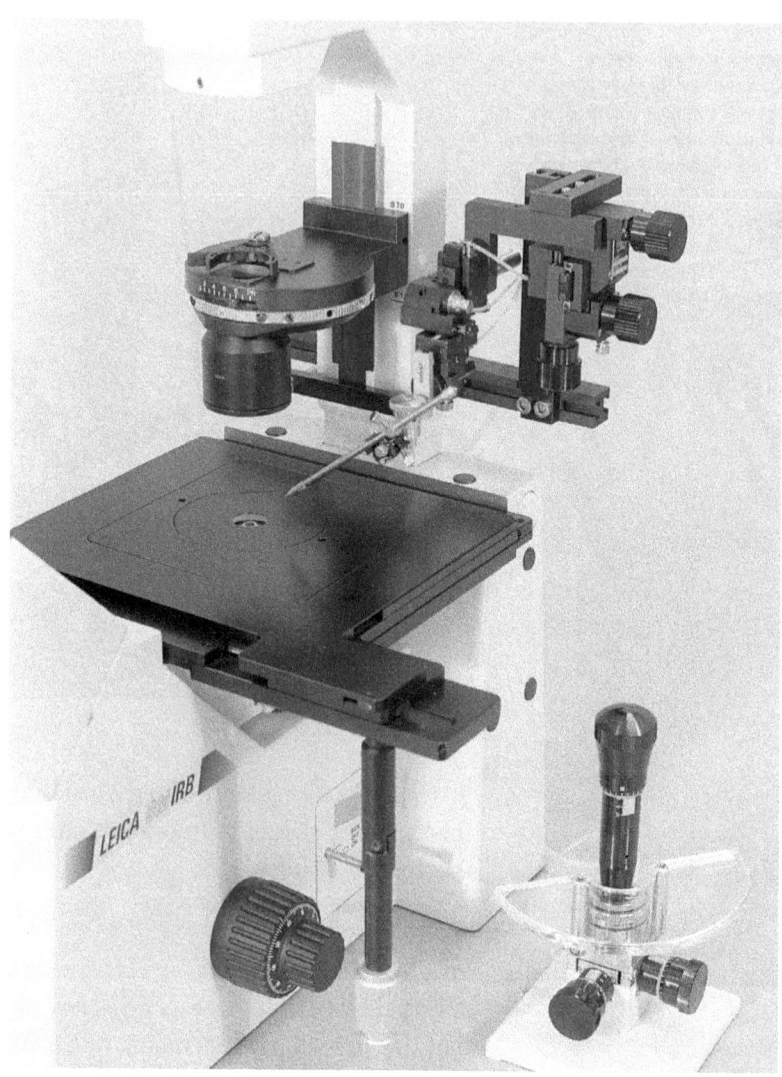

mid-1997, several new universal joints were introduced as optional extras, and by late 1998 they had become standard on all Nikon, Olympus and Narishige-original systems.

The initial setting up of the pipettes can be one of the most difficult aspects of ICSI to master. Achieving the desired angle of the pipette holder, so that the bent portion of the ICSI needle is parallel with the dish, is impossible to achieve by eye, and if one is out by even a few degrees performance of the equipment is compromised. The new Narishige universal joints attempt to get around this problem by isolating the swing and tilt movements (see Figure 3.12). Unlike the B8-C ball joint, the swing (or

Figure 3.11 The completed micromanipulator assembly, including the fitted universal joint and micropipette tool holder.

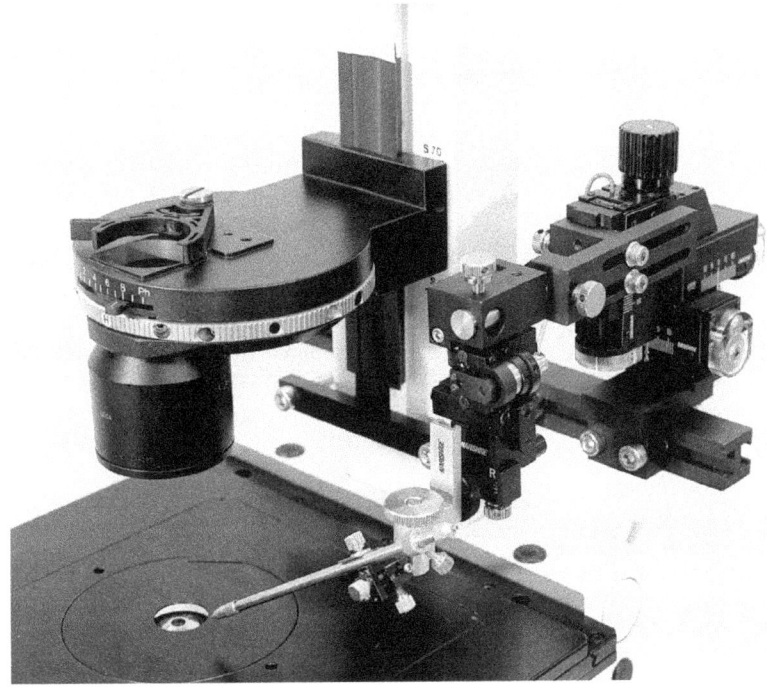

Figure 3.12 The old-style ball joint (left) and the new-style universal joint (right). By isolating the swing and tilt movements of the new-style universal joint, the movements can be set to ensure that their preferred orientation is reproduced.

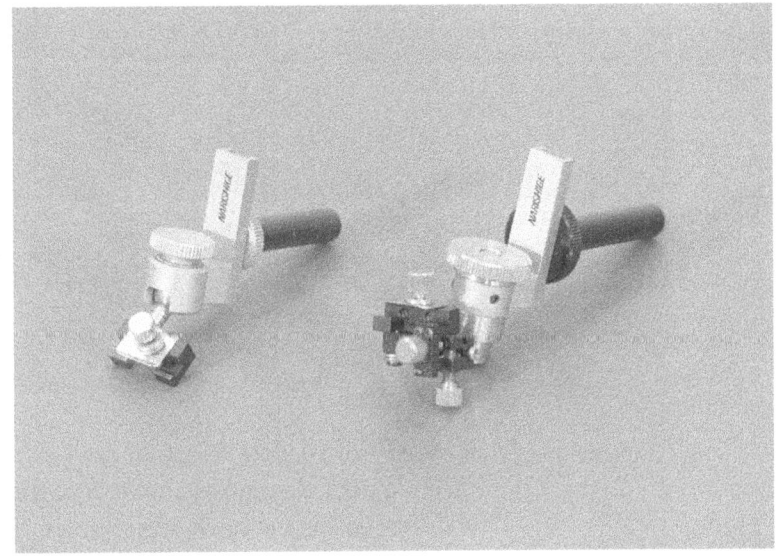

yaw) and tilt (or pitch) can be set so that the joint always returns to the same orientation.

Of the four units available (see Table 3.3), the UT-1 is good, the UT-2 is excellent, and the UT-3 seems somewhat pointless. The UT-1 is useful, but

Table 3.3 *Universal joints*

Part no.	Description
UT-1	A basic swing-and-tilt universal joint with a fine adjustment of the tilt axis only.
UT-2	The same as the UT-1, but with fine control of both swing and tilt.
UT-3	The same as the UT-2, but with a coarse control that allows the pipette to be raised and lowered.
UT-5	The same as the UT-2, but with a hydraulic control that allows the pipette to be raised and lowered.

Universal joint part number UT-4 was also manufactured, but none were ever sold.

Figure 3.13 Narishige fine microinjectors: the older model IM-6 (left), and the newer models IM-60 (centre) and IM-16 (right).

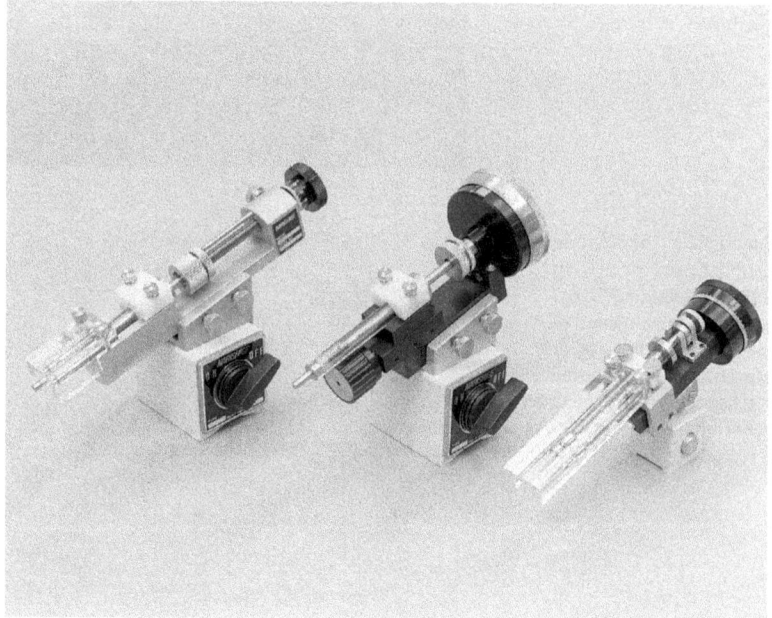

for a few extra dollars the UT-2 offers fine adjustment of both swing and tilt, even when the pipette is in the dish. It is difficult to see the advantage conveyed by the up–down control of the UT-3, since this adjustment is already available through the coarse and fine manipulators.

3.1.5 Microinjectors

The range of Narishige microinjectors is extensive. One of the best-selling microinjectors, the IM-6 (see Figure 3.13), was discontinued in early 1997 and then reintroduced in 2001. Its design is simple, but it is prone to

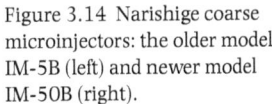

Figure 3.14 Narishige coarse microinjectors: the older model IM-5B (left) and newer model IM-50B (right).

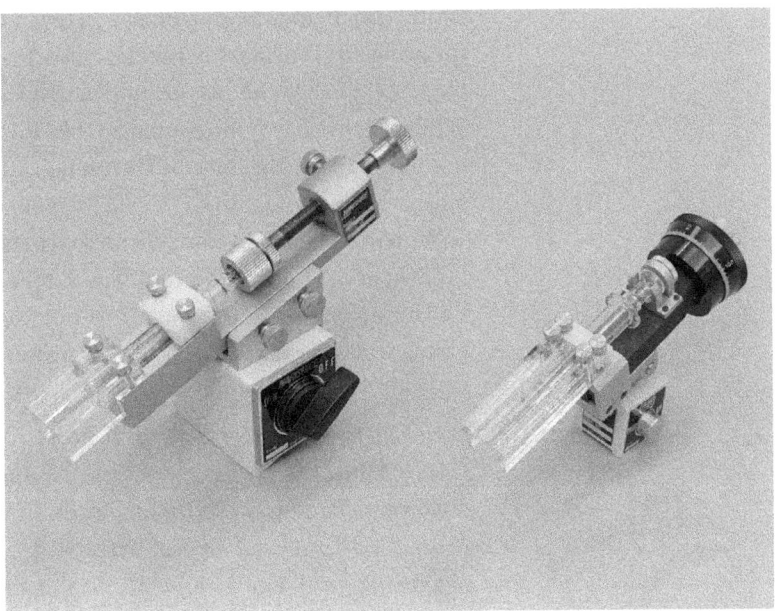

problems during operation. Because its design is that of a simple micrometer screw, driving the plunger of a glass syringe, the centre axes of both micrometer screw and syringe plunger have to be aligned precisely. The syringe plunger is connected to the micrometer screw by means of a clamp ring. If the clamp ring is too loose, the microinjector suffers from backlash[*]; if it is too tight, the syringe plunger can turn with the micrometer screw, affecting the precision of the injector (see section 3.5.4). Indeed, if the clamp screw is too tight and the syringe far enough off the micrometer's axis, the glass syringe can break when the control knob is turned.

After the IM-6 was discontinued in 1997, new models IM-16 (see Figure 3.13) and IM-50B (see Figure 3.14) were introduced as replacements. They circumvented the backlash problem by interposing a slide mechanism between the micrometer screw and the syringe plunger. Basically, the micrometer screw turns, driving the slide forward. On the top of the slide is a slot into which the butt of the syringe plunger fits. The butt is held in place with a locknut. Because the slide is not rotating, the plunger is unaffected by an off-axis micrometer. The problem of backlash in the system is addressed by using a special thrust-race between the

---

[*] In an engineering context, 'backlash' refers to the delay between the turning of a screw and the corresponding movement of the nut in which it turns, as any slack in the system is taken up. It is usually caused by the screw and nut being imperfectly matched, and is most noticeable when the screw movement is suddenly reversed.

control knob and the micrometer screw. This does indeed seem to solve the problem of backlash between control knob and micrometer screw, but there seem to be examples around with backlash in the slide mechanism. While there are ways to minimize this, it is recommended that users do not try to adjust the injector themselves but instead send it to Narishige for servicing.

With this in mind, it was difficult to recommend either the IM-16 or the IM-50B as ICSI microinjectors. The simple fact is that some of the units sold were trouble-free and some were not. Whether this is a quality-control problem at Narishige or a basic design fault is unclear.

3.1.5.1   Narishige microinjectors: a brief history

- *IM-5B:* Fitted with a 3-ml syringe, recommended for the holding pipette, discontinued in June 1997 and reintroduced in 2001 (see Figure 3.14).
- *IM-6:* Fitted with an 800-µl syringe, recommended for the injection pipette, discontinued in June 1997 and reintroduced in 2001 (see Figure 3.13).
- *IM-60:* A very limited production run was made of this instrument, an experimental successor to the IM-6. One of the features was a coarse control to make filling easier. It was introduced at the Middle East Fertility Society meeting in Alexandria in October 1996, and was discontinued shortly after. Only a few were sold (see Figure 3.13).
- *IM-300:* Sold by Narishige but actually manufactured in Taiwan by Micro Data Instrument Inc. of New York. An excellent instrument that features a holding and injecting channel and fully programmable automatic injection sequence. The only disadvantage (apart from a confusing instruction manual) is that it requires an external source of pressurized gas. On balance, this excellent injector is ideal for research but probably too highly specified for routine ICSI.
- *IM-8:* Introduced in June 1997 at the same time as the IM-16 and IM-50B, this injector features both coarse and fine controls and a micrometer slide like the IM-16 and IM-50B. Technical difficulties with the novel coaxial coarse/fine controls suggest that the design of this instrument may be flawed (many of those sold were returned).
- *IM-55:* Coarse version of the IM-26, with a 3-ml syringe. Apparently, it is designed to perform the same function as the IM-50B.

Narishige itself does not make the syringes, but instead buys from an outside supplier in Japan. The original injector, the IM-6, was first supplied with a syringe and an all-metal barrel and plunger. To create a sufficient seal between barrel and plunger, two silicon O-rings were fitted around the plunger tip. These syringes were generally acknowledged to be excellent, but minute irregularities in the inner surface of the barrel would wear down the O-rings over time, until the seal broke. For this reason, the syringes were withdrawn and replaced with glass-barrelled models. The plunger was tipped either with a Teflon™ plug or, like the original all-metal model, with two silicon O-rings. Unfortunately, these were withdrawn suddenly without apparent reason. The syringes that replaced them were again glass-barrelled, but this time with all-metal plungers. These would have been adequate, in theory, had the plungers and barrels been manufactured to high enough tolerances. In practice, however, the seal between the barrel and plunger was frequently poor, and during the injection procedure oil would leak from the plunger–barrel interface. Whether there were problems with quality control at the manufacturer, or whether the syringes were not intended for such pressures, will probably remain a mystery. Eventually, after having to replace a large number of faulty syringes, the problem was addressed and, by early 1997, seemed to have been rectified.

In their latest incarnation, the 800-µl syringes (part number SYR-6) still feature an all-metal plunger, but the quality is much higher. In addition, a resin syringe tip with a Luer-type fitting has replaced the original metal tip, which was also the site of oil leakage. For owners of the older IM-6 injectors, the purchase of the new SYR-6 syringe is a highly recommended upgrade (see section 3.1.6.1).

3.1.6 Accessories and spare parts

At the time of writing, Narishige is in the process of introducing a wide selection of accessories and spares for its ICSI equipment. Some of these have been introduced in response to comments on previous versions, some as upgrades for users of previous models, and some as novel attempts to make the system easier to use. Some of these attempts work and some do not.

3.1.6.1 *Microinjector syringes*

As well as the 3-ml and 800-µl syringes, a 200-µl version, part number SYR-4, is now available, making it possible to upgrade microinjectors to a particularly fine control (see Table 3.4).

3.1.6.2 *Pipette holders*

To date, the Narishige pipette holder has been through three major changes. The original HI-4, the HI-6 and, at the time of writing, the HI-7 (see Figure 3.15). While each instrument has its detractors and its champions, the general consensus seems to be that with the latest configuration

Table 3.4 *Microinjector syringes*

Part no.	Description
SYR-1	A 3-ml all-glass syringe with a plain tip.
SYR-2	Discontinued. An 800-µl capacity glass syringe with a metal barrel.
SYR-3	Discontinued. The same as SYR-2, but with a plastic spacer for mounting on to the IM-6.
SYR-4	A 200-µl capacity syringe with a Luer lock tip.
SYR-5	The same as SYR-4, but with a plastic spacer for mounting on to the IM-6.
SYR-6	An 800-µl capacity syringe with a Luer lock tip.
SYR-7	The same as SYR-6, but with a plastic spacer for mounting on to the IM-6.

Figure 3.15 Narishige micropipette holders: the original model HI-4 (left), the older model HI-6 (centre), and the newer model HI-7 (right).

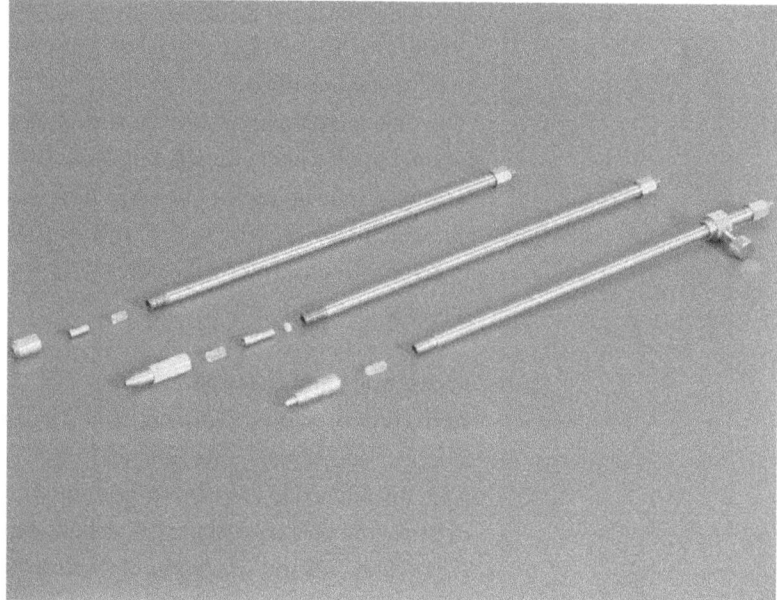

there is an overall improvement. Both HI-4 and HI-6 had small parts that were lost easily; this is less so with the HI-7. In particular, the HI-6 caused problems: there was a production run where the steel bush was made the wrong size, causing oil to leak out of the pipette/holder interface (see section 3.5.4.3).

3.1.6.3   Dual tool holder HD-21

Used primarily for PGD, this dual tool holder allows independent position-ing of the micropipette tips while maintaining control with the hydraulic micromanipulator. The HD-21 fits into the hydraulic headstage of the micromanipulator where the universal joint (B-8C or UT-2, for example) would go. While a reasonably well thought out addition to the range, there have been some complaints of difficulty in positioning the tools relative to each other. This is due to the fiddly screw controls and the poor-quality bearing surfaces used. Hydraulically controlled versions of the dual tool holder are available (HDO-2 and HDO-20), but they are expensive.

3.2 SETTING UP THE MANIPULATORS

It is important to set up the manipulators to ensure they provide the maximum range of movement around the centre of the microscope field of view. This can be achieved by executing the following steps:

1 Fit the mounting adaptor to the microscope as described in the accompanying instructions. Do not tighten the screws until the final positions are achieved.
2 Fit the coarse manipulators to the adaptor.
3 Ensure the coarse manipulators are adjusted so they are in the centre of their movement range.
4 Fit the micromanipulators to the coarse manipulators, and ensure the controls of the micromanipulators are adjusted so they are in the centre of their movement range.
5 Fit the pipettes into the pipette holders of the microinjectors, and fit the pipette holders into the universal joints of the micromanipulators.
6 Place a plastic dish or microscope slide on the microscope stage and, under low power, focus on its upper surface (scratching a small cross on the dish with a sharp object may help). This will be the approximate focal plane when microinjection is performed.
7 Using the freedom of movement of the ball joints, the micromanipulator–coarse positioner joint, and the coarse positioner–mounting adaptor adjustment, position the pipette tips in the centre of the field of view of the microscope, in focus (ensure the coarse manipulator and micromanipulator controls or the microscope focus are not disturbed).

The manipulation equipment is now set up for use, and the relative positions of the mounting adaptor, coarse manipulator mountings, and micromanipulator headstage mountings need not be altered. Any fine adjustments can now be achieved by adjusting the ball joints and, of course, the manipulator controls.

3.3 FILLING THE MICROINJECTORS

The following account describes the filling procedure for the IM-6 microinjector. Later models' procedures will be similar.

It is recommended that Narishige microinjectors be filled with a thin mineral oil to get the best performance (e.g. Sigma mineral oil 0.84 g/ml). Pour a quantity of the oil into a clean container. Unscrew the syringe plunger clamp, the white nylon syringe barrel clamp, and the clear plastic syringe protector. Remove the syringe from the injector. Gently uncouple the syringe from the plastic tubing. You should now be left with the glass syringe with the plunger lockring still attached. Be particularly careful with the syringe in this state, as the plunger will easily drop out if it is held upside down (particularly messy if the syringe is filled with oil!). Carefully dip the syringe tip into the oil, and withdraw the plunger slowly. The plunger will not stop when it is pulled to the base of the barrel, so stop drawing oil before then. Be particularly careful not to draw up any air bubbles. Holding both the syringe barrel and the plunger in one hand, carefully connect the plastic tubing to the tip of the syringe.

Now slowly push home the plunger, and watch the air–oil interface as it passes along the tubing towards the pipette holder. Once oil is flowing freely from the tip of the pipette holder, place the tip into the oil container and, *very slowly*, reverse the plunger, drawing oil into the tubing. Once both the syringe barrel and the tubing are completely full of oil, with no air bubbles, the syringe can be clamped back into its housing.

When filling any oil-hydraulic microinjector, the following points should always be borne in mind:

- Mineral oil is best cleaned up with ethanol, so a bottle of ethanol should always be on hand in case of spills.
- If too much suction is placed on the hydraulic system, the oil can cavitate or degas, and bubbles will form. When filling or operating oil-filled microinjectors, always do things very slowly. It will soon become apparent how fast one can turn the controls without mishap.
- Bubbles, once they have formed in the system, must be bled out before the injector will operate properly. The easiest way to bleed out air bubbles is through the tip of the pipette holder, after which the syringe will be depleted of oil and must be recharged by drawing up more oil. Sometimes, particularly when the air bubbles are in the syringe, it is necessary to detach the tubing from the tip of the syringe, hold the syringe tip-up, and tap the air to the top. After the air bubble is expelled, the tubing can be reattached (being extremely careful, of course, not to reintroduce more bubbles).

The usual convention is to have the holding pipette on the left-hand side and the injecting pipette on the right-hand side of the specimen.

Some workers, while adopting the above convention, reverse the microinjector drives (but not the pipette holders), thus the holding pipette is controlled by the microinjector on the right and the injection pipette by the microinjector on the left. This helps during the sperm-catching process, which is described in section 8.3.

3.4 ALIGNING THE PIPETTES

The micromanipulators and microinjectors are now ready to use. Before commencing the operation with solutions and tissues, place a dry plastic dish under the microscope, switch to the lowest power, and focus on the upper surface of the dish, as when setting up the manipulators initially. This will be the approximate focal plane needed when oocyte injecting. It is important to point out at this stage that to make the process of working under high power easier, one should always focus on the oocyte first. This will invariably lie on the bottom of the dish, and then one can use the z-axis (up–down) controls of the micromanipulator to 'focus' the pipette tips. It is possible, at first, to otherwise miscalculate the positions of the pipettes in relation to the bottom of the dish and accidentally break them off.

With the low-power objective and the microscope focused on the bottom of the dish, you are now ready to set up the pipettes. If you have a microscope whose illumination support limb hinges, and to which the manipulators are attached, then gently tilt back the limb and remove the dish without altering the focus of the microscope. Fit pipettes into the microinjector pipette holders, ensuring that there are no air bubbles in the oil. Very gently, turn the control knobs of the ICSI injector clockwise to push oil down no further than the bend in the pipette. It is very important not to advance the oil too far down the pipette, particularly the injection pipette. If oil is allowed to pass into the very narrow portion of the injection pipette, small bubbles may form in the tip when the oil is drawn back. This has much the same effect as completely blocking the pipette tip and means that considerably more oil pressure is required to inject sperm (see section 3.5.4.6). If any blockages or air bubbles become apparent, replace the pipette immediately. Do not be tempted to try to clear the blockage or remove the air bubbles. Successful ICSI can be performed efficiently only with pristine pipettes! Fit the pipette holders to the micromanipulator headstages so that the bent section of the pipettes will be parallel with the bottom of the dish when the illumination support limb is returned. Try to use the freedom of movement of the universal joints rather than the manipulation controls. Slowly return the illumination support limb to normal. If at any time it seems as if the pipette tips will crash into the objective lens, hinge back the limb and readjust the pipette tips. If the microscope has no hinging illumination support limb facility, then the operation of centring the pipette tips in the field of view is carried out in a similar way but by using the freedom of movement of the micromanipulator ball joints only.

The aim is to get the pipette tips in the field of view of the microscope without having to adjust the manipulator controls or the microscope focus. If the above method is followed, the pipette tips will now be centred and the manipulators will still be in the centre of their tracks, allowing maximum possible movement in any direction. It is now possible to change objective lenses and keep the pipette tips in focus without having to move the manipulators. Turn the z-axis controls of the micromanipulators one turn anticlockwise to raise the pipette tips a fraction and to ensure they do not hit the dish when it is in place.

The workstation is now ready for ICSI. Either tilt back the illumination support limb or raise the pipettes using only the z-axis of the coarse manipulators. Users of MMN-1s must rack up the pipettes by hand until a dish can be fitted underneath. Users of MM-88s or MM-89s should ensure that the speed control is set to minimum then activate the up control along with the yellow over-ride (turbo) button until it is at the top of its movement.

The dish containing the gametes can now be placed on the microscope stage. The illumination support limb should be returned slowly to upright so that the pipettes dip into the dish and return to the field of view. In practice, the pipette tips will now be slightly out of focus, since the optical density of the medium is higher than that of air. Again, focus them with the z-axis of the micromanipulators. If no tilt facility is available, the coarse positioners should be racked down slowly until the pipette tips can be seen in the field of view.

3.5 TROUBLESHOOTING

3.5.1 Manual coarse manipulators

3.5.1.1 *Problem – the z-axis of the mechanical coarse manipulator drifts/runs down*

Probable cause: The vertical (z) axis of the oldest version of the Narishige coarse manipulator, the MN-1 (as opposed to the MMN-1), was particularly prone to running down on its own. A small screw was built in to the instrument so that the axis could be fixed in place once the desired position had been adjusted. With the advent of the next version, the MMN-1, the z-axis was designed as a worm-and-nut array rather than the rack and pinion of the earlier MN-1. Still, if the control knob of the z-axis was not adjusted correctly, the axis was still capable of drifting.

Suggested remedy: To remedy this, the control knob needs to be tightened: Remove the MMN-1 from the ICSI workstation. Locate the grub screw in the end of the control knob. Grip the control in one hand and loosen the grub screw with an appropriate-sized Allen key. Once the grub screw is loosened, the control knob can be unscrewed from its thread. Screw the control knob further on to its thread as far as it will go, without moving the axis (grip the entire manipulator to prevent the movement). Keep turning the control knob clockwise on to its thread until it tightens. Hold the control knob and tighten the grub screw again, locking the knob in place. The whole z-axis movement should now be tighter. If further adjustment is needed, repeat the above steps.

3.5.1.2 *Problem – the control knob is too loose or too tight*
Probable cause: The control has been fitted to the thread incorrectly. This has been known to happen during manufacture.

Suggested remedy: see section 3.5.1.1.

3.5.2 **Motorized coarse manipulators**

3.5.2.1 *Problem – one axis of the motorized manipulator vibrates when activated, or moves intermittently, despite the motor working continuously*

Probable cause: The gear teeth in the motor casing have become unmeshed. Sometimes, the vibrations of the motor in use cause the fixing screws to loosen spontaneously.

Suggested remedy: The motor spindle needs to be realigned and tightened. Remove the clear perspex cover from the top of the motor in question, exposing the gear cog (made of brown plastic) and motor drive cog (which is brass-coloured). It will be possible to see that the teeth of the two cogs no longer mesh, and that the motor cog is possibly loose. Remesh the cogs by pinching them together, but not too tightly otherwise they will not turn. Retighten the motor fixing screws (there are two, cross-headed, located between and to the sides of the two cogs) (see Figure 3.16).

3.5.2.2 *Problem – one of the motorized manipulators does not work in one axis*
Probable cause: In almost all cases, one of the control cables has become jammed between the motor and the mounting adaptor or microscope.

Figure 3.16 The MM-88 motor, which drives the coarse micromanipulators; partially dismantled to show the gear and motor drive cogs.

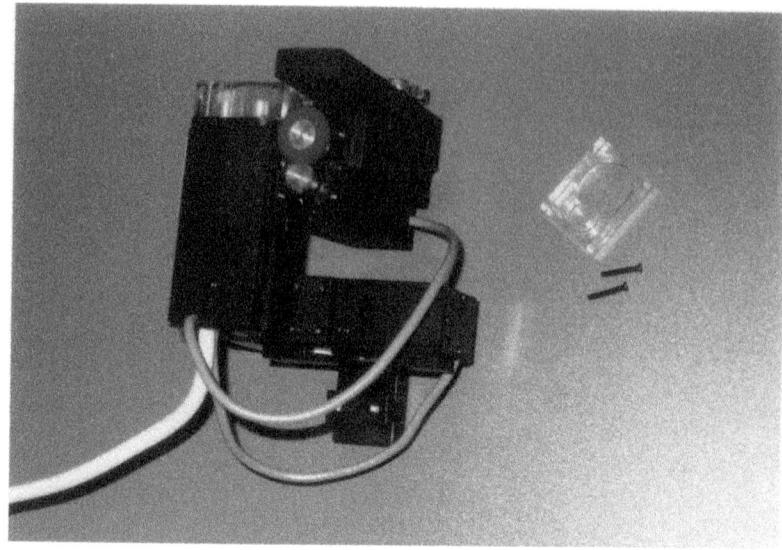

Suggested remedy: Simply switch off the manipulator and gently free the cable, possibly by undoing its fixing screws and removing it from the mounting adaptor. Occasionally, however, this will not correct the problem, in which case the cause is almost certainly of an electrical nature (burned-out motor or faulty control board). In this case, one can determine whether it is motor or controller by swapping the joysticks from one side to the other. Although the problem can be deduced in this way, the only remedy in this instance is to return the unit to Narishige.

3.5.2.3 Problem – one of the motorized manipulators does not work in any axis

Probable cause: There are many potential causes for this problem and, apart from a simple loose wire, most are caused by an electrical fault. As above, a process of elimination can deduce the problem, by swapping controllers from left to right, but the unit will still need to be serviced by a qualified Narishige engineer.

Suggested remedy: Return to your Narishige distributor.

3.5.2.4 Problem – the pipettes vibrate when the motorized manipulator is activated

Probable cause: This is almost always a simple case of a loose fixing screw on the manipulator assembly. The vibrations of the motor then set up sympathetic vibrations in the microscope, affecting the pipettes.

Suggested remedy: Systematically go over the entire micromanipulation assembly, checking and tightening all nuts, bolts and screws.

3.5.3 Hydraulic joystick-operated micromanipulators

3.5.3.1   *Problem – the pipette moves in the opposite direction to the movement of the hydraulic joystick control in the x- and y-axes*

Probable cause: The ratio adjustment of the hydraulic joystick control has been adjusted past the zero position.

Suggested remedy: One of the least utilized features of the Narishige joystick manipulator is the ability to change its range of movement. Directly below the joystick pivot on the hanging-type joysticks (directly above on the upright models) is an adjustment ring with graduations. Loosen the adjacent ring, which allows the joystick to move freely in its socket. Now, holding the joystick so that it does not spin, rotate the ratio ring clockwise (looking from below on hanging models, above on upright) until it will not turn any further. Then, rotate the ring slightly so that the infinity symbol ∝, is below the black line found on the body of the manipulator (just above the ring on hanging versions, below on upright). With a pipette in the holder, any movement of the joystick should produce little or no movement of the pipette tip. Rotating the ring anticlockwise (looking from below on hanging models, above on upright) should result in larger and larger displacements of the tool tip for a given movement of the joystick. The ratios are marked on the ring, which can go two full turns. Starting with the ring tightened all the way in, the ratios are in pairs, the left ratio for the first turn, the right for the second. Unscrewing the ring results in the ratios moving through ∝, $600:1$, $300:1$, $200:1$, $150:1$, $120:1$, $100:1$, $86:1$, $75:1$ and $66:1$. The ratios refer to the movement of the joystick against the movement of the pipette tip, so at $600:1$, a 1-mm movement of the joystick will result in a $1/600$ mm movement of the pipette tip.

The phenomenon of the tip moving opposite to the joystick occurs when the ratio ring has been turned too far past the ∝ ratio. Simply adjust the ratio ring until the movement of the pipette tip at normal working magnification seems appropriate. There is no correct ratio; it is a matter of personal preference. Note that the z-axis cannot be adjusted in this way.

3.5.3.2   *Problem – the pipette moves in the opposite direction to the movement of the hydraulic joystick control in the y-axis only*

Probable cause: In most cases, the heel of the bent microtool rubbing on the bottom of the dish causes this phenomenon. One of the inherent problems of using angled microtools is that if the bent portion is not totally parallel with the bottom of the dish (or at least angled down slightly), it becomes impossible to bring the tip of the microtool into contact with the bottom of the dish. This is necessary, for example, to immobilize and catch the sperm. If the bend is touching the dish, then it acts as a pivot, so that when the joystick is moved one way the pipette holder follows but the microtool bends around the pivot and the tip moves in the opposite direction.

Suggested remedy: To determine whether this is indeed the problem, simply raise the pipette off the bottom of the dish and refocus the microscope on the pipette tip. If this rectifies the problem, then the pipette tip needs to be realigned (see section 3.4).

3.5.3.3 Problem – the pipette moves in an axis at 90 degrees to the one commanded by the hydraulic joystick

Probable cause: The hydraulic headstage has been fitted incorrectly to the coarse manipulator.

Suggested remedy: Since the hydraulic micromanipulators made by Narishige do not come in left- and right-handed versions, the micromanipulators need to be configured for the left or right side of the microscope. The following steps are for setting up the left-hand micromanipulator:

1 Fit the coarse manipulator, whether electric or manual, to the mounting adaptor.
2 Fit the headstage of the hydraulic manipulator to the coarse manipulator. On model numbers MMO-202, MMO-202D, old ONO-121 and MO-188, ensure that the small 'L' on the headstage is facing forwards towards the eyepieces of the microscope.
3 Mount the magnetic base of the joystick to the plate so that the two black dial controls are oriented one towards the operator and one left, away from the microscope.

Do the same for the right-hand side, but make sure the small 'R' is facing forwards, and that the black controls on the joystick point forwards and right. On Narishige's own manipulators, this can be accomplished either by simply rotating the whole joystick through 90 degrees or by detaching the control from the mount, via two Allen bolts on the tip of the cream-coloured body, rotating through 90 degrees and reattaching. If performing the more aesthetic latter adjustment, take extreme care not to pinch the hydraulic lines when reattaching (they are damaged very easily). The newer, curved Olympus–Narishige joysticks have a rotating headpiece, which is simply loosened with a coin, rotated and retightened. (Note that this issue is not a problem for the MO-188NE – the hydraulic micromanipulators are universal for left- and right-handed use.)

3.5.3.4   *Problem – the pipette hardly moves/does not move in response to commands from the hydraulic joystick*
Probable cause: The ratio setting is too fine.

Suggested remedy: Readjust the ratio, as detailed in section 3.5.3.1.

3.5.3.5   *Problem – the pipette hardly moves/fails to move in one axis*
Probable cause: Either the rotary control of the x- or y-axis has been turned out too far, or the cartridge diaphragm for that axis is ruptured.

Suggested remedy: If the rotary controls on the joystick controller have been turned out past their maximum range, then any joystick movements will not affect that axis (the controls should be in the centre of their ranges – see section 3.2). If a diaphragm has ruptured, then the entire micromanipulator must be returned to Narishige for replacement. In most cases, it will be necessary to return the instrument to the nearest Narishige branch office in New York or London or the main office in Japan. Distributors are not usually allowed to make cartridge repairs.

3.5.3.6   *Problem – there is a purple-coloured precipitate in the hydraulic lines of the micromanipulator*
Probable cause: This is usually a mixture of old age and possibly the cumulative effects of ultraviolet light.

Suggested remedy: The official Narishige line here is that the precipitate will not normally cause problems, as long as it is restricted to the middle of the hydraulic lines. They do not say what can happen if these particles enter the cartridge itself, but they recommend a cartridge change if there is any doubt. The cartridge change procedure is simple, although not necessarily rapid, and costs about US$150 per axis.

3.5.4   Microinjectors

3.5.4.1   *Problem – oil leaks from the syringe plunger – barrel interface*
Probable cause: This was a common problem on a particular production run of syringes supplied with the IM-6 model. Since the diameter of the tip of the microtool is narrow, fairly high pressures build up inside the oil reservoir in the syringe. This oil will try to escape at the weakest point, and for some syringes this point was the back of the glass barrel where the plunger inserts. Oil will bleed slowly from the back of the syringe and contaminate the working area. The syringe in question will probably be a glass-barrelled model (800-µl) with a metal tip and metal flange at

the back. The plunger will be all metal, with no O-ring and no plastic tip.

Suggested remedy: These syringes are faulty and should be returned to Narishige for replacement.

3.5.4.2 Problem – oil leaks from the syringe tip – tube connector interface

Probable cause: Caused by a similar problem to that in section 3.5.4.1. This time, the weak point in the system is the point where the metal tube connector joins the metal syringe tip. Again, this is the manufacturer's fault: the metal–metal connection was never a very good idea for a hydraulic system at these pressures. It is exacerbated by the fact that the tube connector is not quite a snug enough fit over the tip of the syringe, resulting in a slow oil leak.

Suggested remedy: In the short term, wind a single layer of plumber's Teflon tape around the syringe tip before reattaching the tube connector. In the long term, purchase a newer, better syringe (SYR-6) from Narishige or a Hamilton syringe (note that adaptors are required to fit Hamilton syringes to Narishige injectors; these are available from Narishige).

3.5.4.3 Problem – oil leaks from the pipette – holder interface

Probable cause: This is almost always due to a damaged silicon seal, found inside the tip of the pipette holder. Take the screw top off to access the seal, but use caution: there is a metal bush (spacer) inside the pipette holder, which can fall out and always rolls under a heavy cabinet! Occasionally, the bush itself is ill-fitting or even missing. The soft silicon seals are particularly easy to damage if pipettes are inserted into the holder when the screw cap is screwed down.

Suggested remedy: For a damaged/missing silicon seal, replacements are available from Narishige. Cutting off the frayed portion with a scalpel blade can extend their lives, but eventually they will need to be replaced. Always loosen off the cap completely before inserting a new pipette.

For a missing bush (HI-4, HI-6 only), replacements are available from Narishige (keep a few spare, as they get lost with surprising frequency). Note that the newer holder (1997 onwards), HI-7, has the bush integrated into the screw cap. For an ill-fitting bush (HI-6 only), with the screw cap off and the bush in place there should be a small gap between the top of the pipette holder screw thread and the wide portion of the bush.

3.5.4.4 Problem – the glass syringe breaks when the control knob is turned

Probable cause: This was possible with the IM-5B (and possible but never documented in the IM-6), when the lockring holding the back of the plunger was overtightened. This could cause the plunger to rotate off-axis when the control was turned. The resulting stress on the IM-5B's all-glass syringe barrel could cause it to break. One or two cases were documented in the Narishige Europe office of the threaded screw portion becoming bent, thus causing the syringe to break, again by turning the plunger off-axis.

Suggested remedy: The lockring holding the back of the syringe plunger should be tightened to a precise amount. Too loose and there will be backlash and poor control of the oil in the pipette; too tight and the plunger may turn off-axis. As a guide, grip the screw with one hand and grip the lockring between finger and thumb of the other, as if holding an eggshell, then tighten the lockring until it just stops turning (it may take some practice to get it just right). A bent screw will need to be replaced by Narishige.

3.5.4.5 *Problem – there is a delay between movement of the injector control and movement of the sperm in the pipette*
Probable cause: This can be caused by backlash in the injector mechanics, but it is due more often simply to poor hydraulics caused by air bubbles in the system.

Suggested remedy: The IM-5B and IM-6 rarely suffer from backlash, since each screw is lapped individually to fit exactly into each thread. This method of manufacture, however, is costly and subsequent versions of Narishige injectors employed different, cheaper mechanisms. Ultimately, backlash problems need to be fixed by Narishige, although a poorly tightened lockring (see section 3.5.4.4) should be ruled out first. For procedures on ensuring the injector is filled properly with oil, see section 3.3.

3.5.4.6 *Problem – there is generally poor control of the oil in the pipette*
Probable cause: This can be due to many causes, all of which need to be explored and eliminated. Among them are air bubbles, backlash, fluctuations in temperature (caused by draughts), leakage of oil, blocked pipette, and poor technique.

Suggested remedy:
   For air bubbles, see section 3.3.
   If there is backlash, see section 3.5.4.5.
   If there are fluctuating temperatures, ensure the workstation is in a constant-temperature environment, away from air-conditioning units,

radiators and draughts, which may raise and lower the temperature, causing the oil in the injector lines to expand and contract.

For oil leaks, see sections 3.5.4.1, 3.5.4.2 and 3.5.4.3.

For a blocked pipette, see Chapter 8.

To remedy poor technique, see Chapter 8.

3.5.5 Micromanipulation workstation in general

3.5.5.1 *Problem – the micromanipulator headstages are too far away to allow the pipette tips to be in the microscope field of view*

Probable cause: This can be for a number of reasons, all of them related to the way the individual components have been assembled in relation to one another. This is the strength and weakness of the Narishige system: the variety of different ways each component can be set up allows the user to tailor the workstation precisely to their needs. The pipette holders can be positioned close to or far away from the microscope stage and can be aligned in a wide variety of angles. However, this means that there is no single set of instructions that apply to every case. Much can be gained from spending time trying different configurations and from talking to other workers who have the Narishige system. Training courses can also be a valuable source of advice.

Suggested remedy: Assuming the guidelines above have been followed (i.e. manipulators are set in the centre of their ranges, etc.), the following adjustments should be attempted, first singly, then in various permutations:

- Slide the mounting adaptor up or down on the illumination support pillar (consider mounting the adaptor above the condenser if a short working distance condenser model is being used; if using the MMN-1 coarse manipulators, the vertical bars can be mounted so that they hang down) (see Figure 3.6).
- Consider mounting the adaptor in front of the illumination support pillar (if originally mounted behind) and vice versa (compare Figures 3.5 and 3.7).
- If using the vertical mounting adaptor bars in conjunction with the MMN-1, consider mounting the vertical bars on the opposite face of the horizontal bar (compare Figures 3.4 and 3.5).
- If using electrical coarse manipulators (MM-88 or MM-89), consider reversing their mounting posts (with two small screws on the front) and mounting them on the opposite side of the horizontal mounting adaptor bar (compare Figures 3.8 and 3.9).

4 Eppendorf micromanipulation workstation systems

Eppendorf AG are relative newcomers to the assisted reproduction technology (ART) market. Recognizing the potential for their instruments, they modified their existing Micromanipulator-5171 (a general-purpose micromanipulator, used mainly for the injection of cultured, adherent cells) in 1995 to a version dedicated to the manipulation of cells in suspension, called the TransferMan (see Figure 4.1). The specific requirements of ART forced the evolution of this instrument into the TransferMan NK (see Figure 4.2 and section 4.3) and then the TransferMan NK2 (see Figure 4.3). To complete the micromanipulation workstation, Eppendorf provides manual microinjectors and micropipettes for both the holding and injection sides.

While other manufacturers' devices maintain some sort of mechanical linkage between the controller and the pipette tip, all Eppendorf manipulators rely on microprocessor control, and the TransferMan models are no exception. The movements of the joystick are sensed, encoded digitally, and passed through a microprocessor and on to the headstage. By this means, an intuitive control of the pipette in all three dimensions can be achieved with these instruments in either a dynamic or proportional mode.

In dynamic mode (TransferMan), the joystick is spring-loaded in all three axes so that it returns to its centre position when released. Furthermore, the position of the joystick controls the speed of the micropipette tip: the further the joystick is displaced from the centre, the faster the tip moves. In proportional mode (TransferMan NK and NK2), similar to mechanical and hydraulic systems, the position of the joystick directly controls the position of the micropipette (see section 6.2.1.1).

The headstage assemblies for all Eppendorf manipulators are three individual precision stepper motors, set at right angles to each other. Each motor originally had a range of movement of approximately 25 mm and

Figure 4.1 Eppendorf's
TransferMan system.

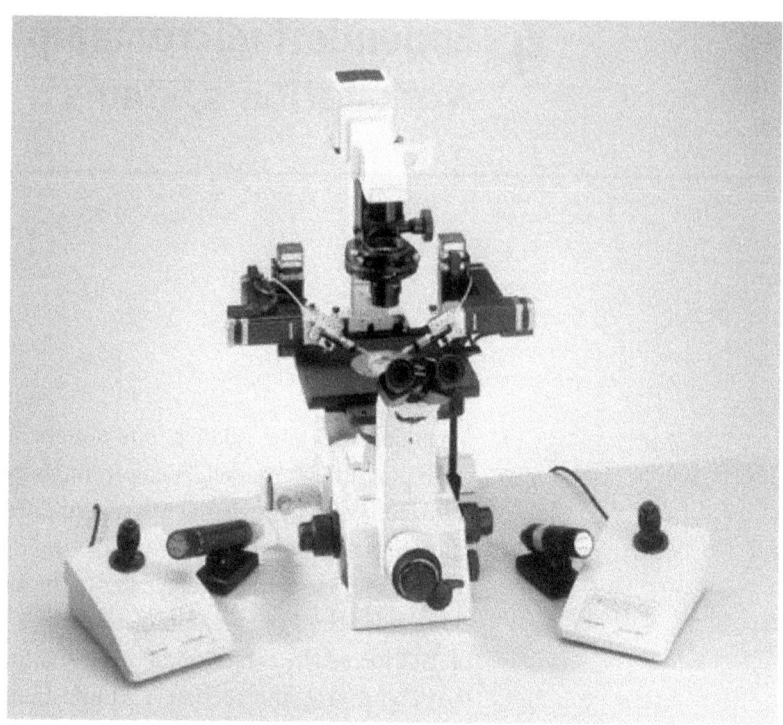

Figure 4.2 Eppendorf's
TransferMan NK system.

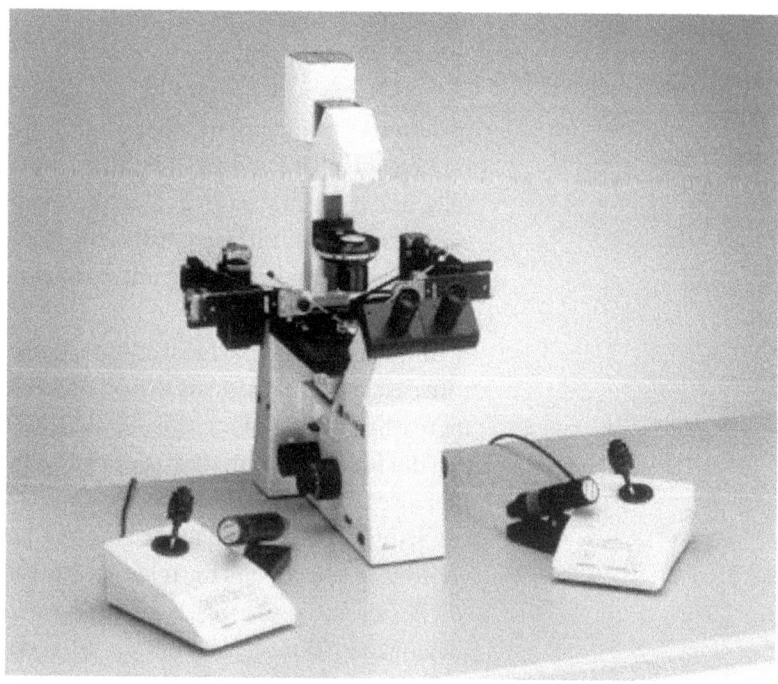

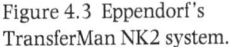

Figure 4.3 Eppendorf's TransferMan NK2 system.

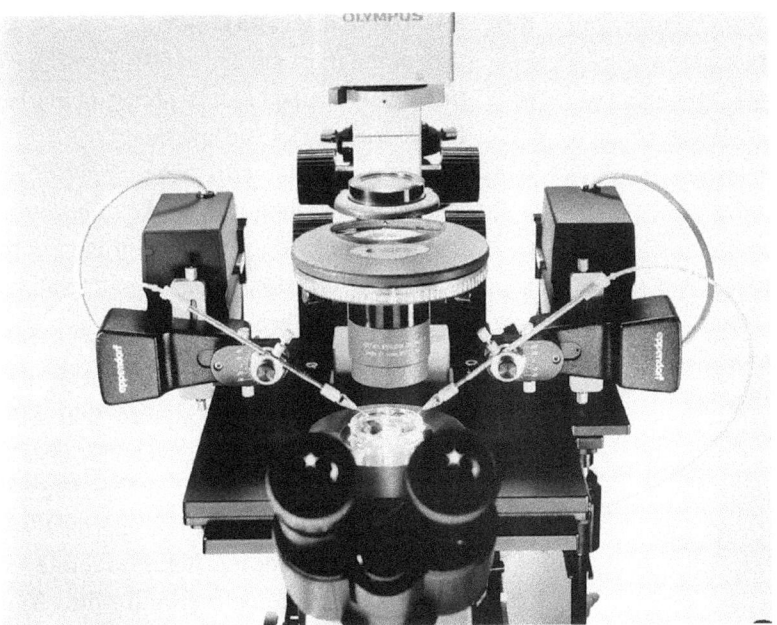

an individual step size of 157 nm. In continuous motion, the steps are so small and so rapid that the movement appears quite smooth. In the latest instrument, the TransferMan NK2, the step size has been narrowed down further for virtually step-free movement.

4.1   TRANSFERMAN FEATURES

4.1.1   Position memory

The microprocessors controlling the positions of the stepper motors are able to store up to two positions in the memory of the machine and then, at any time, and with the touch of a button, return the pipette tip to either of those positions. Typically, users store one position as a 'working' position, close to the bottom of the dish, and one as a 'parked' position, slightly above the working area so that the pipettes do not interfere with the gametes as the dish is moved around the stage.

4.1.2   Home

Since the microprocessors 'know' where the motors are positioned at any time, this makes the Eppendorf home function the most elegant of all. Pressing the home key raises the pipettes to the upper and outer limits of their ranges of movement; when the key is pressed again, they return to the exact same position as they were in originally.

4.2   MICROTOOL ALIGNMENT

One of the most attractive features of the TransferMan manipulators is not apparent upon first reading the marketing literature, nor on seeing the instrument for the first time.

Anyone familiar with the original Narishige universal joint will appreciate just how long it can take to position the pipettes correctly before use. In addition to x, y and z co-ordinates, there are three other degrees of freedom, which need to be taken into account when positioning an ICSI microtool. They are:

- *pitch:* the angle made by the tool holder with the microscope stage – typically 30–40°, so that the bent portion of the microtool is flat against the bottom of the dish or, better, angled down by half a degree;
- *yaw:* the angle at which the two tool holders approach each other; looking down from above, they should approach each other head-on;
- *roll:* the ability of the tool holder to rotate around its own long axis so that the tip of the microtool is pointing directly at its opposite microtool.

If any of these factors is out by more than a few degrees, the microtool can become very difficult to control. Any pipette-holding mechanism, therefore, should isolate each factor so that it can be adjusted independently of the others. This is what the Eppendorf system offers.

The headpiece of the x-motor can pitch, and the pipette holder's tip can roll, even when the pipette is tightly gripped in place. Because each degree of freedom can be adjusted independently, the correct microtool position can be established very quickly. In addition, once the appropriate pitch is determined, their set-screws can be tightened and do not need to be readjusted, even when a new pipette is fitted (assuming the pipettes are similar in construction, as are most prefabricated pipettes).

4.3   NEW KINETICS

In 1997, Eppendorf recognized that while some new users appreciated dynamic control, there were many more that wanted a proportional feel, so they set about redesigning the TransferMan. The project was ambitious: Eppendorf had a manipulator with a proportional mode already on the market, the 5171, but the proportionality was in the x- and y-axes only, and was not as smooth as their mechanical competitors. Working in conjunction with the St Barnabas Medical Center's Gamete and Embryo Research Laboratory in New Jersey, USA, several prototypes were discarded before the final version passed muster.

Based on the TransferMan's existing technology, with the same three motors and a similar joystick interface, the new instrument appears very similar to the older model. It is not until one looks at the movement of the microtool under the microscope that it is possible to appreciate the changes that have been made. The joystick is no longer sprung, and the movement is no longer robotic. Also, the gearing ratio of the joystick to the pipette tip can be altered electronically, effectively allowing a wide movement range at low magnification, and a very small, very fine range at high magnification. The home and preset features are still present. Another innovation is the incorporation of an angle readout and screw adjustment of the pipette angle, a feature that allows for even faster set-up of microtools prior to working.

The result is an instrument that possesses all the advanced features of an electronic manipulator yet moves like a mechanical one (highly experienced users may detect the slightest delay between joystick and pipette tip, but it is barely discernible).

4.4 TRANSFERMAN NK FEATURES

With the new version came the opportunity to redesign the original TransferMan, including the tool holder, and to add features. New features on the TransferMan NK include a lower z-limit and y-lockout.

4.4.1 Lower z-limit

This is designed to prevent the tip of the microtool from inadvertently breaking against the bottom of the dish. The z-limit is set by slowly moving the microtool tip until it is just touching the bottom of the dish (this can be detected by a slight movement to the left of the right-hand tool as it is lowered, and vice versa). The z-limit button is then pressed, and this programmes the manipulator to not allow the tip to move any lower until the limit is cancelled.

4.4.2 y-lockout

This function allows the y-motor to be deactivated, meaning that all left-to-right movements are in the x-axis only (the z-axis can be isolated simply by not touching the control, i.e. holding the lower half of the joystick). All stabbing movements of the pipette are now purely along the axis of the bent portion of the microtool, parallel with the bottom of the dish. The rationale is that without this feature it is possible to tear the hole in the oocyte by slight movements in the y-axis. Whether this feature is of any real value is open to debate and, presumably, study.

4.5 TRANSFERMAN NK2 FEATURES

It is too soon to tell how this newest addition to the market is perceived, but Eppendorf is hoping that it will change the balance in its favour.

By the time this book is in print, the first units will be in place. This latest micromanipulator from Eppendorf has been totally redesigned and upgraded to include the features outlined below.

4.5.1 Mechanics, set-up and adjustment

The motor modules are much smaller and only one cable connects them to their respective joystick. The large power unit of the TransferMan NK is replaced with a small, laptop-like power unit that connects the joystick to the mains supply. Consequently, the TransferMan NK2 is easier to set up. A new feature is the facility for quick adjustment of the micromanipulator in the z-dimension. A useful feature for multiple users is the ability to programme in and store specific user profiles, allowing three independent working positions.

4.5.2 Resolution, range and proportionality of the kinetics

The resolution of the micromanipulators has been narrowed down to approximately 40 nm. These smaller steps, together with new software that translates the movement of the joystick to the stepper motors, ensures that no steps can be seen, even at the highest magnification. The working radius of the TransferMan NK2 micromanipulator has been increased and is easier to control.

4.5.3 Handling and software

Useful new features in the software are the storing of three independent working positions. Also, four different users can store and reload their preferred settings as a profile.

4.6 EPPENDORF INJECTORS

Designed from scratch rather than around an existing syringe, the Eppendorf injectors come in three types: the CellTram Air (see Figure 4.4), recommended for the holding side, and the more sensitive CellTram Oil (see Figure 4.5) for the sperm injection side. As the names suggest, the Cell-Tram Air is a simple air-filled chamber with a large, smooth, micrometer control knob and a weighted base. The CellTram Vario is a recent modification of the CellTram Oil, with a second, much finer transmission ratio (see Figure 4.6). Particularly useful features of the CellTram Air include an angle adjustment for the controls, tubing with screw-fitting that seals very tightly, and a valve (see Figure 4.7) for equilibrating the internal and

Figure 4.4 Eppendorf's
CellTram Air microinjector.

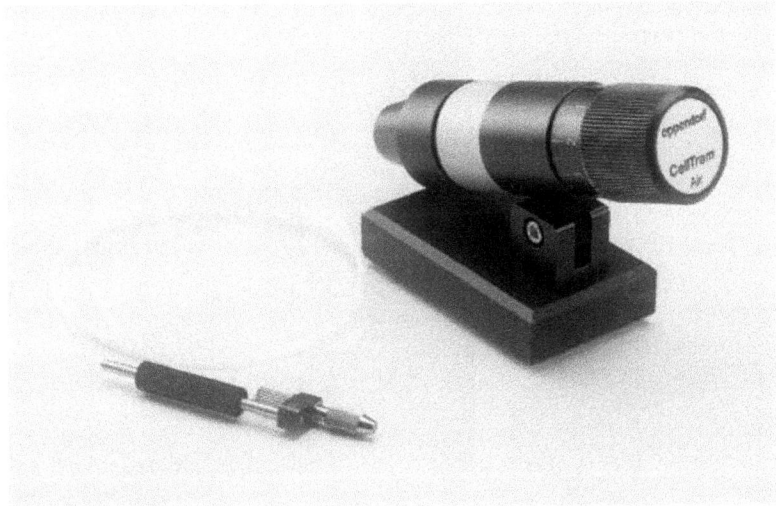

Figure 4.5 Eppendorf's
CellTram Oil microinjector.

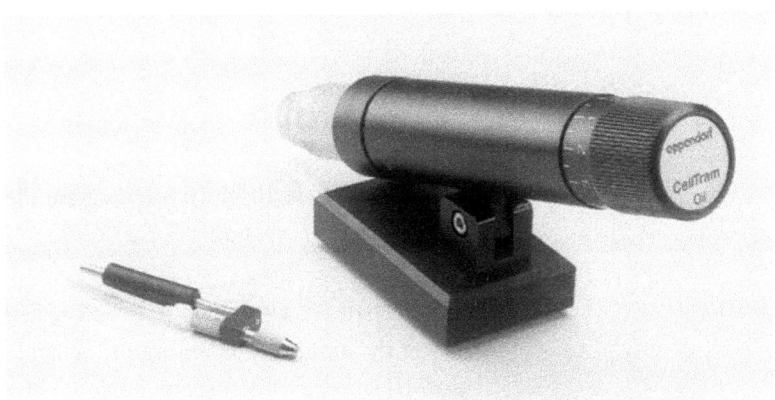

Figure 4.6 Eppendorf's
CellTram Vario microinjector.

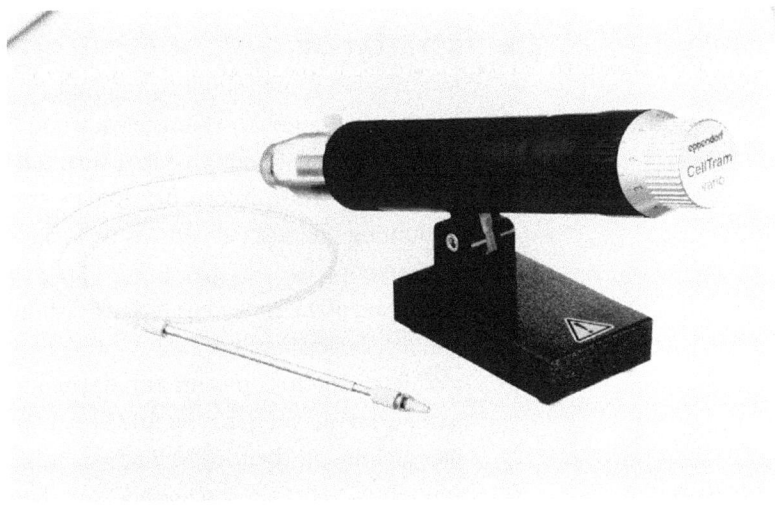

Figure 4.7 Close-up of Eppendorf's CellTram Air microinjector, showing the equilibration valve.

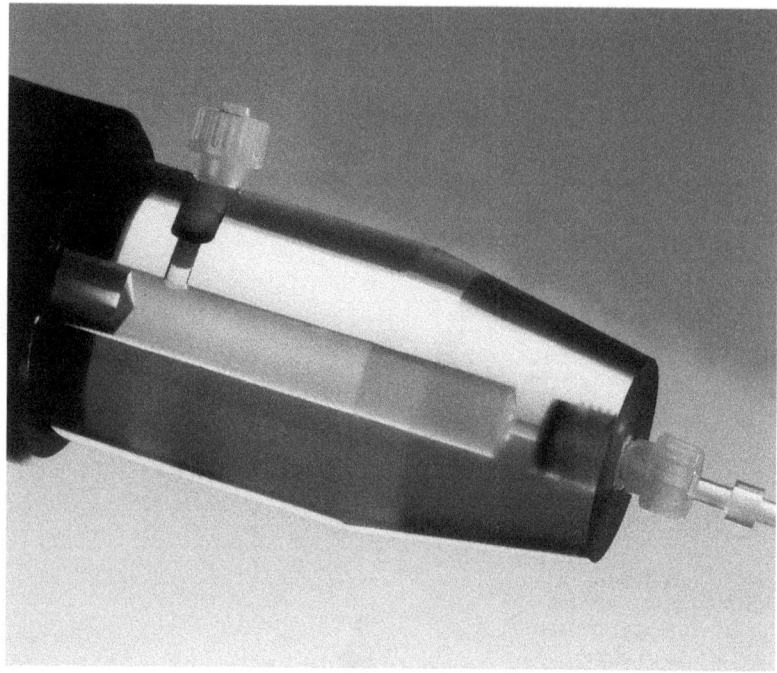

external pressures (useful if you accidentally have the instrument blowing bubbles – see the section 4.9.2.2).

4.7 MOUNTING ADAPTORS

Currently, mounting adaptors are available for all current makes and models of inverted microscope. Table 4.1 outlines the Eppendorf mounting adaptor range.

4.8 INSTALLATION

Since this is a troubleshooting manual, and the installation instructions that come with both the TransferMan and TransferMan NK are excellent, there will be no attempt to duplicate them here. Furthermore, there are no separate parts to order other than two manipulators, two injectors and a mounting adaptor (sometimes two adaptors, depending on the model of microscope used). There is very little that can go wrong during the installation of the Eppendorf ICSI workstation, but some important points should be borne in mind.

While the motor units are unattached to the microscope, they should be treated with care. They should be left on the bench top not on end but laid carefully on their sides. First, the z-motor (vertical control) should be mounted to the microscope adaptor, then the y-motor (backwards and forwards control), and finally the x-motor (left to right control) with its tool

Table 4.1 *Eppendorf microscope mounting adaptors*

Eppendorf part no.	Microscope make/model	No. of adaptors required
5181 200.008	Leica DMIRB/DMIRBE/HC	1
5181 201.004	Leica DMIL/HC	1
5181 202.000	Leica DMIRE 2	1
5181 210.003	Nikon Diaphot/Diaphot TMD	1
5181 211.000	Nikon Diaphot 200/300/ Eclipse TE 200/300	1
5181 212.006	Nikon Eclipse TS 100	1
5181 222.001	Olympus CK 2/CK-30/CK-40	1
5181 221.005	Olympus IMT-2	1
5181 220.009	Olympus IX 50/70	2
5181 232.007	Zeiss Axiovert 25	2
5181 233.003	Zeiss Axiovert 10/35	2
5181 230.004	Zeiss Axiovert 100/135	2
5181 231.000	Zeiss Axiovert 200	2
5181 250.005	Universal Stand	1

holder. The three motors should never be dismounted from the microscope as a single piece. The precision stepper motors can be damaged if they suffer an impact, and this can be manifested as a slight kick of the pipette tip as it moves along one axis (see section 4.9.1.5).

The control pad should never be lifted by its joystick, neither should it be placed upside down on the bench.

The motors and the control pad should be connected to the power supply only when the unit is switched off.

The joystick of the TransferMan NK should always be in the centre of its x- and y-movement range before the unit is switched on (see section 4.9.1.9). Great care should be taken to ensure that the motors will not crash into the microscope stage or condenser when they are at the limits of their movements.

4.8.1 Set-up and optimization of the CellTram Oil

Fresh out of its box, the CellTram Oil needs to be filled with light mineral oil (0.84 g/l, available from Sigma). A small bottle is provided, and operators will find that it is the same oil that is used in most cell culture and IVF procedures.

When setting up the CellTram Oil, it is vital that the system is filled properly, without introducing any bubbles into either the hydraulic line or the cylinder. If it is not already so, turn the micrometer screw clockwise until it will not turn any more. This will expel as much air as possible from the cylinder. Open the small bottle of mineral oil and, using ordinary Sellotape, fasten the bottle to the bench. This is very important. Later, during the filling procedure, the bottle is easily tipped over – a messy clean-up operation will then ensue (it is advisable to have a supply of paper towels and 70% ethanol on hand to clean spills; ethanol can also be used more effectively than soap to clean oily hands).

Attach the short filling tube to the Plexiglas micrometer cylinder, taking care not to cross the screw threads. Slowly begin to turn the micrometer screw anticlockwise, drawing oil along the tube and into the cylinder. It should be possible to follow the advance of the air–oil interface by eye. Keep turning the control anticlockwise until it will no longer turn. The cylinder should now be full of oil.

Carefully detach the screw fitting of the filling tube from the cylinder and lay it on one side. At this point, inspect the cylinder for air bubbles. Point the CellTram Oil upwards (cylinder up, control knob down) and tap the side of the cylinder. Any air bubbles should rise to the top of the cylinder and can be expelled with a small turn of the control knob. Now, keeping the instrument pointing upwards, attach the 1-m length of main tube to the cylinder. Turn the control clockwise, pushing the oil out of the cylinder and into the tubing. Again, it should be possible to follow the air–oil interface by eye. As the air–oil interface reaches the far end of the tube, the cylinder should be almost but not quite empty. The far end of the tube should now be dipped into the oil bottle and the last of the air pushed out by turning the control. Once all the air is expelled from the tube, reverse the control of the injector, turn it anticlockwise, and fill both the tube and the cylinder.

During this filling process, the control should be turned very carefully; the oil can flow into the line only slowly now, and if the control is turned too fast the consequent lowering in pressure can cause the oil in the cylinder to cavitate, or degas, and bubbles to form. If at any time bubbles are seen in the cylinder, stop turning the micrometer, unscrew the hydraulic line, tip up the cylinder, tap the cylinder until the air bubbles float to the top, turn the control clockwise to expel the air, and reattach the hydraulic line. This is important: the CellTram Oil, like any other oil hydraulic system, will not operate optimally if air bubbles are present.

Once the cylinder is full, the hydraulic line can be removed from the bottle, cleaned of oil, and attached to the pipette holder. Oil can be advanced to the tip of the pipette holder and the instrument is then ready for use. Exactly the same procedure is followed for preparing the CellTram Vario injector before use.

4.8.2   **Setting up the manipulators for ICSI**

The following protocol assumes that the micromanipulators have been installed correctly and are working properly.

Set the microscope to the lowest power magnification possible. Switch on the micromanipulators. Activate the coarse (fast) mode (the button on the left-hand side of each keypad). Before commencing pipette set-up, it is important to position each axial motor at the centre of its travel range. This ensures that the full range of movement is available for the final micropositioning of the pipettes, and gives enough travel to allow the pipette to come up clear of the dish when the home button is pressed. Each axial motor is marked with a white bar 2.5 cm long, with a black reference mark in the middle. This is the centre position, and it should be aligned with the centre position of the moving portion of the motor (this is the line where the black body of the motor unit joins the silver motor drive at one end).

Before fitting the pipettes into the holders, place the slide or dish that is to be used on to the microscope stage, select a low-power objective, and focus on the specimen to be injected/manipulated. Now rack up the focus by 0.5–1 mm (i.e. the objective lens should be raised towards the dish by 0.5–1 mm). The focal plane should now be slightly above the specimen. Now, without altering the microscope focus, remove the dish or slide (most inverted microscopes have an illumination support limb that hinges back to facilitate this). Now, when the pipettes are finally aligned in the optical axis of the microscope, they will not crash into the dish or slide when it is replaced.

Fit the first pipette into its holder (it is best to start with the holding pipette since it is larger and thus easier to see unaided). Unscrew the clear perspex griphead until it is loose but does not come off. Insert the blunt end of the holding pipette into the griphead until a slight resistance is felt. This resistance is the rubber O-ring, which will tighten around the pipette when the griphead is screwed down. Push past the O-ring about 4–5 mm, then tighten the griphead firmly.

Fit the pipette holder into the tool block on the x-motor and tighten the fixing screw. Adjust the tilt angle of the pipettes (pitch – see section 4.2). On original TransferMan units shipped before August 1999, this must be done by eye on a trial-and-error basis. On original TransferMan units shipped after August 1999 and on the TransferMan NK, the angle adjustment is a simple matter of turning the angle adjustment screw so that the correct angle reads on the x-motor's protractor.

By loosening the pipette holder fixing screw in the tool block, advance the pipette holder so that the tip of the pipette is just above the microscope stage (take care not to let the pipette tip touch the stage or objective). The x-motor is capable of sliding on its mount. Loosen the set-screw and, assuming the pipette tip is not yet in the optical axis, position the x-motor so that the pipette tip is approximately above the objective.

At this point, consider the following:

- Will the x-motor clear the stage at the limits of its movement?
- Will the tool holder or pipette holder clear the condenser?
- Will the pipette and holder clear the sides of the Petri dish?
- Is the angle of attack (pitch or tilt) precisely correct?

Switch the micromanipulator to fine (slow) mode. The micromanipulator joystick control can now be used to position precisely the holding pipette tip in the microscope's field of view. First, if possible, stop down the microscope field iris, which will give a greater depth of focus. Do not refocus the microscope objective yet – use the z-axis of the micromanipulator to focus the pipette.

Now repeat this procedure for the other micropipette, using the tip of the holding pipette as an approximate guide for the tip of the injection pipette. Both pipettes should now be visible in the microscope's field of view.

Press and hold the home key on the micromanipulator keypad(s). If the pipettes have been set up properly, the micropipettes should retract to the upper and outer limits of their z- and x-axes.

Replace the dish or slide and focus down on the specimen. Press the home keys. The pipette tips will return to their original positions, just above but not interfering with the specimen. Focus on the tips again.

Use the z-axis control on the joystick to lower the pipette tip(s) towards the specimen, following them down with the microscope fine focus. A word of caution here – if the microscope's objectives are not exactly parfocal, the higher-power objectives may protrude slightly above the microscope stage as they are swung into place. This will knock the dish up into the pipettes and break them.

Pipettes, dish and microscope should all now be in correct alignment for microinjection. With practice, some of these steps will become unnecessary and the procedure for setting up pipettes should become second nature.

4.9 TROUBLESHOOTING

4.9.1 Micromanipulators

4.9.1.1 *Problem – the tip of the pipette appears to vibrate excessively when moving*

Probable cause: There are several possibilities here. The first, and most common (particularly if the manipulator has been set up correctly and has worked without problem before), is that the pipette is rubbing against the bottom of the dish. This is particularly apparent when the heel (the bend) is the lower-most part of the pipette, since it will be the first thing to touch the bottom of the dish as the pipette is lowered.

Another possibility (this will occur only with stepper motor actuated manipulators like the Eppendorf) is that the pipette tip is vibrating in harmony with the tiny vibrations of the motors. As mentioned above, the motor steps are very small and fast, but they are steps nonetheless. If one should happen to adjust the pipette holder so that the length in front of the holder's fixing point is a distance of 35 mm, the pipette holder and the pipette will resonate in harmony.

An unlikely but remotely possible cause is that the power box for an original TransferMan has been shipped instead of the box for a Transfer-Man NK. The software of the NK has been modified considerably from the version installed on the original TransferMan. This mistake can be confirmed by looking at the back of the control box, by the cooling fins. In the case of the TransferMan, there should be a small label specifying model number 5177; with the NK, there should be two labels, one reading 5171 and one reading 5178.

Suggested remedy: In any event, all the screws fixing the motors to each other and to the mounting adaptor, and holding the pipette, should be tightened.

If the pipette is rubbing on the bottom of the dish, then the pitch angle of the pipette holder should be increased slightly so that the bent portion of the microtool is slightly toe-down.

If the vibrations are as a result of harmonic resonance from the motors, then the distance from the pipette tip to the holder's fixing point should be reduced as much as possible below 35 mm.

In the case of an incorrect power supply being shipped, there is no alternative but to return the power supply and ask for the correct version to be supplied.

4.9.1.2   *Problem – the x-motor stops moving inboard before it reaches the end of its travel*

Probable cause: In a situation like this, the motor has almost certainly come up against an obstacle, either the microscope condenser array or the edge of the stage.

Suggested remedy: The motor should be backed off a safe distance until it is clear of the obstruction. Ideally, the motors should be reconfigured, according to the instructions, so that this does not happen (the motors can be damaged). If the motor is hitting the stage, it should be raised. If it is hitting the condenser, it should be slid away using the dovetail slide and the pipette holder extended to bring it back into the field of view.

4.9.1.3 Problem – the z-motor stops moving upwards before it reaches the end of its travel

Probable cause: As with the problem in section 4.9.1.2, the motor is coming into contact with an obstacle, almost certainly the condenser.

Suggested remedy: Slide the x-motor away from the condenser so that when the manipulator is raised it does not interfere.

4.9.1.4 Problem – the z-motor stops moving downwards before it reaches the end of its travel

Probable cause: Either the manipulator is touching the microscope stage (see sections 4.9.1.2 and 4.9.1.3) or, in the case of the TransferMan NK, the z-limit has been activated and reached.

Suggested remedy: Reconfigure the motors as described above (see section 4.9.1.2), or deactivate the z-limit and reset it at the correct level (i.e. at the bottom of the dish).

4.9.1.5 Problem – the pipette appears to jump slightly at a single point in its range of travel

Probable cause: If this jumping is part of some general underlying vibration, then see section 4.9.1.1. If, however, the kick is isolated and in the same place in the range of travel, then some damage has probably occurred to the motor.

Suggested remedy: The motor should be isolated carefully and returned to the distributor with an explicit description of the problem. It will probably need to be replaced.

4.9.1.6 Problem – when the home key is pressed, the pipette moves too short a distance to clear the sides of the dish

Probable cause: If the home function is activated when the micromanipulator is already near the top of its range of travel, it will go no further. On the original TransferMan (but not on the NK), a brief press of the home key activates the 'clean' function, which moves the pipette a shorter distance out of the dish. The purpose of this feature is to clean the pipette tip of any debris, by allowing it to pass through the meniscus of the fluid in the dish. Unfortunately, it does not work well with bent pipettes,which is probably why the feature was discontinued in the later NK model.

Suggested remedy: Before commencing ICSI, the pipettes should be placed within the field of view of the microscope, while ensuring the x- and z-motors are set at the centres of their ranges of travel (see section 4.8.2). On the original TransferMan, be sure to depress the 'Home/Clean' key for more than one second to activate the home function.

4.9.1.7   *Problem – the motor moves the pipette in the opposite direction to the joystick*
Probable cause: When the manipulator is shipped, it is always configured as a right-handed device. Therefore, when mounting a TransferMan on the left-hand side of the microscope, the x-axis movement will need to be inverted.

Suggested remedy: Looking at the TransferMan or TransferMan NK keypad, there are four buttons along the top. Press the first and second buttons from the left simultaneously until both of the green LEDs on the first button light together. Each axis can now be inverted by pressing the corresponding button on the keypad once, the second, third and fourth buttons corresponding to the x-, y- and z-axes, respectively. Once the appropriate axis has been inverted, press the first button once. Only one green LED should now be lit on the first button, and each axis should work in the direction that the joystick is pushed/twisted.

4.9.1.8   *Problem – the joystick button will not depress*
Probable cause: This occurs very occasionally when the manipulator is first unpacked.

Suggested remedy: Simply loosen the two cross headed screws on top of the joystick until the button is freed.

4.9.1.9   *Problem – the micromanipulator bleeps continually and will not respond to commands from the joystick*
Probable cause: This is a sign that the joystick and the power supply are not communicating properly, usually because the joystick was not in its centre position when the unit was turned on.

Suggested remedy: Switch off the manipulator with the main switch at the back of the power supply. Align the joystick so that it is in the centre of its range of travel. Switch the unit back on, and the problem should be rectified. If it is not, it will be necessary to perform a 'factory reset': press the

'Pos 1' and 'Pos 2' buttons simultaneously, then release the 'Pos 1' button and hold down the 'Pos 2' button for a further two seconds. This restores the settings that were programmed in during manufacture and will cancel any axis inversions that may have been programmed (see section 4.9.1.7). A factory reset will usually restore communications between the joystick and the power supply. If it does not after several tries, it is necessary to enlist the help of the Eppendorf distributor.

4.9.1.10 *Problem – the home setting of the NK2 micromanipulator automatically cancels itself and has to be reset*
Probable cause: The operator has inadvertently touched the joystick during the home manoeuvre. This feature was deliberately added to the Transfer-Man NK2 to allow a means of rapidly stopping the movement and thereby preventing damage to a micropipette that might otherwise crash on to the bottom or side of the microinjection dish.

Suggested remedy: Store the home and working positions as positions 1, 2 or 3, and use this memory as a back-up in the event of the home function cancelling itself.

4.9.2 Injectors

4.9.2.1 *Problem – the griphead will not grip the pipette, no matter how hard it is tightened*
Probable cause: If there is an insufficient number of O-rings in the griphead, the griphead will not bite on to the metal part of the tool holder and consequently will not grip the pipette shaft. The sequence of O-rings, counting from the tip of the griphead back, should be two black and one white.
Occasionally, the threads on the perspex griphead are not long enough to allow the griphead to be screwed down to bite on the O-rings.

Suggested remedy: Add O-rings as necessary. Either insert another (supplied) black O-ring or discard the griphead (save the O-rings, though) and use the spare supplied.

4.9.2.2 *Problem – the CellTram Air is sucking medium out of the dish, and it is hard to find the equilibrium point*
Probable cause: The control on the CellTram Air has simply been turned too far anticlockwise, and now medium is being sucked into the holding pipette.

Suggested remedy: Unscrew the equilibration valve, found on the tip of the CellTram Air, leave for two seconds or so, then retighten it. The equilibrium point (neither aspirating nor blowing) should now be reset at wherever the control knob is currently.

4.9.2.3 Problem – the CellTram Oil has a black deposit on the inside of the cylinder

Probable cause: This is something that can happen over time, as the O-ring on the end of the CellTram Oil's plunger rubs back and forth over the inside of the cylinder.

Suggested remedy: Newer O-rings have been introduced that do not leave a black deposit, but if it has already occurred the unit must be dismantled and cleaned and a new O-ring put in. Note that dismantling the unit may invalidate the instrument's warranty. However, if the instrument is over a year old and not under extended warranty, then it is an easy task. Great care should be taken, however, when unscrewing the restraining collar from the barrel. The unit is under spring tension and the chamber will fly off once the restraining collar is removed. Therefore, hold it tight while unscrewing the collar.

4.9.2.4 Problem – there is poor control of the sperm in the injection pipette (see also section 8.2.3)

Probable cause: The Eppendorf injectors are not known to suffer from back-lash, but if all other causes have been eliminated, then the unit should be returned to the dealer for servicing. In most cases, however, poor control can be attributed to hydraulic problems.

Suggested remedy: Poor hydraulic control can usually be attributed to one of the following: a blockage, a leakage, or air bubbles in the system. Blockages occur most often at the pipette tip, which can become clogged with cellular debris after manipulating tissue (particularly after using a microinjection pipette to sort sperm from epididymal aspirate). A blockage of the pipette will be particularly difficult to clear, since this type of tissue sticks rather well to the glass from which the pipette is made. The best remedy is to load a fresh pipette.

Air bubbles can mimic blockages, especially when the bubbles are at the tip of the pipette. If the oil is allowed to go right to the pipette tip, tiny bubbles will form as the oil is drawn back up. Successful manipulation will then be impossible, and the pipette will need to be exchanged. It is inadvisable to allow the air–oil interface to get any further than halfway down the pipette. Air bubbles in the hydraulic lines must be purged by following the instructions for filling the system with oil (see section 4.8.1).

The CellTram Oil was designed specifically to avoid leakage problems (primarily by listening to complaints about the Narishige systems). As such, leakage is rare and can be attributed to one or more of the following:

- a crossed thread where the hydraulic tubing joins the syringe or the pipette holder;
- a missing or split O-ring in the griphead of the pipette holder (see also section 4.9.2.1);
- broken glass in the tip of the pipette holder;
- a damaged O-ring in the syringe plunger (see also section 4.9.2.3).

5 Research Instruments micromanipulation workstation systems

Established in 1964 by Mike Lee and Vince Grispo, Research Instruments developed a range of mechanical micromanipulators for the microelectronics market for electrical testing of integrated circuits. The early micromanipulators, e.g. the TCV500 produced in 1964, had three axes of movement from one lever and a range of movement reduction from 500 : 1 to 100 : 1. Offering a price advantage and simplicity, these manipulators were purchased by large research organizations, such as the microelectronics giant GEC.

In the 1980s, Research Instruments developed the TLO500, an early derivative of the current TDU500 model, which incorporated the use of flexural hinges, giving the important advantages of stability and relatively low maintenance needs.

Approached by Simon Fishel, Research Instruments expanded into the IVF market in the early 1980s, developing micromanipulators that could be mounted on to an inverted microscope. The TDU500 was thus developed, and the Sonic Sword was designed to improve the ease of cell-wall penetration for the up and coming SUZI technique. During this period, Research Instruments concentrated on the IVF market and developed systems that responded to embryologists' needs.

With the advent of the ICSI technique, Research Instruments continued to develop innovative features to help the novice embryologist get to grips with micromanipulation. In the early 1990s, Research Instruments introduced a home function, which allowed the user to set up the micropipettes above the Petri dish and then to lower them into the dish rapidly without incurring accidental damage. In 1994, the company announced the laser setting-up device (LASU), where, when the micropipettes were set to the correct position, the tips entered a fixed beam of red light, which caused them to glow brightly.

A range of other features were introduced in the 1990s, including angle adjustments for overbent premade needles and a range of accurately

Figure 5.1 Research Instruments' Integra Ti system.

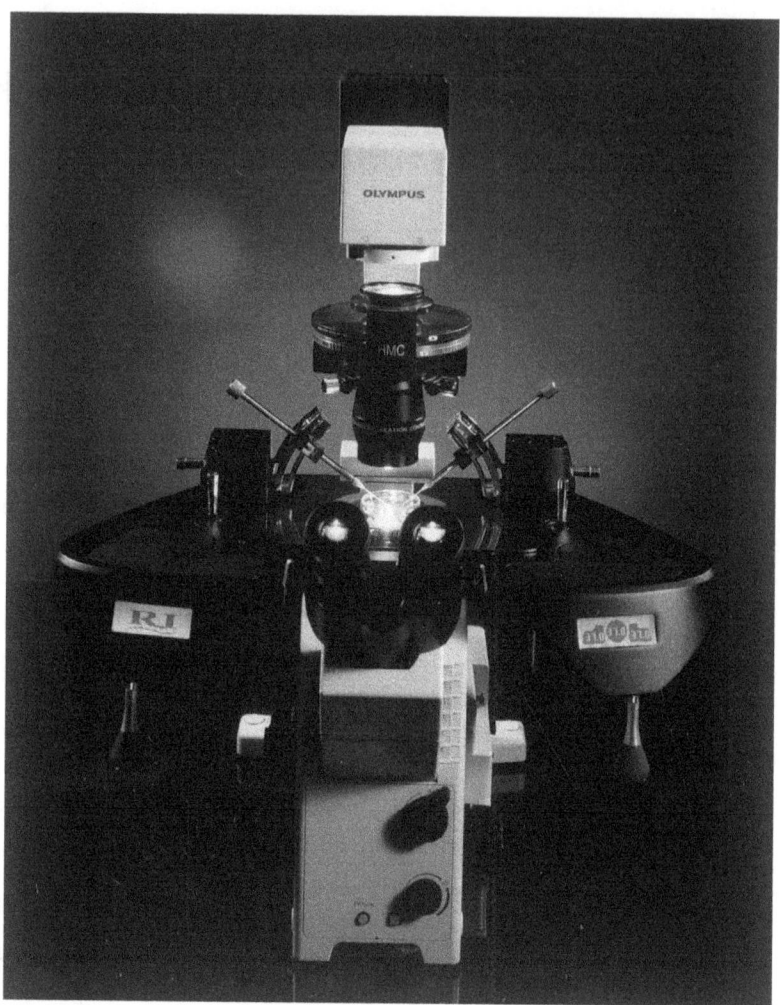

controlled heated stages. Research Instruments launched the Integra micromanipulator system in 1999 (see Figure 5.1).

5.1 THE INTEGRA

The Integra Ti is the latest model to be offered by Research Instruments and represents a move towards a more integrated design (see Figure 5.1).

5.1.1 Micromanipulators

Movement of the micropipettes is provided by Research Instruments' TDU500 purely mechanical micromanipulators. They incorporate both coarse and fine controls in one compact unit. Unlike the Narishige or Eppendorf manipulators, the Research Instruments units are not controlled remotely. The manipulator joysticks extend downwards from the Integra stage. Semicircular handrests are supplied, which greatly assist ergonomics. Like the Narishige and Eppendorf micromanipulators, rotating the fine control knob actuates the z-axis movement.

The movement is proportional, and very similar in feel to Narishige. Being based on simple mechanical components, the Research Instruments micromanipulators are also highly reliable and do not require routine servicing or maintenance.

The reduction ratio can be altered from $100:1$ down to $500:1$, the total maximum displacement being 5 mm.

5.1.2 Quadruple heated stage

The Integra Ti is supplied with four independently controlled heated surfaces or, as an upgrade option, a glass heated central stage (see Figure 5.2). The second and third additional heated stages are designed to maintain the temperature of additional Petri dishes while others are being worked on. The fourth heating channel can be used to heat an external plate such as a stereo microscope.

5.1.3 Pipette angle adjustment

The PL30 tool holder allows the user to make one degree adjustments to the angle of the micropipettes without the tip ever moving out of focus, ensuring that the micropipette is slightly toe-down during sperm manipulation and horizontal during injection (see Figure 5.3). This feature helps to minimize any damage to the oocyte.

5.1.4 Damage-free visible pipette set-up

All Research Instruments tool holders have a special function to instantly move the micropipette vertically by 16 mm. The home function, consisting of a special objective and spacer, allows the micropipette to be set up 16 mm above the Petri dish and then lowered rapidly to the desired position. This system is extremely quick, taking just ten seconds to load a pipette and locate it within the microscope's field of view.

5.1.5 Screw-actuated syringe injectors

The Screw-actuated syringe (SAS) air injectors are the only air syringes designed specifically for air injection of sperm, eliminating the need for oil. Due to their distinctive design, some users have nicknamed them 'the mushroom' (see Figure 5.4). The addition of an equilibration button allows the micropipettes to be equilibrated with the external atmospheric

Figure 5.2 Research Instruments' ITO glass heated stage provides a uniform heated working area while allowing complete viewing of the petri dish.

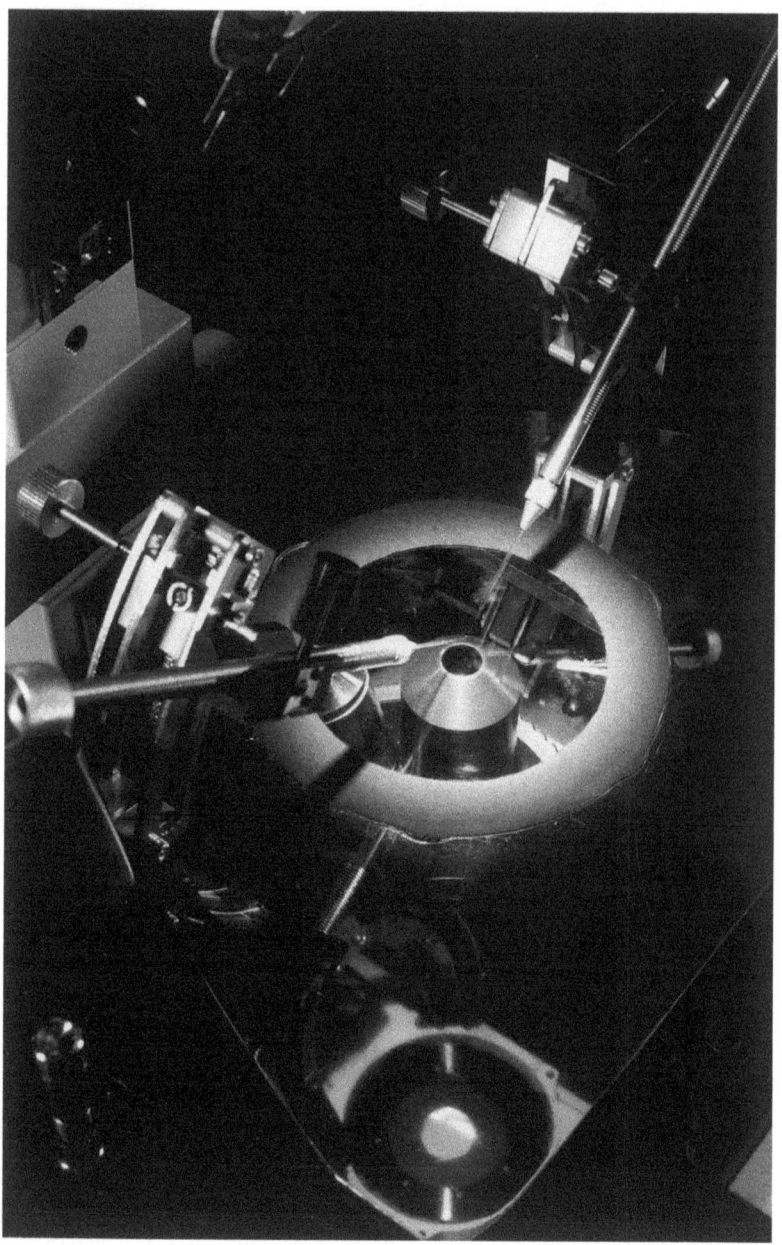

pressure at any time, a very useful feature. The SAS-SE has very smooth rotation.

5.1.6 Dual variable-reduction lever stage

The Research Instruments system is not compatible with standard microscope-branded xy stages. To overcome this, Research Instruments has designed its own xy stage incorporated in the Integra Ti.

Figure 5.3 Research Instruments' MPH microtool holder mounted upon a PL30 tool holder. This set-up allows the angle of the pipette to be changed while the pipette is *in situ* in the petri dish, to achieve a 'toe-down' approach for ease of sperm immobilisation.

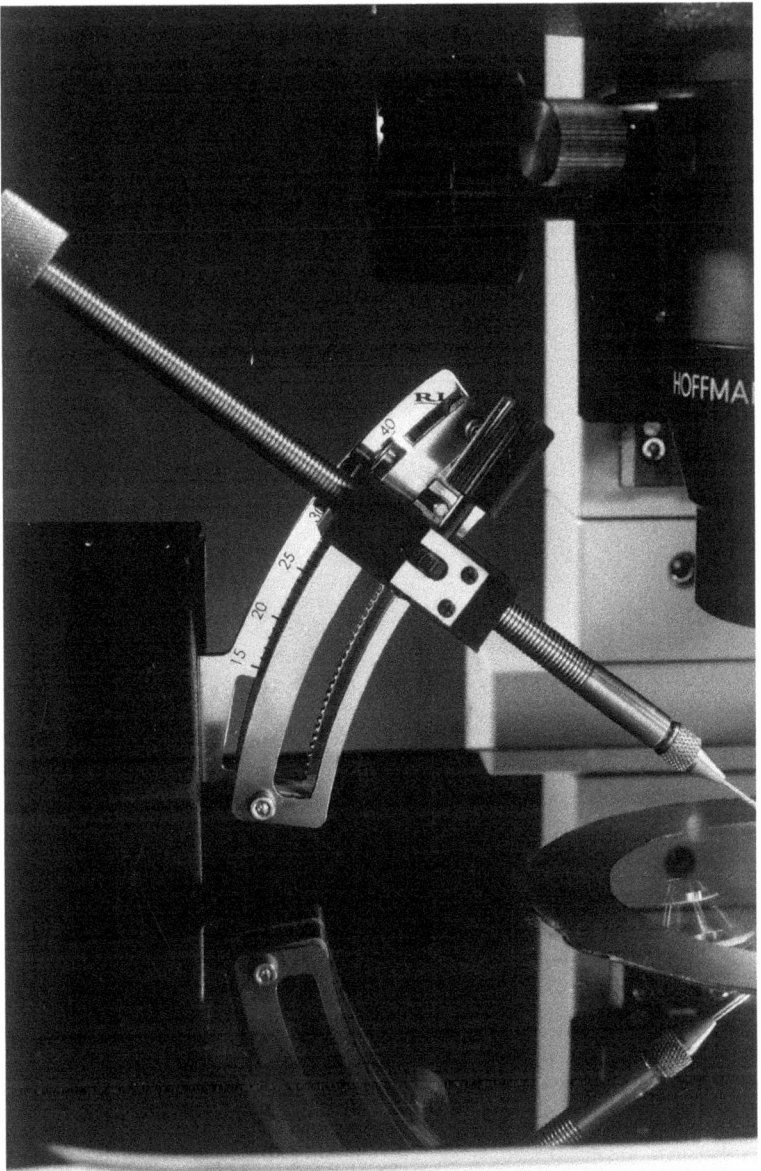

5.1.7 Microscopes

The Research Instruments manipulators are adaptable to all available inverted microscopes, and it is even possible to obtain microscopes indirectly from Research Instruments.

5.1.8 Installation

On purchasing a Research Instruments Integra Ti micromanipulator system, the end user need specify only to which microscope the system is to be

Figure 5.4 Research Instruments' special edition SAS air injector, originally nicknamed 'the mushroom' due to its characteristic shape. The equilibration button on top of the SAS-SE air injector can be pressed during aspiration or injection to immediately halt the flow of media within the micropipette.

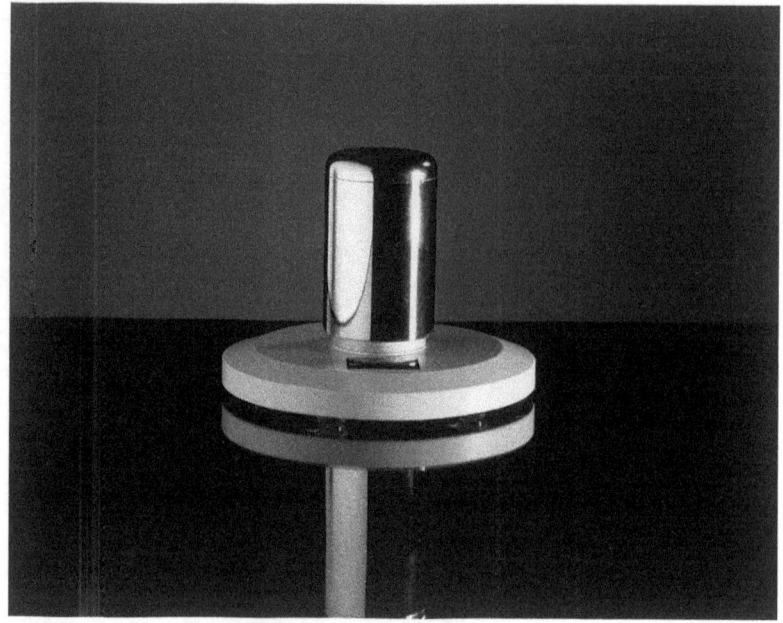

attached. All items that are necessary for micromanipulation, including heated stages and injectors, are included in the package. In the past, Research Instruments' installation manuals were functional and produced in-house, and lacked the polish of professionally produced literature. However, written by native English speakers, the manuals were at least correct and easy to follow. Recently, the installation manuals and troubleshooting guides have been updated and are available in Adobe Acrobat format on CD or can be downloaded from the Company's website, www.research-instruments.com. Also, Research Instruments has a dedicated technical support department to deal with any difficulties found during the installation or operation; this department can be contacted by telephone (+44 1326 372 753) or by email (techsupp@research-instruments.com).

The latest Integra system comes pre-assembled in a purpose-built despatch case. Installation involves attachment to the microscope with just four screws (see Figure 5.5). Care should be taken when removing the Integra from its despatch case, as any severe shock could damage the mechanism of the micromanipulators. Apart from this precaution, installation of the Integra Ti is a simple, quick and easy process.

5.1.9 Set-up

Set-up of the tool holders is a one-off procedure. The following protocol demonstrates the microtool set-up of a Research Instruments system. It assumes that installation is complete and that the PL30 tool holders

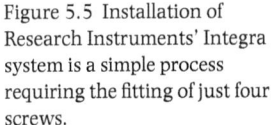

Figure 5.5 Installation of Research Instruments' Integra system is a simple process requiring the fitting of just four screws.

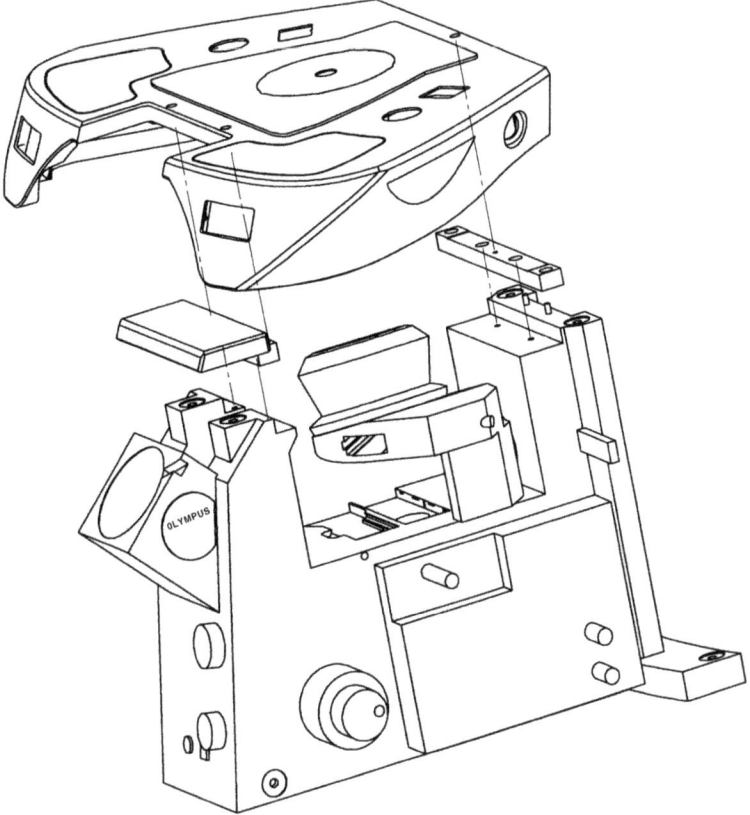

are attached and adjusted to the bend angles of the micropipettes in use.

Make a scratch on the inner surface of a Petri dish and place on to the stage. Focus on the scratch using the 4× objective lens. During the set-up procedure, do not adjust the microscope focus again.

With the holding pipette in the pipette holder and the yellow vertical movement lever in the fully up position, move to the 4× objective with spacer. This spacer allows the user to focus on the pipette in this upper position. Ensure that the manipulator is in the middle of its vertical travel by rotating the fine control lever so that the height gauges on the surface of the Integra are at their middle position, i.e. in the centre of the green division, not in the red divisions. Both the fine and coarse control levers should be in their vertical positions.

Loosen the bottom securing screw of the PL30 (see Figure 5.6) and place into the silver output of the TDU 500. Drive the micropipette forward until it is over the objective, and then by eye look along the pipette and rotate the microtool holder so that it bisects the objective path. Tighten

Figure 5.6 The bottom,
securing screw of the PL30 tool
holder.

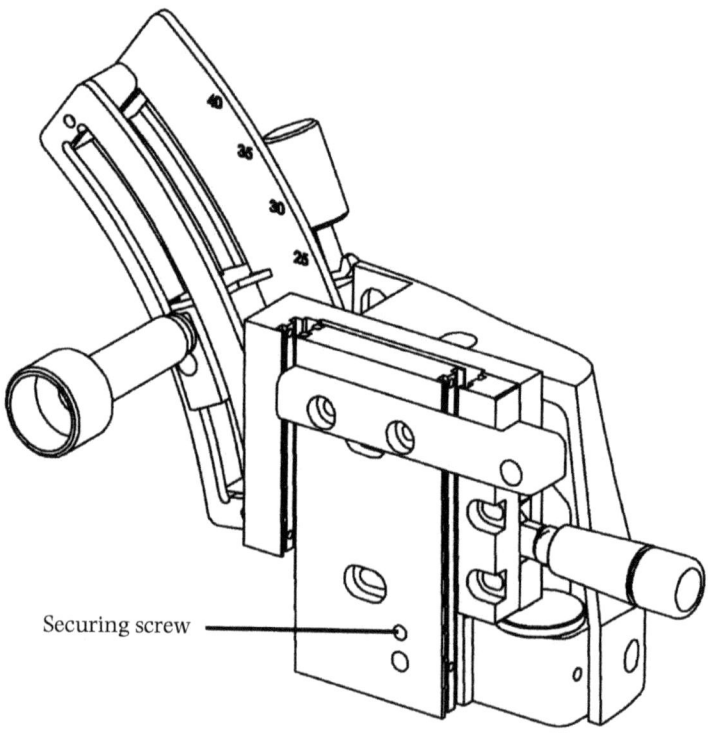

Securing screw

the securing screw. This is a one-off requirement to centralize the detent
position of the microtool holder. Using the special axial-drive mechanism,
position the pipette so that it is in the centre of the field of view. Rotate the
pipette axially using the rotating wheel at the end of the pipette holder so
that the tip is in the correct orientation (see section 8.2.2). Use the fine
control lever to focus the pipette.

Move back to the 4× objective and lower the vertical lever on the PL 30
fully. The scratch on the Petri dish should still be in focus, and the pipette
should be slightly out of focus. This is because the pipette is positioned
slightly above the surface of the Petri dish. If the pipette is repeatedly
found to be too high or too low, the distance of travel in the height can
be adjusted using a small silver thumbwheel located on the side of each
PL30. (N.B. The thumbwheel adjusts only in the down position.) Repeat
the above steps to set up the injection pipette.

5.1.9.1   Injector set-up

The air syringes of the Integra system must be equilibrated before sperm
injection. The holding side is not so critical, but it should be equilibrated
nonetheless. To equilibrate the sperm injector SAS, place a drop of medium

or PVP in the Petri dish. It is not necessary to cover this drop of medium with oil, providing that you are working in an aseptic environment. Lower the micropipette into the equilibrating drop. From its lowest position, rotate the SAS anticlockwise (i.e. upwards) a number of turns (approximately 75% of its travel). Leave to equilibrate for approximately five minutes; the PVP/media should rise up the micropipette until it almost reaches the unpulled shank of the micropipette. Press the equilibration button to neutralize the air pressure (see Figure 5.4). For older models without an equilibration button, to equilibrate the pressure within and outside the micropipette it is necessary to disconnect and reconnect the tubing between the SAS and tool holder. Lift the pipette using the PL30 vertical movement lever and exchange the equilibration dish for the injection dish.

5.2 TROUBLESHOOTING

5.2.1 Micromanipulators

5.2.1.1 *Problem – cannot focus on to the pipette tip*
Probable cause: The pipettes are heel-down on the Petri dish, such that their tips are out of range of the microscope's focus. Attempting to raise the focus merely pushes up the pipettes further until they break (note that this tends to happen only at high magnification).

Suggested remedy: Wind the objective lens back down and use the PL30 angle compensator screw to adjust the pitch angle (see Figure 5.3).

5.2.1.2 *Problem – the pipette does not move smoothly in the xy planes*
Probable cause: The tip of the pipette is touching the Petri dish.

Suggested remedy: Raise the pipette by rotating the fine control lever.

5.2.1.3 *Problem – no fine movement (up and down) on the micromanipulator*
Probable cause: The z movement fine control has been rotated too much either up or down.

Suggested remedy: Rotate the fine control clockwise or anticlockwise (depending on whether the micromanipulator has been locked in the upper or lower position) to free the locked movement.

5.2.1.4 *Problem – joysticks and levers are too stiff/too loose*
Probable cause: This problem typically applies to control levers (fine and coarse) that have a ball joint retained by a plate fixed by three screws.

Figure 5.7 Tightening or loosening the three securing screws that hold the ball joint retaining plate in place will stiffen or loosen the movement of the joystick, respectively.

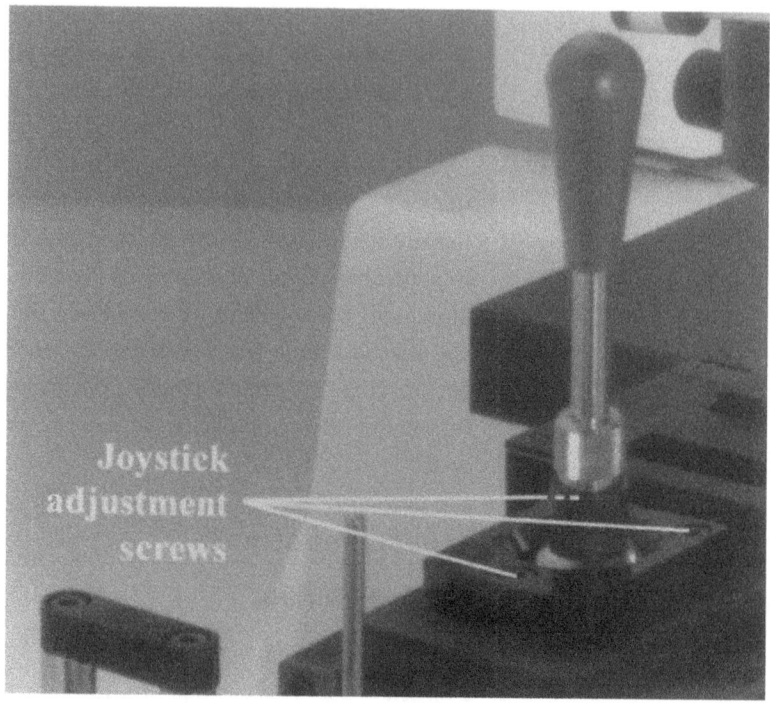

Suggested remedy: Use the correct-sized hexagonal wrench supplied with the system to tighten or loosen the three screws shown in Figure 5.7.

5.2.1.5   *Problem – S16 yellow lever does not stay in the up position (pre-Integra systems only)*
Probable cause: An internal screw has become loose.

Suggested remedy: Contact Research Instruments for self-repair instructions.

5.2.1.6   *Problem – micropipette holder axial drive is not driven axially (pre-Integra systems only)*
Probable cause: Wear in the drive wheel.

Suggested remedy: Contact Research Instruments for a free-of-charge replacement unit.

5.2.2   Heated stage

5.2.2.1   *Problem – the display shows a '?' message*
Probable cause: Heated plate malfunction.

Suggested remedy: Requires repair/replacement by Research Instruments.

5.2.3   SAS air syringe

5.2.3.1   *Problem – Poor control of the sperm*
Probable cause: This problem usually occurs with an incorrectly equilibrated syringe.

Suggested remedy: To equilibrate the syringe, follow the equilibration protocol described in section 5.1.9.1.

5.2.3.2   *Problem – the sperm drift inside the injection needle after equilibration*
Probable cause: Air leak within the injection system.

Suggested remedy: Check that the seals are tight on both the micropipette holder and syringe. If this is not the problem, replace the O-ring inside the SAS barrel. Remove the top of the SAS to reveal the O-ring. Replace the O-ring and relubricate with special lubricant supplied by Research Instruments and its distributors (only applies to SAS11/2-E). If the problem still exists, return the unit for repair.

6 Instrument selection

6.1 SELECTING THE MICROSCOPE

The microinjection is carried out on an inverted microscope at a magnification of 200–400×. It is essential to equip the microscope with some form of contrast optics. Originally, only differential interference contrast (DIC) optics (Nomarski) was available. One of the most widely used optics systems is now Hoffman Optics' Modulation Contrast Optics, although Carl Zeiss introduced its low-cost 'Varel' system in 1996. The advantage of the latter two optical systems is that they can be used with plastic dishes, whereas DIC optics are optimized for working with glass. Dishes with a glass base are now available from, for example, WillCo Wells B.V. in Amsterdam, allowing DIC to be used as originally intended.

The microscope itself should be of the inverted type. The IX-71 from Olympus, the DM IRB/E from Leica, the Axiovert 200 from Zeiss, and the TE 2000 from Nikon are all good examples. These microscopes are available with a bewildering array of accessories and options. Those options considered important would be a camera port, allowing a simple camera and monitor to be attached (useful for teaching), and a movable stage.

Essential specifications for the microscope are:

- inverted microscope (Zeiss Axiovert series, Olympus IX series, Nikon TE series, Leica DM-IR series);
- 10×, 20× and 40× objectives;
- Nomarski (DIC) or Hoffman optics (note that Nomarski optics are not optimized for use with plastic dishes);
- long or ultra-long working distance condenser;
- mechanical stage, with a long-arm coaxial control;
- heated stage insert.

Recommended options include:

- camera port;
- basic closed-circuit TV camera and monitor;
- anti-vibration plate or table (depending on the level of ambient vibration).

6.2 SELECTING THE MICROMANIPULATORS

While there are advantages and disadvantages to all the different systems available, no one system comes out ahead on all aspects, which can make it very difficult to make a choice. However, the systems are all very different in the way they go about achieving the same ends – manipulating a fine microtool in three-dimensional space. The Research Instruments offering is purely mechanical, the Eppendorf is electronic, and the Narishige offers oil hydraulics for fine movement and a choice of electrical or mechanical for coarse positioning.

There is no doubt that the Narishige-based system is by far the most popular. Whether this is because it is better than the rest is open to debate. Narishige certainly has the best coverage in terms of its distributors, choosing to supply all of the four microscope dealers. Research Instruments does have a network of distributors that is worldwide, but its style of business seems to rely very much on dealing directly from its offices in Cornwall, UK. Eppendorf is a relative newcomer to the field and so has not achieved a particularly high market share, although in some countries it has been adopted by independent microscope dealers (in the USA in particular). Narishige has been selling its systems through the big four microscope manufacturers since 1985, and so has been able to utilize the considerable resources of those companies – their marketing skills, salesforces, and so on. There is little doubt that Narishige owes its success in the ICSI market to Nikon and to Nikon's dedication to selling its tremendously successful TMD and Diaphot microscopes.

While hardly exhaustive, the following sections try to draw attention to the kinds of features that the various manipulation systems offer, and their relevance to ICSI.

6.2.1 Micromanipulation Workstation Features

6.2.1.1 *The feel*

The way the instrument feels during use is arguably the most important consideration to be made when comparing micromanipulation systems. In general, different users with differing backgrounds and experience with micromanipulation will have different perceptions of the feel of any given system.

For basic quality of engineering and smoothness of use, the old-fashioned Leitz manipulators must come out on top. These instruments are mentioned here because they are one of the original micromanipulators and found their place in many transgenics laboratories. The degree of resistance of the joystick movement can be altered to create just the right feel, but only in the x- and y-axes. The other purely mechanical system on the market, made by Research Instruments, also boasts extremely smooth movement, this time in all three axes. Research Instruments' claims that the bearing surfaces never wear out and so never need servicing are hard to understand, however.

The hydraulic system utilized by Narishige is also extremely smooth and responsive. By altering the pivot point of the joystick, it is possible to adjust the radius of movement in the x- and y-axes only. The hydraulic system has one weak spot, however: if the rubber diaphragms at either end of the oil line are damaged and oil leaks out, movement in that axis will be lost to some degree.

The original Eppendorf TransferMan is different to the traditional mechanical manipulators. Its 'dynamic' action is not to everyone's taste (although it should not be discounted – clinics are still using older TransferMan systems rather than the newer, proportional TransferMan NK and NK2).

Something as subtle as the feel of a micromanipulation system is difficult to describe on paper, and no suggestion is made here as to which mechanism is better. The user is advised to try the systems before buying, and not to accept the statements made by any manipulator company unless they are willing to back them up with a demonstration. Both authors have heard from users who wished they had bought something different after it was too late.

Basically, the proportional systems feel more intuitive, as if the pipette is an extension of the user's own hand, whereas the dynamic systems are more robotic.

Acceptance of a particular system tends to be based largely on what the technician is used to, the technician's level of experience, and the features offered.

6.2.1.2 *Home function*

All the available manipulators possess a home function of some sort. The purpose is to be able to lift the microtools from their working positions in the field of view, replace the dish, and return the microtools to the field of view without breaking them or having to laboriously find them again under low power.

Table 6.1 *Comparison of the manipulators' home functions*

	Research Instruments	Narishige	Eppendorf
Mechanism	Lever	Coarse z-axis	Stepper motors
Location of controls	Headstage	Headstage	Joystick keypad
Direction of movement	z only	z only	z and x
Resolution of return	High, c. 2 µm	Medium, c. 5 µm	Very high, 160 nm

The Research Instruments home is an excellent lever-actuated mechanism that simply lifts the tool holder out of the dish and returns it, but only in the z-axis. The Narishige offering involves either a coarse control on the top of the headstage (which must be wound up laboriously, then wound down again) or a separate hydraulic control on the side of the joystick. Table 6.1 summarizes the different aspects of the three manipulators' home features.

6.2.1.3 Ergonomics

Neither the Research Instruments system nor the Leitz system is truly a remote-controlled system. The joysticks, control instrumentation and housing are all fixed, or very close, to the microscope stage. In certain circumstances (i.e. users with a short reach), it could be necessary to stretch further than is normally comfortable. Prolonged work in this position can result in repetitive strain injuries. The Narishige manipulators have joystick controls that can be placed up to 1 m away from their slave units, the Eppendorf up to 4 m away.

Overall, the latest Narishige units, whether from Narishige directly or whether their OEM systems from Olympus or Nikon, are probably the most versatile ergonomically. The control units are capable of being mounted magnetically anywhere there is a suitable base, and raised or lowered, and the length of the joysticks can be altered for really fine-tuning comfort.

The Eppendorf system is the only one that provides both coarse and fine positioning from a single joystick control. For laboratories that have a high turnover of injections, this can save considerable time over the course of an ICSI session.

6.2.1.4 Ease of use

As with the feel of the system, the perception of ease of use will depend largely on the user. Some of the more common difficulties experienced include a lengthy pipette set–up time, loss of the microtool tip from the field of view, and breakage of the microtool on the bottom of the dish. A recent study found that the memory positions of the Eppendorf systems allowed users to work faster, presumably because the set-up, loss and breakage incidents were fewer (Al-Hasani *et al.*, 1999).

6.2.1.5 *Pipette set-up and exchange*

For busy clinics with a high throughput of cases, pipette set-up can be one of the most critical aspects of a manipulation system since it is almost always the most time-consuming. Bearing in mind the number of steps required to position microtools accurately, it can take several minutes to position the pipettes in the slightly toe-down aspect that will allow the gametes to be moved around with ease. The original Narishige ball joints were difficult and time-consuming to use, even for an experienced practitioner, but the advent of their newer models, such as the UT-2 with its isolated pitch and yaw adjustment, has made life a little easier. Nevertheless, the fact that the whole hydraulic headstage array can move while these adjustments are being made makes accurate adjustment something that requires some practice. The Research Instruments units are better since it is easier to roll, pitch and yaw the pipette holder, and the holders are sturdier than the Narishige, allowing the process to be watched down the microscope. The Eppendorf instruments probably come out best in this aspect, though. Firstly, the *x*-axis is already perpendicular to the optical axis of the microscope, meaning there is no need for a yaw control. The pitch is achieved with a simple screw, like the Narishige, but because the manipulators are inherently more sturdy it is far easier to watch the adjustment through the microscope, and there is even an angle readout on the side of the tool holder. It is probably not surprising that the Eppendorf is superior to the others in this aspect, since it is the instrument launched on to the market most recently (not counting Research Instruments' Integra, the manipulators of which are essentially the same as Research Instruments' previous models; see section 5.1).

In the final analysis, this is an aspect of the micromanipulation workstation that should be scrutinized carefully during the sales demonstration.

6.2.1.6 *Double tool holders*

For clinics that want to perform PGD, the ability to fit a double tool holder, usually on to the right-hand manipulator, is essential. Fortunately, all the manufacturers supply such accessories, although, as may be expected, not all are equal in their ease of use. The Narishige HD-21 is the simplest and cheapest, although it is not the best in their range (see section 3.1.6.3). Research Instruments' axial-drive double tool holder is simple and effective, providing independent movement of both micropipettes in each axis.

The Eppendorf Twin-Tip holder can be fitted to the x-motor of either the right- or left-hand manipulator and has a simple cable control that allows either, both pipette or neither to be lowered into the dish. Coupled with the TransferMan's two preset memory positions, it provides probably the greatest combination of versatility and stability of all the systems for PGD.

6.2.1.7 Injectors

Another important aspect of the manipulation system is the quality of the injectors. However, this is something that the user can gain considerable control over, since all three manufacturers' injectors are, to some degree, able to fit on any of the three manufacturers' manipulators (note that Research Instruments' tool holders only fit Research Instruments' manipulators).

The Research Instruments SAS (affectionately known as 'the mushroom') is very nearly a perfect design of an air-filled microinjector. Simple, easy to operate, and with a very small footprint, it incorporates a feature that allows the internal and external pressures to be equalized in case too much suction has been applied. There are clinics where, because of its precision, this injector is being used as a sperm injector, negating the use of hydraulic oil. Should this injector be required to work with anything other than the Research Instruments tool holder, the user must find a way of attaching the tubing to the Eppendorf or Narishige (or Leitz) tool holder, which can be a difficult task. All the SAS units appear to suffer from static friction, or 'stiction', a phenomenon where it takes slightly more effort to start the control knob turning than it does to keep it turning; however, this does not seem to be a cause for complaint, nor does it affect its operation. Research Instruments also manufactures a simple micrometer-controlled syringe microinjector, which should be used with oil (part number MSHD).

The extent of the range of Narishige injectors available varies from time to time, but there are usually ten or so different models available at any moment. New models are constantly released and old models discontinued. While there seems to be no reason for such a rapid turnover in instrument design, one would hope that they are constantly striving for better instruments. Unfortunately, this is not always so. One of the best injectors Narishige ever produced, the original IM-6 with the metal-barrelled syringe, was discontinued after only a year or so and replaced with an inferior glass-barrelled model (see section 3.1.5). True, it was an inherently flawed design, in that the rubber O-ring on the tip of the plunger wore out rubbing against the inside of the metal cylinder, but the control it gave over the sperm in the pipette was excellent. This behaviour not only makes for a confusing marketing campaign, but also makes it almost impossible to write an up-to-date review of the instruments currently available, so no attempt is made here. Instead, prospective buyers are advised to trial any Narishige microinjector before buying it, return any faulty injectors they have bought already (warranty permitting), see section 3.5.4 for fixing problems not covered by warranty, or finally give up and buy something else. Microinjectors are comparatively inexpensive, and a good one can be a valuable addition to the ICSI workstation.

Finally, there are the Eppendorf CellTram Air and CellTram Oil devices, which have been available for several years. Designed from scratch, without using Hamilton or similar syringes, they work extremely well when installed properly and also appear to have been received well by the market.

6.2.1.8 *Ease of installation*

For truly effort-free set-up, the new Research Instruments Integra system is definitely worth considering. It is delivered in one single piece; the micromanipulators, injectors and tool holders are all attached to a large microscope stage with a built-in heating plate. Of course, this means that one's options for choosing different accessories are limited: you have to have Research Instruments' injectors, heated stage, moving stage and tool holders, and experienced users may wish to pass up this unit in favour of a more versatile set-up, such as the Eppendorf or Narishige.

Narishige is slowly working towards making its systems easier to install. The new Olympus–Narishige and Nikon–Narishige systems now come partially assembled – a far cry from the 1980s and early 1990s when everything came individually in little plastic bags with a set of poorly written instructions!

The Eppendorf systems, TransferMan, TransferMan NK and NK2, are similar in their set-up, with minor differences in the attachment of the pipette holder. While no means as simple to install as the Integra, they do come with the benefit of a good instruction manual.

Overall, for the price most companies ask, set-up and training should be included, but this service varies wildly from one company to another, and in different parts of the world. Installation and training should be negotiated in advance of the purchase.

6.2.1.9 *Upgrades*

The various micromanipulation companies are, understandably, cagey about their 'next thing' in micromanipulation. The purely mechanical systems have probably reached their peak in the Leitz and Research Instruments devices. If Narishige stays with an hydraulically based format, they are also unlikely to surpass themselves. If their hydraulic control lines get any longer (they are currently about a metre long), then the joystick controllers will become less responsive.

Only the electronic systems seem capable of pushing forward the technology. Eppendorf's TransferMan is an electronic stepper motor, using digital signalling to control motorized headstages, and Burleigh now have a proportional piezoelectric manipulator, which seems to be improving with every new version. Sutter, which has long had a presence in the market for electrophysiology micropositioning, is now manufacturing a micromanipulator for suspended cell injection, to be marketed by Bio-Rad Laboratories.

6.2.1.10   Service

As with installation and training, one would expect that getting a micromanipulation workstation serviced would be a simple matter, but this is not necessarily so. In general, the bigger the company, the better the network of regional offices around the world, and the greater the chances that one of those offices can do the service work locally. Narishige has offices in London and New York that are capable of carrying out limited service and repairs, but for complicated work, especially electronic repairs, the unit may need to be returned to Japan. Eppendorf has sales offices in most major markets, which are capable of doing extensive repair work, and this work will be free if the instrument in question is still under warranty. One thorny issue that needs to be broached is that of loan instruments. If part or all of your microinjection workstation needs to be sent away to be serviced or repaired, then your ICSI programme will grind to a halt, which can be catastrophic to a clinic that has paying patients waiting. This is worth mentioning to the representative before deciding on a system, just so that all parties concerned are aware of the issues.

6.2.1.11   Price

So, if the choice of equipment itself is not the most important factor, what is? Price is always a consideration, and the most expensive system is not always the best. Prices of equipment will vary wildly, depending on what is bought, from whom and from where. It is important to realize that although a third-party dealer will add on its own margin, the dealer will already be receiving a dealer discount. This could make the price from a dealer equal to, or even cheaper than, the price direct from the manufacturer. Indeed, the microscope manufacturers are in business to sell microscopes. They may be able to supply micromanipulation and microinjection equipment at cost prices if it gets them the sale of a microscope.

6.2.1.12 *Discounts*

Naturally, scientific equipment dealers are in business to cover their costs and to make a certain margin to keep their businesses profitable. The size of the margin and the subsequent discount that a dealer will be prepared to give depends on the culture of the particular region. Suffice to say that there is usually some flexibility in the price quoted, and that discounts, sometimes considerable, can be negotiated.

6.3 **SUMMARY**

In many ways, the final decision may depend not on the various features of the systems themselves but on the attitudes of the companies selling them. The user may decide to deal directly with the manufacturer, or through a distributor, but in either case the questions to be asked are:

1 How quickly do they respond to your requests?
2 Will they arrange a demonstration?
3 Does the company representative have the necessary technical knowledge to advise the user on the system in question?
4 Do the manufacturers in question convey the attitude that they are dedicated to consistently improving their products over time?
5 Do you feel that the distributor is actually interested in solving your problems, or just after a quick sale?
6 What sort of after-sales service do you think you'll receive?
7 Do any of your contacts in other clinics have any opinions on a particular supplier?
8 Most importantly, taking into account the price you are being asked to pay and the level of service offered, do you feel like you are getting value for money?

To sum up, then:

• It does not necessarily matter what mechanism is interposed between the joystick and the pipette tip – even though there are considerable differences.
• Weigh up obvious considerations like price and delivery time against the seller's long-term commitment to support, i.e. are you getting value for money?

- Be reasonable: the dealers are human too and you won't endear yourself to them by arranging a demonstration by all competitors simultaneously!
- Most trained sales staff are aware that if they treat the customer with courtesy and consideration, then they are more likely to get the sale. This works the other way too, though. If you want to get the best possible service, you have to understand the pressures that the dealers are under.

This may sound a little surprising, but the market for micromanipulation in assisted reproduction is growing and becoming more competitive. At the time of writing, all three major systems are equally good. The future, however, belongs to the company that understands that it is not just selling instruments to a customer, but that it is selling solutions to the customer's problems.

If the obvious considerations are not the most important, how does one decide on a specific system? The simple answer is that the most important consideration when choosing a micromanipulation system is the commitment of the manufacturer or its agents to helping the embryologist solve his or her problems. While research institutions often have time to learn all the delicate intricacies of their instruments, more often than not a working assisted conception unit views a micromanipulation system as just another tool. Because this particular tool is complex, inherently bug-ridden and often temperamental, effective ongoing support from the supplier is an essential, if somewhat intangible, part of the package sold. Obviously, if you can negotiate a service contract, then you have that commitment in writing, but this is probably the exception rather than the rule.

It is time for all manufacturers, distributors and agents to realize that they are not selling scientific instruments; they are selling solutions to their customers' problem. The customer's problem is not 'I have no micromanipulation system'; it is 'I need an effective ICSI programme that helps my patients achieve pregnancy'. In all fairness, some distributors have already realized this, and do all they can to satisfy their customers' needs.

7 Preparation of gametes for micromanipulation

Spermatozoa and spermatids can be found within the ejaculate as well as in aspirates and biopsies taken from the epididymis and testis. Therefore, the method of preparation employed is influenced more by the condition of the sample rather than by the maturational stage of the spermatozoa, although some approaches have been developed for the enrichment of specific stages of spermatid. The procedure and requirements for the preparation of oocytes vary only according to whether immature or mature oocytes have been aspirated.

7.1 SEMEN ANALYSIS

Technical details concerning the routine production, collection and analysis of semen are outside the remit of this book. Therefore knowledge of these aspects is assumed and, in any case, may be gleaned from several already established sources (Fleming *et al.*, 1997; Mortimer, 1994; World Health Organization, 1999).

If no spermatozoa are observed on a Makler chamber (Sefi Medical Instruments Ltd) during semen analysis, then a drop of the ejaculate should be placed under a coverslip on a glass microscope slide as a wet preparation and examined under $200\times$ magnification using a compound microscope with phase-contrast optics. If one or more spermatozoa are then visible, then it should be possible to obtain sufficient spermatazoa for micromanipulation following standard preparation, providing the volume of the ejaculate is adequate (i.e. at least 1 ml). Even if no sperm are visible on a wet preparation, it is still worthwhile centrifuging the ejaculate over a density gradient or in medium (1 : 1, v/v) at 500 g for 10 min in order to concentrate whatever spermatozoa may be present at the bottom of the tube. Subsequently, if spermatozoa are seen on a wet preparation, then the patient is presenting with cryptozoospermia; if spermatozoa are still not evident, then the patient is most probably azoospermic. In either case, it is usually necessary to resort to surgical sperm recovery, although sometimes it is possible to collect sufficient spermatozoa for micromanipulation from the edges of a large drop of the centrifuged concentrate, overlaid with oil, from those patients presenting with cryptozoospermia (Ron-El *et al.*, 1997). However, it is always worthwhile asking the patient to produce a second sample if spermatozoa have been seen on a previous semen analysis, even if they are all immotile (Ron-El *et al.*, 1998), as the second sample often exhibits improved sperm motility and morphology.

7.2 PREPARATION OF SPERMATOZOA FROM THE EJACULATE

All sperm preparation is performed in a laminar flow hood or, better still, in a class II safety cabinet, because this ensures two-way control of contamination. Even though the semen is not sterile initially, it may be thought of as semi-sterile once it has been passed through a gradient of sterile centrifugation medium.

There is a case for simplifying the preparation of spermatozoa for micromanipulation, even to the point where a drop of ejaculate may be placed straight into a large drop of medium and overlaid with oil. In this instance, the spermatozoa are allowed to swim out to the edges of the medium, from where they may be aspirated. This has the advantage of being both quick and easy to perform, although the spermatozoa so collected still have to be transferred to a drop of PVP before injection. However, it could be argued that omitting a purification step such as density gradient centrifugation increases the likelihood of bacterial contamination or injection of poor-quality spermatozoa. Indeed, recent data suggest that density gradient centrifugation removes spermatozoa with damaged DNA (Larson *et al.*, 1999). On the contrary, there are data that suggest that omission of such procedures does not have any adverse effect on either fertilization or embryogenesis (De Vos *et al.*, 1997). Nevertheless, there are ejaculates that do merit more rigorous preparation. These include those of low density and those that are particularly contaminated with leucocytes and other cell debris that could otherwise compromise the micromanipulation procedure. In particular, if bacterial contamination is present within the semen sample to a significant degree, then sperm viability will be reduced rapidly, especially if a sample of the ejaculate is stored in medium at 37 °C. In such instances, it is preferable to concentrate the available spermatozoa free of contaminants by employing a density gradient purification step.

7.2.1 Preparation and use of density gradient centrifugation media

The volume of density gradient media to be prepared depends on the laboratory workload; any unused media can be refrigerated and brought out the next morning to warm up to room temperature on the bench or in a 37 °C incubator. Alternatively, gradients sufficient to requirements may be prepared aseptically in advance and left out on the bench overnight to ensure that they are at room temperature first thing in the morning, when the preparation of spermatozoa usually begins. Different concentrations of Percoll have been employed by various workers in the past, but a discontinuous 45–90% gradient achieves satisfactory separation of living, motile, morphologically normal spermatozoa from other constituents of semen (Fleming *et al.*, 1997). Indeed, the manufacturers of PureSperm and Isolate have suggested the use of a similar concentration gradient. Hence PureSperm, as an example, can be used for sperm preparation as described in the following protocol:

1. PureSperm is diluted with Hepes-buffered culture medium in a ratio of 8 : 1 in order to obtain an 80% solution. An aliquot of the 80% solution is then diluted with an equal volume of culture medium to produce a 40% solution.

2. To prepare the gradient, dispense 1 ml of 80% PureSperm solution into a 15-ml centrifuge tube using a Pasteur pipette. Holding the centrifuge tube at a 45-degree angle, with another pipette gently layer 1 ml of the 40% PureSperm solution over the 80% solution in the tube. Take care to minimize mixing of the two solutions.

3. Overlay up to 1 ml of semen on to the discontinuous gradient in the tube. (The precise volume of semen to load on to the gradient depends upon the sperm density, but overloading of gradients should be avoided as this can result in a dirty preparation. If the density of spermatozoa in the ejaculate is low enough to demand the concentration of more than 1 ml of semen, then it is better to use several gradients.)

4. Being careful not to disturb the gradient, recap the centrifuge tube and transfer it to a bench centrifuge. Balance as appropriate and spin at 300 g for 20 min.

5. When the first spin has finished, remove the centrifuge tube and then, using a sterile Pasteur pipette, carefully remove all but the bottom 0.5 ml of the supernatant from the gradient, so as not to disturb the sperm pellet. Using a clean sterile Pasteur pipette, pass it rapidly through the remaining 0.5 ml of the supernatant from the gradient and remove the very bottom 0.25 ml which constitutes the sperm pellet, to a clean sterile centrifuge tube. Dispense 2–5 ml of fresh culture media over the sperm pellet. Draw the solution slowly up and down with the pipette to mix the contents thoroughly (without creating bubbles). Cap the tube and recentrifuge the washed pellet at 250 g for 5 min.

6   When the centrifuge has stopped, remove the centrifuge tube and gently remove the supernatant, leaving about 50–200 μl of the washed pellet at the bottom.

7   The remainder of the preparation depends upon the size of the pellet:

i.   If the pellet is of a reasonable size (i.e. visible), approximately 0.5 ml of Hepes-buffered culture medium may then be dispensed over the pellet of sperm remaining in the bottom of the centrifuge tube. With a sterile pipette, draw the solution slowly up and down to mix the contents thoroughly (without creating bubbles) and sample approximately 5 μl of this to roughly determine the sperm concentration. Then dilute the sample using the same culture medium until a density of around 10^6/ml is achieved. This can then be used as a stock solution, a small volume of which (1–5 μl) can be added to a drop of PVP (1 : 5, v/v) placed in a Petri dish used for micromanipulation.

ii. If the density of the pellet is less than that required to prepare a stock solution of around 10^6/ml spermatozoa, then resuspend it using approximately 1 ml of Hepes-buffered culture medium and transfer the entire volume to a sterile 1.5-ml Eppendorf tube. This may then be centrifuged at 1800 g for 5 min in a microfuge just before use. The spermatozoa at the bottom of the tube are removed in a microvolume using a pulled-glass Pasteur pipette and added straight to a drop of PVP placed in a Petri dish used for micromanipulation.

7.3   PREPARATION OF SURGICALLY RECOVERED SPERMATOZOA AND SPERMATIDS

Surgical sperm recovery is necessary for patients with obstructive or non-obstructive azoospermia. Azoospermia may be encountered due to various disorders, such as agenesis, aplasia, infection and trauma, some of which originate within the testis, others of which result from obstructions within the genital tract. However, even in very severe cases, such as hypospermatogenesis, Sertoli cell-only syndrome and spermatogenic arrest, pockets of spermatogenic activity not identified by previous biopsy may exist (Silber *et al.*, 1995). With the advent of ICSI, different techniques have been applied for the recovery of spermatozoa from the epididymis or, failing that, from the testis. PESA has been adopted widely as a front-line approach due to its simplicity and less invasive nature. However, some patients, such as those with high follicle-stimulating hormone (FSH) concentrations or patients with Sertoli cell-only syndrome, may not possess spermatozoa within their entire ejaculatory duct. In these instances, sperm may be recovered from the testis using TESA or TESE, the former being the preferred approach as it causes less testicular trauma.

Clearly, spermatozoa recovered surgically may have fewer requirements for preparation than those recovered by masturbation, the former not having to be separated from seminal plasma. However, in practice it is rare to recover spermatozoa that are free of blood cells and other contaminating debris, especially in TESA and TESE cases. Therefore, if sufficient numbers are recovered, it is often worthwhile employing a gravity sedimentation or density gradient centrifugation step to separate viable spermatozoa from other contaminants.

Fluid aspirates from the epididymis or testis may be washed out from the collection needle and tubing into drops of culture medium. At this stage, it is good practice to place a small volume of any aspirate containing spermatozoa under mineral oil in reserve, as an insurance policy in the event of severe loss of sperm motility or recovery during subsequent preparation. As with ejaculates of very poor quality, providing the sperm concentration is sufficient the remainder of the aspirate may be placed on to a discontinuous density gradient and prepared for ICSI (see section 7.2.1). Alternatively, the aspirate may be allowed to stand to remove red blood cells and other debris by density gravity sedimentation. An erythrocyte-lysing buffer can be used to remove red blood cells if these constitute the main source of contamination of the aspirate (Verheyen et al., 1995; Nagy et al., 1997). If there is insignificant contamination of the aspirate by blood and cellular debris, then these purification steps can be omitted and the sample simply washed with culture medium or placed straight under oil. Hence, the purity of the aspirate collected and the density of spermatozoa present tend to dictate the preparation method employed.

With TESA and TESE cases, it is necessary to macerate the tissue. To achieve this, shredding, mincing, vortexing or crushing may be employed (Verheyen et al., 1995), but shredding with fine needles or mincing with scalpel blades in a drop of culture medium usually produces satisfactory results (see Figure 7.1). The aim here is to dissociate the tissue into short lengths of separated seminiferous tubules and, if possible, to extrude their contents on to the bottom of the Petri dish. The macerate can then be sampled in peripheral areas devoid of larger pieces of tissue, placed under mineral oil, and observed for motile spermatozoa that are able to migrate to the edge of the droplet, from where they may be collected using microinjection pipettes. Unfortunately, the application of these methods for retrieving spermatozoa from biopsied testicular tissue does not always yield success, particularly in those patients suffering from hypospermatogenesis, Sertoli cell-only syndrome or spermatogenic arrest, where the failure rate can be 30–50%. One of the reasons for this failure to recover

Figure 7.1 TESA macerate obtained by running a scalpel blade along the length of the seminiferous tubules, held in place at one end with a fine needle, in order to extrude their contents.

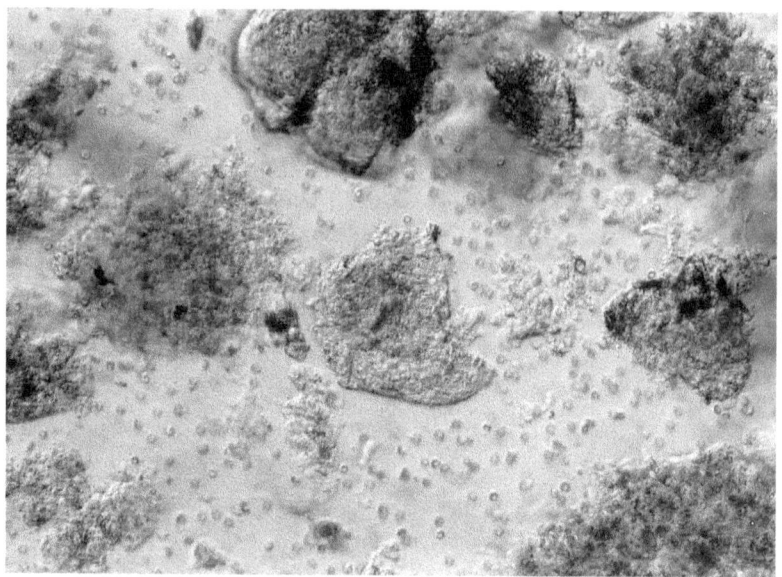

spermatozoa from testicular biopsies can be that the tissue is simply not disaggregated to a sufficient extent. In such instances, it has been found that the use of enzymes such as trypsin and collagenase (types I and IV) can improve the chances of recovering spermatozoa (Blanchard *et al.*, 1991; Salzbrunn *et al.*, 1996; Crabbe *et al.*, 1997). Indeed, it appears that the best yield is achieved using an enzymatic solution containing collagenase IV (see Table 7.1).

There may be some concern for the integrity of spermatozoa retrieved via enzymatic digestion of testicular biopsies. One way to limit continued digestion is to add 1 ml of serum to the digests immediately upon collection, so saturating any binding sites for the enzyme.

Spermatids can be found within the ejaculate and within epididymal aspirates, but it is usually from testicular biopsies that they are recovered, this often being the last option after failure to locate spermatozoa elsewhere. Spermatid identification is not an easy process, and reference to the different cell types in situ is strongly advised (Johnson *et al.*, 1999; Johnson *et al.*, 2001). The more advanced the stage of spermiogenesis, the easier it is to identify spermatids, elongated spermatids appearing not unlike spermatozoa (see Figure 7.2). They are identified most readily soon after preparation of the biopsy macerate, and it is good practice to collect those required for micromanipulation as soon as possible. (N.B. It should be appreciated that some regulatory bodies, such as the Human Fertilisation and Embryology Authority in the UK, do not permit ELSI and ROSI.)

Table 7.1 *Formulation for the preparation of enzymatic dissociation medium*

Constituent	Supplier	Product no.
Hepes-buffered EBSS (HEBSS)	Merck	
5% HSA	Sigma	A8763
1.6 mM CaCl$_2$	Sigma	C5670
25 g/ml DNase	Sigma	DN25
1000 IU/ml collagenase IV	Sigma	C5138

The tissue is exposed to this medium for one hour at 37 °C, the sample being shaken every 10–15 min. The digest is then centrifuged at 50 g for 5 min, the supernatant being washed twice in HEBSS and centrifuged at 1000 g for 5 min. The supernatant is removed and the pellet is resuspended in 50–100 µl of HEBSS.

Based on Crabbe *et al.* (1997) and Crabbe *et al.* (1998).

Figure 7.2 Spermiogenesis: the maturation of a round spermatid into a spermatozoon. (a) Round spermatid. (b) Elongating spermatid. (c) Elongated spermatid. (d) Spermatozoon.

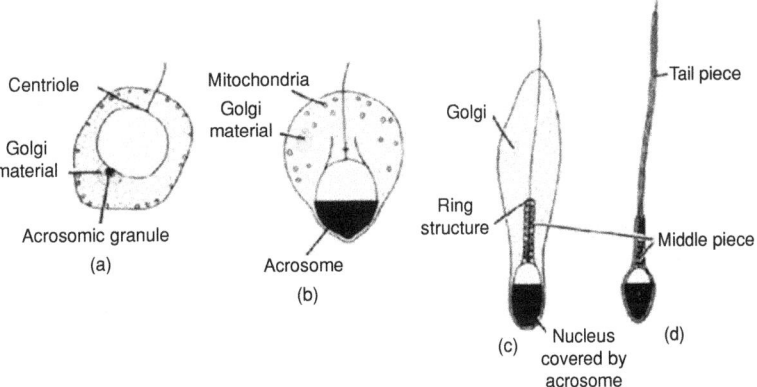

The yield of spermatids from testicular biopsy macerates is minimal, and this is not improved greatly following enzymatic dissociation of the tissue. Therefore, various purification methods are currently under investigation to enhance the recovery of spermatids and thereby facilitate their identification. One approach is based upon the use of sequential purification using velocity sedimentation under unit gravity (VSUG) and density gradient centrifugation of enzymatic digests (Shepherd *et al.*, 1981; Bellve, 1993; Aslam *et al.*, 1998). Essentially, this method employs the following protocol, using reagents supplied by Sigma (Aslam *et al.*, 1998):

1   Biopsied tissue is placed into an enriched Krebs–Ringer bicarbonate (EKRB) medium (for the formulation of EKRB, see O'Brien, 1993), dissected into 1–2-mm^3 pieces, and washed three times to remove blood cells.

2 The tissue is minced and added to 10 ml EKRB containing 2 mg/ml trypsin type III in a glass flask gassed with humidified 5% CO_2 in air, and incubated in a shaking water bath at 32 °C for 15 min.

3 The digest is filtered through a nylon mesh (80 μm), and the filtrate is added to 10 ml EKRB containing a final concentration of 2 mg/ml DNase-I.

4 Steps 2 and 3 are repeated with the tissue retained by the mesh, and the resulting filtrate is added to the initial one.

5 The combined filtrates are centrifuged at 500 g for 10 min at 4 °C, and the cell pellet is resuspended in 10 ml EKRB containing 0.5% HSA.

6 Step 5 is repeated, and the washed cell suspension is filtered through a nylon mesh (80 μm), the filtrate being made up to a final volume of 10 ml using EKRB containing 0.5% HSA.

7 The final cell suspension is loaded into a small, clean, sterile STA-PUT chamber (John Scientific Co.), and the cells are allowed to sediment through 450 ml of 2–4% HSA gradients for 160 min at 4 °C, 5-ml fractions being collected using a fraction collector.

8 Each fraction is centrifuged and resuspended in 2.5 ml of PBS containing 0.7% (w/v) HSA, Hepes (25 mM), 100 IU/ml of penicillin (potassium salt), 50 mg/ml of streptomycin sulphate and glutamine (100 mM).

9 Using the PBS solution above as diluent, 90%, 68%, 45%, 23% and 0% discontinuous isotonic Percoll gradients are prepared in 15-ml glass centrifuge tubes, comprising 2.5 ml of each concentration.

10 Each cell suspension is mixed with the top layer of each gradient and centrifuged at 2670 g for 50 min at 4 °C, the second of four bands down the gradient containing the purified spermatids. These are aspirated using a needle and syringe for washing and resuspension in EKRB.

An alternative approach to enhance the recovery of spermatids is based upon the use of fluorescence-activated cell sorting (FACS) using light in the visible range (Mays-Hoopes *et al.*, 1995; Coskun *et al.*, 2002). This technique has been reported to produce a more rapid and higher yield of round and elongated spermatids from enzymatic digests than that achieved with VSUG and density gradient centrifugation (Aslam *et al.*, 1998), but the expense of the equipment required prohibits its use for many centres. Spermatids might be identified more easily and more likely to result in viable pregnancies following their IVM in medium containing 25 mIU/ml FSH (Tesarik *et al.*, 1998). However, these very recent developments require confirmation by other workers in the field and further refinement prior to their clinical application. Indeed, it is only very recently that IVM of spermatids, resulting in fertilization and pregnancy following injection into oocytes, has been reported (Tesarik *et al.*, 1999).

Figure 7.3 Spermatozoa placed into a hypo-osmotic medium absorb water by osmosis, which causes their tails to curl in order to accommodate their increased volume.

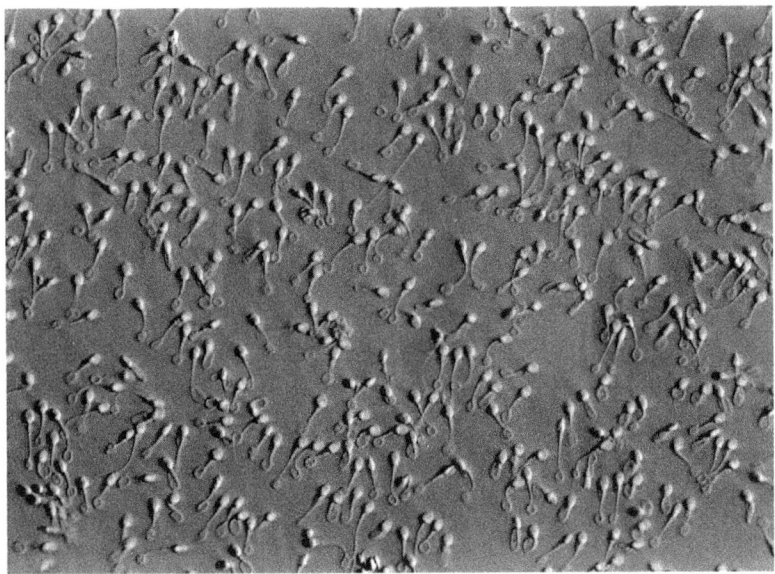

7.4 PREPARATION AND SELECTION OF VIABLE IMMOTILE SPERMATOZOA

In some instances, such as with immotile cilia syndrome or following the thawing of some frozen epididymal sperm samples, all the spermatozoa are completely immotile. In such cases, any viable spermatozoa may be identified using the HOST. This has the advantage over methods employing vital stains or dye exclusion in that the spermatozoa are not exposed to potentially harmful agents and, therefore, may be injected into oocytes. Spermatozoa prepared for ICSI, as described earlier in this chapter (see section 7.2), are incubated in a hypo-osmotic medium (see Table 2.5) for one hour in an incubator at 37 °C. The tails of viable spermatozoa, which possess an intact plasmalemma, curl in order to accommodate their increased volume in the hypo-osmotic medium (see Figure 7.3). These may be washed in ICSI medium using a micropipette and then injected using the same methods employed for motile spermatozoa (see Chapter 8).

7.5 PREPARATION OF OOCYTES

Similar to classical IVF, it is probably important to allow retrieved oocytes a sufficient period of time in which to complete their nuclear and cytoplasmic maturation, albeit in vitro. In this respect, it is likely that their maturation enclosed within their cumulus mass is more physiological than that in their denuded state (Coticchio and Fleming, 1998). Therefore,

Figure 7.4 Three different pipettes are used consecutively for oocyte denudation: a flame-polished bevelled pipette (left), a wide-bore flame-pulled pipette (centre-left) and a narrow-bore flame-pulled pipette (centre-right). Once denuded, the oocytes may be rolled along the bottom of the culture dish using a flame-sealed, narrow-bore pulled pipette (right) as a probe to check for extrusion of the first polar body.

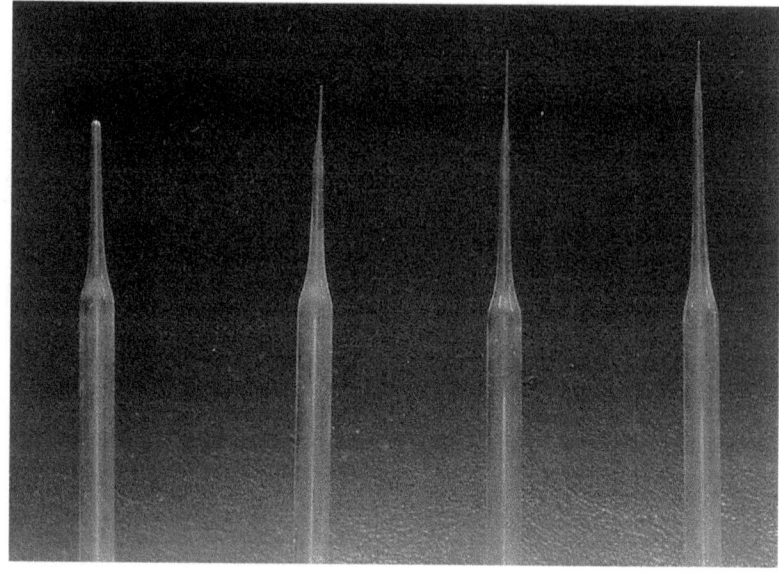

it is recommended that the COC be left in bicarbonate-buffered culture medium for at least two hours following oocyte retrieval, although it has been reported that this may not be necessary (Jacobs *et al.*, 2001).

7.5.1 Oocyte denudation

Essentially, three different types of glass Pasteur pipette are required for the entire procedure (see Figure 7.4):

- An ordinary pipette with a bevel at its tip is necessary for transferring the large COCs to a dish for cumulus removal.
- A slowly pulled pipette with a fairly wide diameter is necessary for removing the oocyte with its intact zona radiata from the surrounding cumulus oophorus.
- A quickly pulled pipette with a fairly narrow diameter but a squared-off tip is necessary for the dispersal of the corona radiata.

The pulling of pipettes requires practice to acquire the necessary skills, but there are also some tricks of the trade. One is far more likely to obtain a pipette with a squared-off rather than a jagged tip if the pipette is first pulled over a flame without breaking, allowed to cool for a second or two, and then pulled to breaking without twisting. In essence, this follows the process adopted by an electromechanical pipette puller. If the tip of the pipette is jagged, although it may be of the required diameter it will prove difficult, if not impossible, to aspirate oocytes into it as they will become caught up on its jagged sides. Commercially prepared glass pipettes for human oocyte denudation are available from a few companies (e.g. COOK), but these have received a mixed reception from the end users. Although they might avoid the necessity to pull a pipette, they do not always perform well.

The efficient denudation of oocytes depends initially upon their rapid removal from their surrounding cumulus mass using a medium containing the enzyme hyaluronidase. One reason why this procedure must be carried out quickly is that hyaluronidase is toxic to oocytes upon prolonged exposure. However, this enzyme is extremely useful for degrading the extracellular matrix that holds the cumulus cells together. Therefore, the objective is to remove the oocytes (with their corona radiata still intact) from their surrounding cumulus oophorus and transfer them without delay into culture medium devoid of hyaluronidase. Hence, it is recommended that large numbers of oocytes be processed in batches (e.g. five or six at a time). The medium employed for this purpose may be buffered with either bicarbonate or Hepes (e.g. see Table 2.8) but must be prewarmed to $37\,°C$ for the enzyme to work efficiently. Hepes-buffered media have the advantage in that they are excellent for maintaining pH outside of an incubator environment, but unfortunately they can also be toxic to oocytes upon prolonged exposure. Bicarbonate-buffered media are equally appropriate, as the duration of exposure to ambient conditions should be limited to less than a minute or so. Besides, using bicarbonate-buffered medium overlaid with oil that has been equilibrated in a CO_2 incubator will minimize any elevation of pH and has the added advantage of buffering against any fall in temperature.

The denudation of oocytes relies upon the mechanical dispersal of the cumulus cells that comprise the corona radiata. This can be achieved using gentle but rapid aspiration in and out of glass Pasteur pipettes pulled to a diameter of $130–150\,\mu m$, slightly larger than the diameter of the oocyte itself ($\sim125\,\mu m$). The key to success in all of this is the ability to pull pipettes to appropriate dimensions, as a pipette that is too wide will be ineffective whereas one that is too small will be damaging to the cytoskeleton of the oocyte. However, it should be realized that it is only necessary to remove sufficient cumulus cells to enable observation of the oocyte to determine its maturity and monitor the flow of ooplasm within the injection micropipette during the ICSI procedure. In fact, since one of the functions of cumulus cells is to transfer nutrients to the oocyte, it may confer a physiological advantage to leave as many as possible intact, and there is some evidence to support this concept (Lars Hamberger, personal communication, 1994). The disaggregation of the corona radiata also needs to be performed rapidly to minimize the duration of exposure of the oocytes outside of an incubator environment. Again, the use of media overlaid with oil is therefore recommended. Aspirating groups of two to four oocytes at a time usually facilitates the process. It is important to monitor the length of time that any oocytes are maintained outside of the incubator during denudation, and it is good practice to limit this to periods of less than five minutes. If many oocytes have to be denuded, then they can be split between several dishes, alternating between them so that they can be returned to an incubator when not in use. Also, it is advised to finally transfer the denuded oocytes to freshly equilibrated media that has been maintained in an incubator throughout the entire process. A suggested protocol for oocyte denudation would be as follows:

1 Place a large drop of warmed bicarbonate-buffered medium containing 80 IU/ml of hyaluronidase into a small Petri dish and overlay it with equilibrated oil.
2 Transfer five or six COCs to the medium containing hyaluronidase, returning any remaining COCs to the incubator.
3 Quickly aspirate each oocyte with its corona radiata intact from the surrounding cumulus, and transfer them together to fresh equilibrated medium devoid of hyaluronidase. Return them to the incubator.
4 Repeat steps 2 and 3 until all the COCs have been processed for a given case.
5 As quickly as possible, denude the oocytes as groups of two to four at a time, until it appears possible to determine their stage of nuclear maturation (see section 7.5.2).
6 Once all of the oocytes have been denuded sufficiently, wash them through two washes of medium into freshly equilibrated medium that has been maintained in an incubator during the entire process.

7.5.2 Assessing oocyte maturation and quality

It will save time during the injection procedure if the denuded oocytes are examined beforehand to determine their stage of nuclear maturation. In this way, it can be ensured that only mature oocytes are loaded into the microinjection dish. Providing the oocytes have been denuded adequately, it will be possible to assess the oocytes with the aid of a dissecting stereomicroscope under high power ($\sim 80\times$) magnification. During examination of the oocytes, it is necessary to roll them along the bottom of the dish while focusing on different areas, so as to differentiate cumulus cells from the first polar body (see Figure 7.5). This can be achieved using a pulled glass Pasteur pipette slightly larger than that used for denudation.

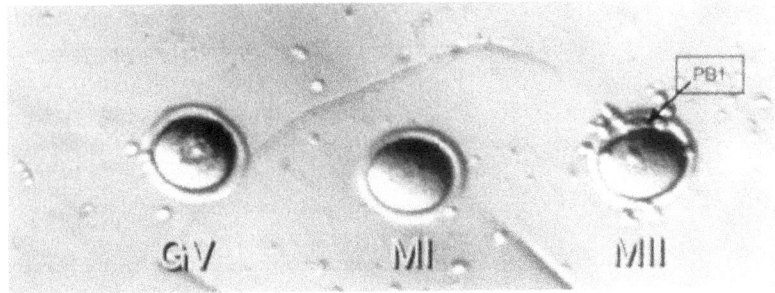

Figure 7.5 Immature oocytes are identified by the presence of a germinal vesicle (GV) either at the centre or periphery of the ooplasm. Oocytes that commence maturation undergo GV breakdown, progressing from the GV stage to the metaphase I (MI) stage. Oocytes that have completed their meiotic maturation have progressed to the metaphase II (MII) stage, characterized by the extrusion of the first polar body into the perivitelline space.

However, it is easier to use a glass Pasteur pipette pulled to form a fine rounded probe (see Figure 7.4). To create one of these, simply pull the pipette over a flame without breaking, allow to cool, and then introduce the thinned section to a flame whilst applying gentle tension. The result will be that the pipette breaks and becomes closed off by the heat at the same time, so forming a fine rounded probe. This can then be used safely to quickly roll the oocytes along the bottom of the dish without any risk of damaging them.

On examination, the oocytes will be at one of three stages of maturation (see Figure 7.5). Oocyte maturation follows oocyte growth and encompasses the transition of an immature to a mature oocyte capable of being fertilized and supporting embryogenesis. If an oocyte is immature, it can be identified as such by the presence of an organelle within the ooplasm, termed the germinal vesicle (GV), the oocyte being at prophase I of the first meiotic division. If an oocyte is undergoing maturation, the GV will have undergone germinal vesicle breakdown (GVBD), the oocyte being at metaphase I (MI) of the first meiotic division. If an oocyte is mature, it will have extruded a polar body (PB), the oocyte being at metaphase II (MII) of the second meiotic division. Usually, more than 85% of the oocytes should be mature. However, there will be cases where many oocytes prove to be immature. For example, patients with polycystic ovarian disease (PCOD) can respond to stimulation with the production of a large number of immature oocytes. Also, it is sometimes necessary to administer human chorionic gonadotrophin (hCG) to a patient before all of their follicles are fully grown, so as to minimize the risk of ovarian hyperstimulation syndrome (OHSS). Therefore, it is quite possible that the smaller follicles will yield immature oocytes. Occasionally, abnormal oocytes will also be observed (see Table 7.2).

Occasionally, mature oocytes will possess two PBs, but this is not necessarily an abnormality as it is possible for the PB that is extruded to divide

Table 7.2 *Different types of abnormal human oocytes*

Oocytes with a dark central and light peripheral ooplasm
Oocytes containing refractile bodies or vesicles
Oocytes with an irregular outline to their oolemma
'Giant' or irregularly shaped oocytes
Oocytes with 'giant' or multiple polar bodies
Oocytes devoid of a zona pellucida

These irregularities are found in both mature and immature oocytes, although more frequently in the latter. Vesicles should not be confused with vacuoles, the latter being a normal organelle for osmoregulation. Giant oocytes should not be used for clinical treatment as they may be digynic, which would yield triploid embryos following ICSI (Balakier *et al.*, 2002; Rosenbusch *et al.*, 2002).

or fragment. However, interesting recent evidence does suggest that the quality of the first PB is indicative of the oocyte's viability and reproductive potential (Ebner *et al.*, 1999). Once the oocytes have been graded, they can be separated into their different categories. This ensures that only mature oocytes are loaded into the microinjection dish, and provides a means for monitoring the further maturation of immature and maturing oocytes. Furthermore, if any of the mature oocytes prove to be abnormal, these too should be separated out. Some centres prefer not to inject abnormal oocytes, whereas others may opt to do so but will usually maintain them separate from the normal injected oocytes.

7.5.3 In vitro maturation of oocytes

It has long been known that oocytes that prove to be immature following denudation can undergo maturation spontaneously in vitro (Edwards, 1965). However, not all oocytes will have developed sufficient meiotic competence to achieve maturation, particularly those at the GV stage. Nevertheless, those that do undergo IVM represent a potentially valuable source of clinical material, particularly for those patients who would otherwise fail to reach embryo transfer. Essentially, oocytes age rapidly only once they have matured. Therefore, oocytes may be injected once they have undergone IVM even though this is usually not until the day after oocyte retrieval. In fact, it may be detrimental to fertilization outcome to inject them too soon following extrusion of the PB as they may not have

Table 7.3 *Different types of oocyte maturation media*

Cha and Chian (1998)	Trounson *et al.* (1994)	Russell *et al.* (1997)
TCM 199	EMEM	TCM 199
20% FBS	10% FCS	10% FCS
10 IU/ml PMSG	0.075 IU/ml hMG	0.075 IU/ml hMG
10 IU/ml hCG	0.5 IU hCG	0.5 IU hCG
	1 g/ml Oestradiol	1 g/ml Oestradiol

EMEM, Eagle's modified minimal essential medium with Earle's salts (Flow Laboratories); FBS, fetal bovine serum; FCS, fetal calf serum; hMG, human menopausal gonadotrophin (Serono); PMSG, pregnant mare's serum gonadotrophin; TCM, tissue culture medium. (N.B. restrictions apply on FBS, FCS and PMSG for human usage in some countries.)

acquired the full potential to respond to the activating stimulus provided by the spermatozoon. On the other hand, successful fertilization has been achieved following the injection of MI oocytes (Hamberger *et al.*, 1995). However, there is concern with this practice in that abnormal zygotes with a diploid female nucleus may be created (i.e. if the oocyte that has undergone GVBD has not yet reached MI). Of course, embryos created by the injection of oocytes maturing later than the remainder of the cohort may have a lower implantation potential, not least because they will be one day out of phase with the endometrium. Therefore, it may be worthwhile cryopreserving such embryos for transfer in a later cycle.

It is quite possible that our practice of assisted conception will undergo a revolutionary change in the near future, whereby immature oocytes are retrieved and then matured in vitro without recourse to ovarian stimulation with high doses of gonadotrophins. This could have numerous benefits, including the transfer of fresh embryos to an endometrium during a 'natural' cycle. Various types of oocyte maturation media have been developed for this purpose (see Table 7.3).

The concept behind the development of oocyte maturation media is to recreate the follicular environment that the immature oocytes would otherwise be exposed to. However, in practice it appears that human immature oocytes may be matured in vitro in the absence of gonadotrophins (e.g. using Chang's medium from Irvine Scientific; Trounson *et al.*, 1996). Although pregnancies from IVM oocytes have been reported in humans (Cha *et al.*, 1991; Trounson *et al.*, 1994; Barnes *et al.*, 1995; Russell *et al.*, 1997), the developmental competence of the embryos so produced is currently low. The most likely explanation for this is some defect in the cytoplasmic maturation of the immature oocytes retrieved. Therefore, we must assume that the selection of oocytes for IVM or the culture conditions require some refinement. Once these aspects have been investigated more fully, the IVM of oocytes will become a more widespread technique in assisted reproduction.

7.6 TROUBLESHOOTING

7.6.1 Sperm preparation

7.6.1.1 *Problem – no spermatozoa are recovered following density gradient purification*

Probable cause: Providing a sufficient volume has been loaded on to the gradient, and that there is an adequate concentration of sperm within this, it is quite possible that the gradient is not isotonic with the semen. Alternatively, it may be that the sample is particularly viscous, causing entrapment and 'rafting' of the spermatozoa, preventing their release through the gradient.

Suggested remedy: Prepare fresh gradients, ensuring that culture medium is mixed with the separation medium so as to make it isotonic. Before density gradient purification, either incubate the semen at $37\,^{\circ}\text{C}$ or treat it with chymotrypsin so as to reduce its viscosity.

7.6.1.2 *Problem – no spermatozoa are recovered following preparation and washing*

Probable cause: Poor recovery of spermatozoa is indicative of loss at one or more steps during preparation, most likely during the washes. Alternatively, it is possible that the spermatozoa have been resuspended in too great a volume of medium, causing overdilution and giving the appearance of poor recovery.

Suggested remedy: Check the supernatants removed from the sperm pellet at each stage of preparation to identify where the loss is occurring. Those containing spermatozoa may be combined and centrifuged once more, taking extra care not to disturb the pellet when removing the supernatant (this can be achieved more easily using a pulled Pasteur pipette). Resuspend the final pellet in a minimal volume (e.g. 50–100 µl) and place the entire volume in a Petri dish overlaid with oil for examination under an inverted microscope. Spermatozoa should now be visible and can be collected during the micromanipulation procedure.

7.6.1.3   *Problem – all of the spermatozoa are immotile or dead*
following preparation
Probable cause: There may be several explanations for this. If the spermatozoa appear dead immediately following preparation, it is possible that they
have been exposed to toxic media (e.g. it has been known for some batches
of HSA to have this effect when added to media used to prepare spermatozoa). If they become immotile or dead some time after preparation, they
may have been killed by bacteria or they may have an intrinsically limited
lifespan.

Suggested remedy: Test the media used for preparing the spermatozoa with
a different sample. If this has the same effect, then use a different media
and employ quality control to identify the causative constituent within
the toxic medium. Check the prepared sperm sample under high-power
magnification for evidence of bacterial contamination and culture a sample for confirmation. If there is significant contamination of the prepared
sample, then prepare a fresh sample just before the microinjection procedure, storing it at room temperature until use. The same policy should be
adopted for spermatozoa with a short lifespan.

7.6.1.4   *Problem – the sperm preparation from a surgically recovered sample*
forms a sticky and viscous interface between the medium and the
overlying oil
Probable cause: This is more typical with TESA and TESE cases, and it
appears to be associated with specific individuals. Presumably, proteins are
released into the medium during disaggregation of the biopsied sample,
creating a colloid-like solution.

Suggested remedy: Aspiration of the media from under the oil and washing
with fresh culture medium usually resolves this problem. Once washed,
centrifuged and resuspended, the sample can be plated out again in a
microinjection dish overlaid with oil.

7.6.2   Oocyte preparation

7.6.2.1   *Problem – using hyaluronidase, it proves difficult to remove the oocyte*
from the cumulus mass
Probable cause: The hyaluronidase may be cold. Nevertheless, the cumulus
mass can be sticky or compacted, the latter problem being more typical of
immature COCs.

Suggested remedy: Ensure that the hyaluronidase has been warmed to 37 °C before use. If the cumulus mass is sticky, repeatedly aspirating the oocyte and lifting the pulled glass Pasteur pipette free of the cumulus usually has the desired effect. If the cumulus mass is compacted, then it will be necessary to resort to the use of hypodermic needles to gently tease the cumulus free of the oocyte, taking care not to damage it.

7.6.2.2   *Problem – it proves difficult to pull a glass Pasteur pipette to a diameter appropriate for denuding oocytes*
Probable cause: If the pipettes are too wide, then the heating is insufficient and/or the speed of the pull is too slow. If they are too narrow, then the converse is true.

Suggested remedy: If attempts to directly pull a pipette to the correct size are repeatedly in vain, pull a very long and narrow pipette, rapidly breaking it at increasing widths along its length until the desired diameter is achieved.

7.6.2.3   *Problem – during denudation, an oocyte becomes stuck to the end of a pulled Pasteur pipette*
Probable cause: The pipette may not have a cleanly squared-off tip, or the corona radiata may be particularly sticky.

Suggested remedy: Using a pulled glass probe or a hypodermic needle, gently prise the oocyte free from the tip of the pipette.

7.6.2.4   *Problem – despite using a pulled pipette of the correct diameter, it proves impossible to denude an oocyte adequately*
Probable cause: This problem is typical of immature oocytes, which may have a particularly compacted corona radiata.

Suggested remedy: Aspirating the oocyte gently on to a holding micropipette, turn the oocyte with the injection micropipette and try to determine its maturity. If identified positively as mature, it may be injected as it is.

8 Intracytoplasmic sperm injection

The successful introduction of ICSI for the alleviation of male-factor infertility must surely be one of the most significant advances in reproductive medicine since the birth of Louise Brown back in 1978 (Palermo *et al.*, 1992). Patients presenting with semen containing either too few sperm and/or sperm with poor progressive motility are obviously good candidates for ICSI. Also, it is well known that sperm that have a normal shape, as determined by morphological criteria, are more likely to bind to and therefore fertilize eggs; therefore, ICSI may be warranted where there is a very low percentage of morphologically normal sperm within the semen. However, routine IVF can also fail despite apparently excellent semen parameters, presumably for biochemical reasons. Again, ICSI offers a suitable remedy should this prove to be a consistent problem that cannot be attributed to poor egg quality alone. Nevertheless, ICSI must still mimic the latter stages of fertilization in vivo if it is to prove successful.

Essentially, as with gamete fusion, both cell membranes (i.e. the oolemma of the egg and the plasmalemma of the sperm) should be temporarily breached, so it is necessary to ensure that the oolemma has been penetrated, as is evident by a sudden free flow of ooplasm, and that the plasmalemma has been ruptured, as is evident by permanent immobility of the sperm tail. Considering these requirements, ICSI is technically demanding and there is substantial potential for damage to the egg, which can cause it to degenerate. For example, if the egg is aspirated too strongly on to the holding micropipette, the egg can be distorted, possibly resulting in damage to its cytoskeleton, the network of filaments that control cell shape and cell division. Similarly, excessive aspiration of ooplasm during injection may also distort the cytoskeleton, resulting in compromised embryogenesis (Dumoulin *et al.*, 2001). If the injection micropipette is allowed to pierce the oolemma opposite the initial injection site, any stabilization of ooplasm within the egg is lost, allowing it to leak out. Similarly, other aspects of poor microinjection technique can result in degeneration of the egg. Even if the oocyte should survive injection, ICSI can still result in failure for a variety of reasons. For example, there may be insufficient egg activation, which in turn can lead to incomplete decondensation, or unpackaging, of the sperm nucleus. Injection of an egg close to where the spindle normally resides, adjacent to the first PB, may result in failure to complete fertilization. Damage to the spindle, the part of the cytoskeleton concerned with cell division, may result in the egg being arrested at MII of meiosis rather than progressing to the first cleavage division. Hence, the reasons for fertilization failure can be technical or biochemical. The oolemma may not be actually ruptured, in effect resulting in SUZI, which we know has poor success rates even with motile sperm. If the plasmalemma of the sperm has not been fully ruptured, then residual motility of the sperm within the ooplasm may cause damage or the egg may fail to sufficiently detect the activating stimulus of the sperm in a timely fashion. These and other factors can lead to poor embryogenesis or even failed cleavage.

Despite the intricate physiological basis of fertilization and the technical demands of ICSI, it is nevertheless still just a technique. As such, providing some basic concepts are understood and the key requirements of the procedure are satisfied, there is no reason why it should not be mastered. Indeed, it is now considered routine, and fully trained clinical embryologists are usually expected to have attained this skill. However, the heterogeneity of gamete quality and the severity of some forms of male-factor infertility impose a variety of demands that can be extremely challenging to the novice. The experienced practitioner will usually have learnt to cope with such problem cases. Unfortunately, not all novices have immediate access to the advice and assistance of a more experienced colleague. The objective of this chapter, therefore, is to provide a clear guide to the essentials of the ICSI technique along with suggestions as to how best to troubleshoot the most commonly encountered problems.

8.1 MEDIA AND MICROINJECTION DISH PREPARATION

Since ICSI is routinely performed using an inverted microscope situated on a laboratory bench, it is advisable to use a Hepes-buffered medium that can maintain physiological pH independent of a CO_2 incubator (see Table 2.1). The ICSI medium of choice may need to be supplemented with antibiotics, protein (HSA) and a nutrient source such as pyruvate (see Table 2.2 as an example). The same medium, with hyaluronidase added, can be used for oocyte denudation (see Table 2.9). These media are best stored in a refrigerator and aliquoted for use as required. However, it is essential to prewarm all media to 37 °C in an incubator before use. In the case of denudation medium, all that is necessary is simply to place an aliquot into the incubator an hour before intended use. For ICSI, small droplets of medium are usually placed into a microinjection dish and overlaid with light mineral oil. These will rapidly reach the required temperature, especially if the oil used for this purpose is normally maintained at 37 °C in an incubator. Therefore, preparation of the microinjection dishes before oocyte denudation allows sufficient time for the droplets of medium to warm up during their storage in an incubator. PVP, used to slow down sperm progression and facilitate the ICSI procedure, is also best stored in a refrigerator. Since this is also usually prepared as a droplet in the microinjection dish, it can be handled similarly to the ICSI medium, but it is much more viscous. PVP can be prepared in-house, but since the process is somewhat laborious it is usually deemed more expedient to obtain it ready for use from a commercial distributor (see Table 2.11). Dishes suitable for microinjection include all plastic Petri dishes used routinely for the handling of oocytes and embryos (see Chapter 2). However, shallow Petri dishes (such as those available from Falcon; product number 1006) are particularly recommended for those that prefer to work with micropipettes at a 25-degree angle.

The most important consideration when preparing dishes for microinjection is that the droplets of medium should be stable and covered completely with oil. Otherwise, there is risk of confusion over what has been injected should droplets coalesce, or oocytes may inadvertently be subjected to detrimental fluctuations in temperature and osmolarity. Therefore, it is best to place small droplets of medium (10–50 μl) and PVP into the microinjection dishes first, and then overlay them with oil. This way, the droplets lie flatter on the bottom of the dish and are therefore more stable and more easily covered with oil. Another practical consideration is where to place the droplets in the dish. To avoid 'grounding out' of the micropipettes on the sides of the dish, it is advisable to place the droplets towards the centre and away from the periphery (see Figure 8.1). Also, it can make it easier to keep track of which oocyte is in which drop of medium if the droplets are placed asymmetrically, rather than all in a straight line or circle (see Figure 8.1). Since the droplet of PVP is where spermatozoa are manipulated, it is central to the procedure and will be used frequently. Therefore, it is helpful if it can be located easily and quickly. One way to ensure this is to place it in the dish as a long and narrow line of medium (see Figure 8.1). A larger droplet of ICSI medium (50–200μl) may also need to be placed into the microinjection dish as a reservoir for spermatozoa in cases where the number available is very few or the preparation is particularly 'dirty'. This droplet is often referred to as the 'sperm drop'

Figure 8.1 This dish has been prepared for microinjection by placing small and large drops of Hepes-buffered media and PVP under oil. The large drops at the top and on the left-hand side of the dish may be used for equilibration of the micropipettes and as a reservoir for prepared spermatozoa prior to ICSI. The small drops at the bottom of the dish may be used for microinjection, a single oocyte being placed into each drop. The long drop of PVP in the centre of the dish can also be used as a reservoir for prepared spermatozoa to swim out into, but it is used primarily to slow down sperm progression to facilitate their manipulation.

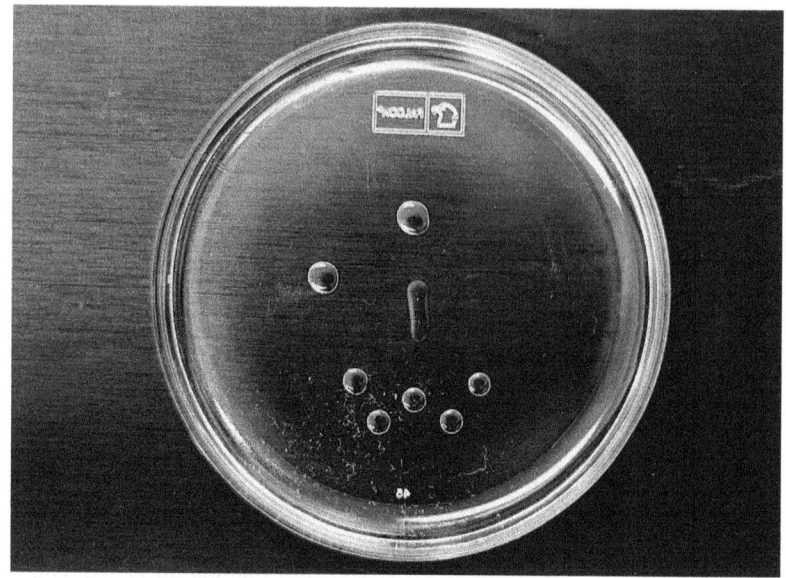

(see Figure 8.1). The only other requirement is another large droplet of ICSI medium (50–200 µl) for equilibration of the micropipettes, often referred to as the 'equilibration drop'. This can be placed either in a separate dish or in the microinjection dish itself (see Figure 8.1). It can be convenient to have an equilibration drop in the microinjection dish should it prove necessary to re-equilibrate one of the micropipettes during the ICSI procedure. Some practitioners prefer to equilibrate the injection micropipette with PVP, in which case it is necessary to have a droplet of PVP separate to that used for sperm manipulation.

Before placing droplets of medium and oil into the microinjection dish, it is important to write identifying details (name and date of birth) of the patient whose oocytes are to be injected on the underside of the dish. This can either be written using a non-toxic indelible marker pen or, better, be scratched with a hypodermic needle or diamond pen. Also, it may be desirable to identify the different drops of medium, especially while learning to navigate the microinjection dish as a trainee or novice. It is considered good practice not to inject more than three to five oocytes at any one sitting, so as to minimize the total exposure of each oocyte to the relatively unfavourable conditions outside the incubator. For example, excessive cooling of the oocyte may result in failure to extrude the second PB, failure to cleave, or poor embryo quality (i.e. fragmentation) and viability. So, up to five droplets of ICSI medium may be placed into the microinjection dish (see Figure 8.1). Therefore, if a patient has more than five mature oocytes for injection, it will be necessary to prepare two microinjection dishes. The rationale for this is that while one dish is being used for microinjection, the other can be kept warm inside an incubator. Otherwise, the practice of injecting only up to five oocytes at any one sitting would be partly negated. Also, the use of two dishes allows an assistant to 'load' oocytes ready for injection and wash oocytes following injection, to speed up the procedure. Likewise, an assistant can locate and prepare spermatozoa for injection using the 'spare' dish, an approach that is particularly of benefit when dealing with extremely difficult cases. To place small droplets of ICSI medium on to the bottom of the microinjection dish, it is easier to use either a sterile pulled Pasteur pipette or micropipettor using non-toxic sterile pipette tips. On the other hand, because PVP is viscous, the use of either a bevelled sterile Pasteur pipette that has not been pulled to a narrow diameter or a micropipettor using larger non-toxic sterile pipette tips is necessary. Once the appropriate number of droplets of ICSI medium and PVP have been placed into the microinjection dish, oil can be poured or pipetted over them until they are completely covered. This can be observed by watching the interface between the medium and oil as the dish fills. It is advisable not to overfill the dish with oil as this can lead to spillage, which can result in smearing of the underside of the dish with oil and distortion of the microscope optics. Indeed, any oil contaminating the underside of the microinjection dish must be wiped away using a tissue lightly soaked with 70% alcohol. Once prepared, the microinjection dish may be placed into an incubator until required.

8.2   FITTING, ALIGNMENT AND EQUILIBRATION OF MICROPIPETTES

The setting up of the micropipettes is best done well before commencing the ICSI procedure. It is assumed here that in the meantime the gametes have been prepared for injection (see Chapter 7). Indeed, some practitioners consider it beneficial to allow the oocytes sufficient time ($\sim$2 h) to recover following denudation. Correct preparation of the micropipettes is crucial to the micromanipulation technique. Essentially, the better they are fitted and equilibrated, the greater is the control achieved during the procedure. This requires care and attention to detail, which are time-consuming. Indeed, gametes can be manipulated gently and rapidly only if the micropipettes have been set up properly, and the ease and speed of handling will influence ICSI outcome. Since the holding pipette is much larger in diameter than the injection pipette, it is advisable to use the holding pipette as a guide for positioning and equilibrating the latter; hence, the holding pipette will be dealt with first in each of the following subsections.

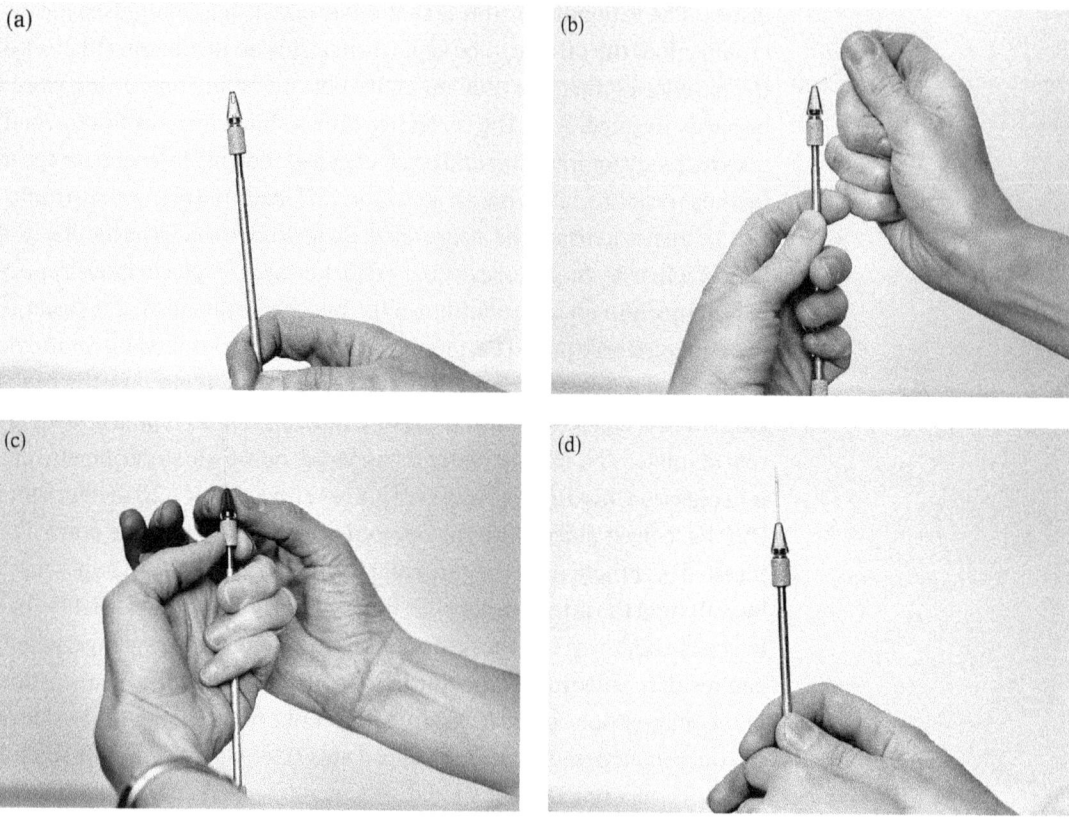

Figure 8.2 (a) The microtool holder of an oil microinjector is primed by forcing oil out of its tip until all traces of any air bubbles have been removed. (b) In order to avoid the introduction of any air bubbles, the base of the micropipette is introduced into the tool holder through the convex layer of oil protruding from its tip. (c) The ferrule is tightened down gently. (d) To ensure that good control is achieved with an oil injector, the micropipette is primed by forcing oil approximately halfway along its length, ensuring that a large air gap remains between the leading edge of the oil and its tip.

8.2.1 Fitting micropipettes to their tool holders

If the tool holder is attached to an oil injector, it will be necessary to check first that no air bubbles remain in the dead space left following removal of the previous micropipette that was used. To do this, turn the injector screw clockwise to force oil along the tubing and tool holder while holding the latter vertically, with its open tip uppermost (see Figure 8.2a). Oil and bubbles of air should eventually begin to exit the tool holder. Continue this for a short period to ensure that no air remains trapped inside. While the oil still forms a convex layer over the tip of the tool holder, check that the locking ferrule at its tip is loosened off a few turns and carefully introduce the base of the holding pipette into the tool holder (see Figure 8.2b). It is important here to try and avoid creating any gaps of air between columns of oil, as this may impair control during microinjection. Gently push the micropipette just past the sealing ring inside the tool holder (this will be felt as a slight and temporary resistance to the passage of the pipette). Leaving an ample length of the micropipette outside of the tool holder, gently tighten the locking ferrule to hold the micropipette in place (see Figure 8.2c). Slowly turn the injector screw clockwise to force oil along the micropipette until it has travelled approximately halfway along its length (see Figure 8.2d). Essentially, the larger the gap between the meniscus of the oil and the tip of the micropipette, the easier the control during microinjection. Therefore, avoid taking the oil too close to the end of the micropipette. This stage of the procedure provides a good opportunity at which to confirm fine control of the oil inside the micropipette in response to minute turns of the injector screw, both clockwise and anticlockwise. The tool holder and micropipette may now be attached to the retaining clip of the universal joint, but do not tighten down the lockscrew fully until alignment has been completed. Repeat the same procedure with the injection pipette to attach it to the tool holder on the other side of the micromanipulation rig. If the tool holder is attached to an air injector, the procedure is the same except that there is no need to touch the injector at any stage as there is no oil to be concerned with.

8.2.2 Aligning the micropipettes

Once the micropipettes have been fitted to the tool holders and attached to the universal joints, their alignment can be checked and, if necessary, adjusted. Approximate alignment of the holding pipette can be achieved by eye, but precise alignment requires the aid of an inverted microscope. Alignment of an injection pipette containing a 25- or 35-degree bend depends almost entirely upon the use of the microscope because it is extremely difficult to see the angle of its tip by eye alone. Therefore, it is easier to align the holding pipette first. Then, the position of the holding pipette can be used as a landmark for initial alignment of the injection pipette. If the micropipette tips are straight (e.g. Z-shaped micropipettes), then alignment in the vertical plane has to be achieved by eye alone, by sighting along the length of the pipette to verify that it is aligned vertically. The same approximation may be made for a holding pipette containing a 25- or 35-degree bend. In this instance, however, further fine adjustment can be made, viewing the pipette using the $4\times$ or $10\times$ objective of the inverted microscope (see Figure 8.3a–c). To do this, first rotate the tool holder along its long axis so that the straight tip of the holding pipette, following the bend, is lowermost and approximately horizontal. Then, use the coarse manipulators to position the holding pipette just above the microscope stage, over the objective lens. With the microscope light source switched on, the tip of the micropipette will glow in the beam of light when in approximately the right position over the lens. Looking down the eyepieces of the microscope, if necessary use the coarse manipulators and focus to bring the micropipette into view. It will probably appear to be at a slight diagonal, either upwards or downwards (see Figure 8.3a and b). This is because it is not lying precisely within the exact vertical plane, so the angled bend in the micropipette will offset the tip in the horizontal plane when viewed from below through the inverted microscope. Still looking down the eyepieces, rotate the tool holder along its long axis until the angled tip of the holding pipette appears straight in the field of view (see Figure 8.3c). This confirms that the micropipette is aligned in a precisely vertical position, as viewed via the objective lens directly below. Using the fine manipulator, withdraw the holding pipette to the perimeter of the field of view to allow sufficient space in which to similarly align the injection pipette. To locate the tip of the injection pipette, use the coarse manipulators to position it as close as possible to the tip of the holding pipette, but without making contact, which would otherwise snap it off. Then, for the injection pipette, repeat the procedure employed to align the holding pipette. Again, the injection pipette is aligned precisely in the vertical plane when its tip appears horizontal in the field of view of the microscope (see Figure 8.3f).

Once the micropipettes have been aligned in their vertical planes, it is then necessary to align them accurately in their horizontal planes. This step is more important and more exacting than the previous one, as it will determine the angle of contact made between the pipette tips and the bottom of the microinjection dish. Again, the holding pipette is aligned more easily than the injection pipette. To do this, view the straight tip of the holding pipette using the $10\times$ objective of the inverted microscope. Focusing along the length of the straight end of the holding pipette, establish its horizontal alignment. If the focus needs to be altered to maintain a sharp image along the pipette, then it is not lying in an exactly horizontal plane. If the focal plane is higher at the very tip of the pipette than at its heel (i.e. at the bend), then it is tilted upwards (see Figure 8.4a). Conversely, if the focal plane is lower at its tip, then it is tilted downwards (see Figure 8.4b). As necessary, adjust the tilt of the tool holder using the universal joint to bring the pipette into its horizontal plane. This can be verified when the straight tip of the holding pipette remains in sharp focus along its length without having to alter the focal plane at which the microscope focus is set (see Figure 8.4c). The tilt of the injection pipette may be established and adjusted in a similar fashion. However, for ICSI, the alignment requirements of the holding and injection pipettes differ. With

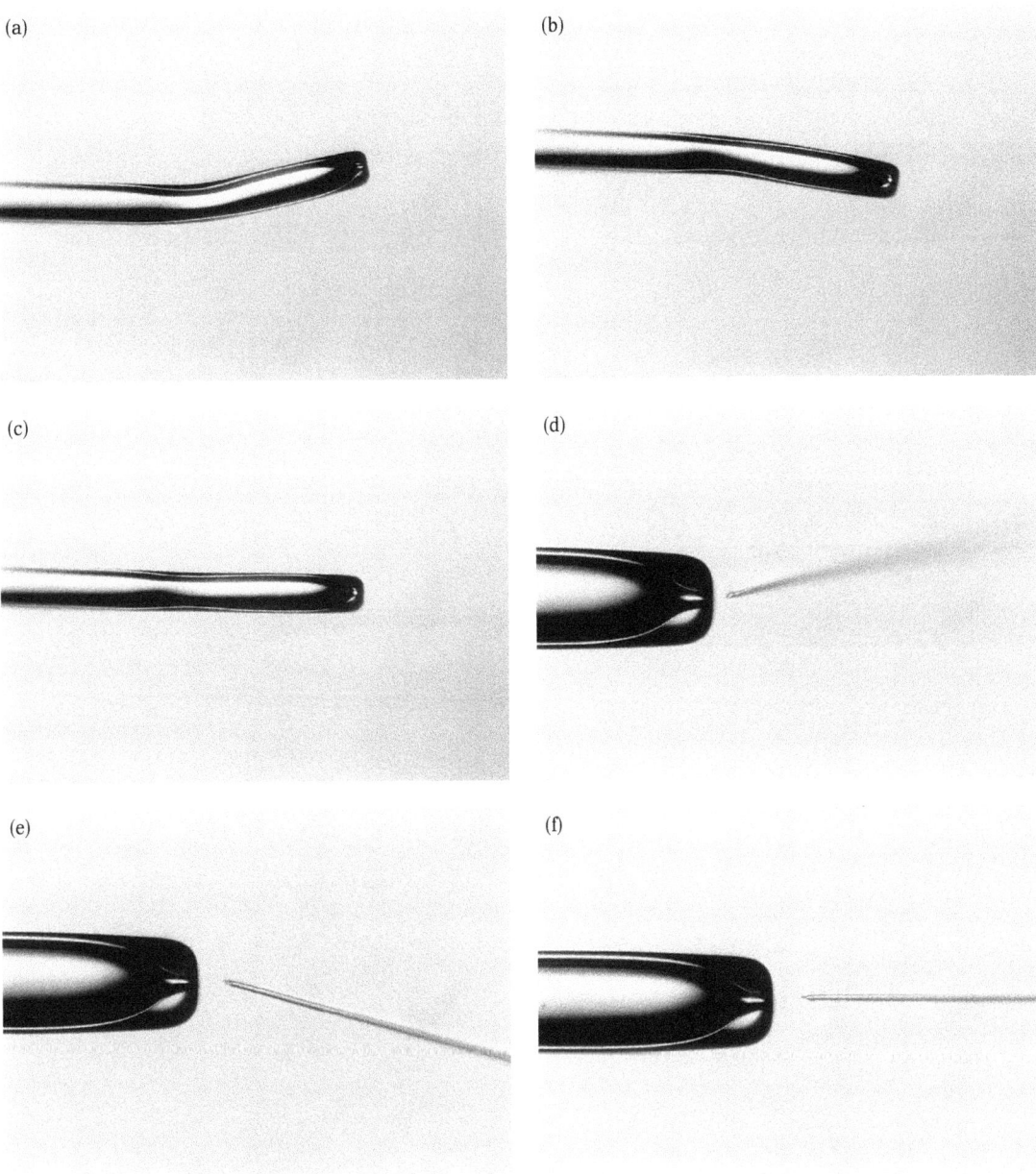

Figure 8.3 (a) Viewed under the inverted microscope, the 25-degree holding pipette bends upwards, indicating that it is not aligned correctly in the vertical plane but is angled away from the operator. (b) Viewed under the inverted microscope, the 25-degree holding pipette bends downwards, indicating that it is not aligned correctly in the vertical plane but is angled towards the operator. (c) Viewed under the inverted microscope, the 25-degree holding pipette appears straight, indicating that it is correctly aligned in the vertical plane. (d) Viewed under the inverted microscope, the 25-degree injection pipette bends downwards, indicating that it is not aligned correctly in the vertical plane but is angled towards the operator. (e) Viewed under the inverted microscope, the 25-degree pipette bends upwards, indicating that it is not aligned correctly in the vertical plane but is angled away from the operator. (f) Viewed under the inverted microscope, the tip of the 25-degree injection pipette appears straight, indicating that it is aligned correctly in the vertical plane.

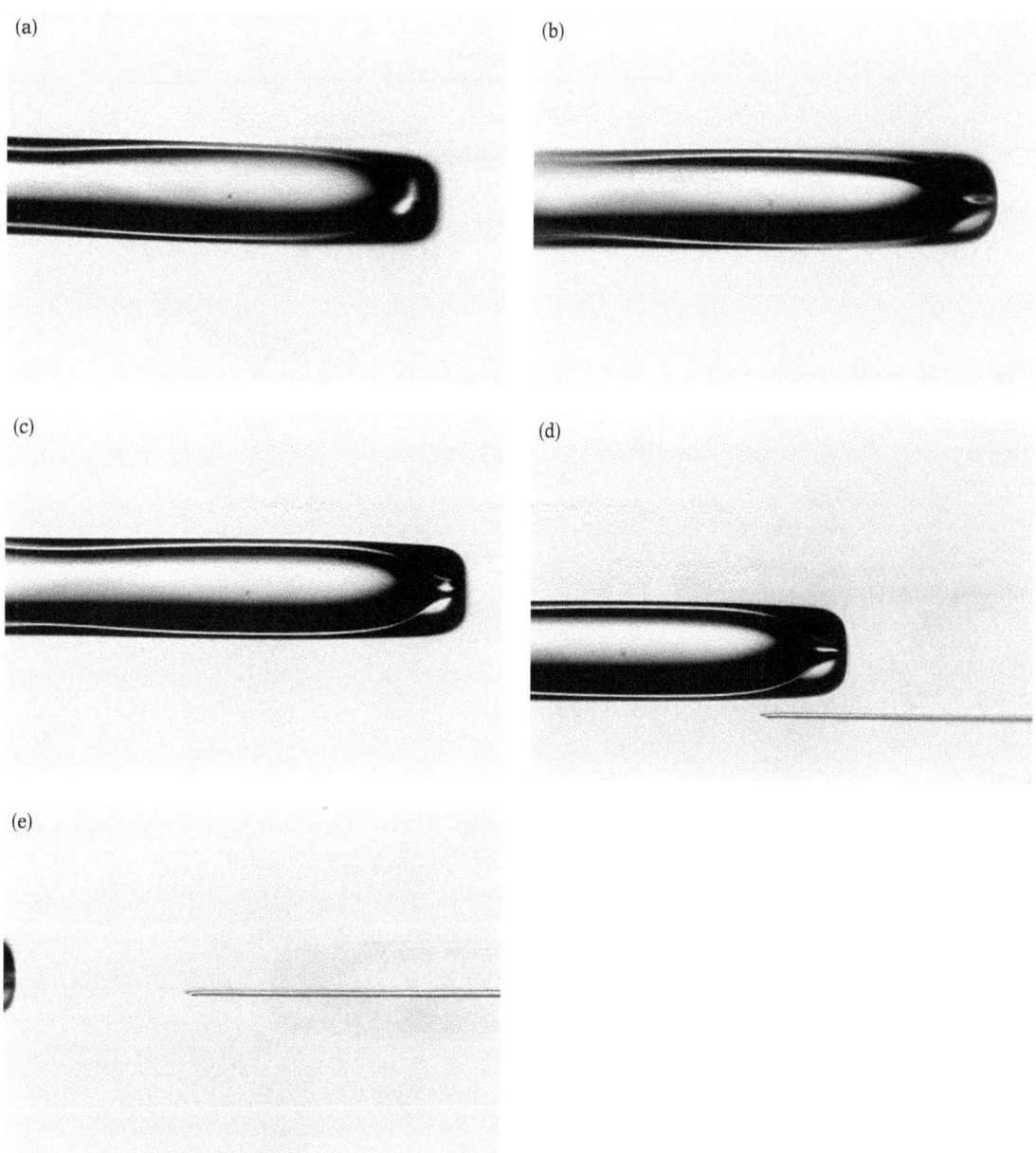

Figure 8.4 (a) Viewed under the inverted microscope, the focal plane of the tip of the holding pipette is higher, indicating that it is not aligned correctly in the horizontal plane but is tilted upwards. (b) Viewed under the inverted microscope, the focal plane of the tip of the holding pipette is lower, indicating that it is not aligned correctly in the horizontal plane but is tilted downwards. (c) Viewed under the inverted microscope, the focal plane of the tip of the holding pipette is the same as at its heel, indicating that it is aligned correctly in the horizontal plane. (d) Viewed under the inverted microscope, the focal plane of the tip of the injection pipette is higher, indicating that it is not aligned correctly in the horizontal plane but is tilted upwards. (e) Viewed under the inverted microscope, the focal plane of the tip of the injection pipette is lower, indicating that it is not aligned exactly in the horizontal plane but is tilted slightly downwards, which is necessary to enable the tip of the pipette to make contact with the tail of the spermatozoon.

the holding pipette, it is necessary to align it without tilt in the horizontal plane, as it needs to lie flat on the bottom of the dish to aspirate the oocyte in a controlled manner. However, the injection pipette needs to be tilted downwards slightly towards its tip in the horizontal plane, so that the tail of the spermatozoon can be effectively damaged and easily aspirated. Therefore, final alignment of the injection pipette is best established by using the bottom of the dish against which to obtain flexion. Then it becomes apparent exactly where the initial point of contact between the micropipette and bottom of the dish lies. However, it is more convenient to do this after equilibration of the micropipettes (see section 8.2.3).

8.2.3   Equilibrating the micropipettes

It is necessary to prime or equilibrate micropipettes with medium before use so that the gametes subsequently manipulated never come into contact with any air or oil. Micropipettes can become primed spontaneously by capillary action alone, but some aspiration is often required, especially when equilibrating the injection pipette. Usually, equilibration is achieved using ICSI media. This procedure is fairly simple, but again it is better to prime the holding pipette first as this is easier to locate within the equilibration drop of medium. To do this, using the coarse manipulators raise the micropipettes well above the microscope stage. This ensures that there is no risk of them being broken on the bottom of the microinjection dish when lowered for equilibration. Place the dish containing the equilibration drop of medium on to the heated stage of the microscope and locate the edge of the droplet using the 10× objective lens. Focus on the interface between the edge of the droplet and the oil to establish the focal plane of the bottom of the dish. Without changing the focal plane at which the microscope is set, locate the centre of the equilibration drop and, using the coarse manipulator, slowly lower the holding pipette until it comes into focus. If the holding pipette moves forward as it is coming into focus, this indicates that it has touched the bottom of the dish. In this case, raise it slightly off the bottom of the dish using the fine manipulator and refocus. If the internal diameter of the holding pipette is quite large, then it is quite likely to have primed itself by capillary action. On the other hand, holding pipettes with a fairly narrow internal diameter often require equilibrating manually. This will be evident by the appearance of an interface between the meniscus of medium at the entrance to the pipette and the air inside it. Turn the injector screw very slowly in an anticlockwise direction so as to draw medium into the holding pipette. Initially, medium will resist entering the holding pipette but all of a sudden it will rush in. Therefore, it is necessary to immediately neutralize the negative pressure, otherwise too much media will enter the holding pipette and the equilibration drop will be emptied. With an oil injector, this can be achieved only by reversing the flow, by turning the injector screw slightly clockwise. With air injectors, the negative pressure can be neutralized immediately by temporarily 'opening' the line, either at the injector itself or at the connection between it and the tubing. The injection pipette is equilibrated in exactly the same way. However, the position of the holding pipette above the bottom of the dish can now be used as a landmark to prevent accidental breakage of the injection pipette on the bottom of the dish when lowering it for equilibration. Also, because the internal diameter of the injection pipette is much narrower than that of the holding pipette, equilibration is slower and neutralization of any negative pressure does not have to be effected so rapidly. It is best to leave the micropipettes in the equilibration drop or in oil until ready to begin microinjecting so as to prevent them drying out and consequently becoming blocked.

Once equilibrated, the injection pipette may be lowered gently to the bottom of the dish whilst moving it from side to side using the fine manipulator. As it makes contact with the bottom of the dish, the pipette will flex about the point of contact between them. Hence, it becomes possible to determine the degree of tilt of the injection pipette in the horizontal plane. If the flexion is back from the tip of the injection pipette, then the angle is too shallow, the tilt being above horizontal. In this case, it will be necessary to raise the injection pipette using the coarse manipulator, increase the downward tilt using the universal joint, relocate the pipette, and recheck its alignment on the bottom of the dish. Once it can be seen to flex at its very tip, it can be assumed that the angle of downward tilt of the injection pipette is sufficient for sperm manipulation (see Figure 8.4e).

8.3 MANIPULATION OF SPERMATOZOA

Microinjection is quicker if the spermatozoa to be manipulated are already within the PVP rather than having first to be transferred from the 'sperm drop'. Therefore, it is preferable to load the PVP drop with a sample of prepared spermatozoa whenever possible. However, sperm manipulation can be hindered if the PVP is cluttered with too many spermatozoa. In this respect, it is better to load too few than too many, as more spermatozoa can be added in the former case. Alternatively, the prepared spermatozoa may be diluted to a concentration of 10^6/ml and added to the PVP at a ratio of 1 : 5 using non-toxic sterile pipette tips. This preparation of spermatozoa in PVP can then be used as the PVP drop in the microinjection dish, and should yield a reasonably good working concentration of spermatozoa. If the density of spermatozoa is very low, first microcentrifuge the prepared sperm sample at $1800\,g$ for 5 min. Then, allow a minimal volume of the pellet to enter a sterile pulled Pasteur pipette by capillary action, and deposit this minute volume into the PVP drop in each microinjection dish to be used for that patient. It will be necessary to do this under the high power of a stereo dissecting microscope, so as to monitor the flow to ensure that only a relatively small number of spermatozoa are deposited into the drop. An alternative to centrifuging sperm preparations of low density is to prepare them as drops under oil, from which the few spermatozoa available can be retrieved and transferred to the PVP drop for ICSI.

Some practitioners prefer to perform all sperm manipulation before injection, to minimize the duration for which the oocytes remain outside the incubator. Others prefer to inject each oocyte immediately after manipulating each spermatozoon. Either of these approaches is probably quite acceptable, and which is chosen may be determined by personal preference. However, it might be argued that it is better to inject a spermatozoon immediately after it has been damaged so as to maximize its potential for activating the oocyte. Clearly, if this is the approach adopted, then it is necessary to load the oocytes for injection into the droplets of ICSI medium before commencing sperm manipulation. To locate and manipulate spermatozoa in the PVP drop, it is preferable to switch to a $20\times$ objective lens and refocus upon the injection pipette. However, make this change only following equilibration/alignment of the injection pipette on the bottom of the dish using the $10\times$ objective lens. This way, the injection pipette is less likely to get broken and will be easier to locate under higher power if having been previously visible under lower-power magnification. If the prepared spermatozoa have been added directly to the PVP, then the most motile, and therefore probably the most viable, individuals will be found at the periphery of the droplet. If the prepared sperm are so low in number that they have to be added to the 'sperm drop' of ICSI medium in the microinjection dish, then it will be necessary to harvest them and transfer them to the PVP drop. Again, the most motile individuals will be found at the periphery of the droplet. Therefore, the injection pipette can be lowered to the edge of the sperm drop so that its open end faces into it. Spermatozoa will then either swim into the injection pipette or be aspirated into it by capillary action. Sometimes, in order to aspirate the spermatozoa successfully, it is necessary to apply very slight negative pressure to the injection pipette by turning the injector screw marginally anticlockwise. Once sufficient spermatozoa for injection have entered the injection pipette, they may be deposited into the PVP drop by turning the injector screw slowly clockwise. Care needs to be taken at this juncture not to introduce too much medium or, worse, bubbles of air into the PVP while forcing the spermatozoa from the injection pipette. Otherwise, the spermatozoa will be flooded to the top of the PVP drop or obscured by numerous air bubbles.

It is absolutely vital to damage the plasmalemma of the spermatozoon and so immobilize it, and this has been shown to markedly enhance fertilization rates following ICSI (Dozortsev *et al.*, 1994; Payne *et al.*, 1994). Immobilization of the spermatozoon may prevent undue disruption of ooplasm and ensure oocyte activation (Tesarik *et al.*, 1994). In turn, oocyte activation is a prerequisite for decondensation of the sperm nucleus and formation of the male pronucleus (Tesarik and Kopecny, 1989). The use of Hoffman modulation contrast optics makes the spermatozoa much easier to visualize if using plastic ICSI dishes. To immobilize a spermatozoon, locate a suitable individual and, using the fine manipulator joystick, isolate it on the bottom of the dish with the injection pipette tip. The spermatozoon should be immobilized by holding it against the bottom of the dish until it stops moving. Most practitioners prefer to immobilize the sperm with a quick movement of the pipette from left to right, or vice versa, crushing the tail against the bottom of the dish. A fairly reliable and simple way in which to achieve this is to align the spermatozoon so that its tail lies at right angles to the injection pipette (see Figure 8.5a). Then, raise the injection pipette slightly above the bottom of the dish, pass its tip over the sperm tail, lower it until it makes contact with the bottom of the dish, and draw it rapidly across the sperm tail (see Figure 8.5a and b). This way, the injection pipette cannot fail to make contact with the sperm tail and should result in permanent damage and immobility. This can be confirmed most easily if the tail of the spermatozoon is clearly kinked following the procedure (see Figure 8.5b). More sophisticated techniques for immobilizing spermatozoa and damaging the plasmalemma have been suggested, including the use of lasers (Montag *et al.*, 2000). However, there may be safety concerns with the use of lasers for such purposes. It is better to damage the sperm tail well away from its midpiece region, as this contains the proximal centriole and there could otherwise be some risk of damaging it. The sperm's proximal centriole is required by the oocyte to participate in bipolar spindle formation for the first mitotic division. Likewise, injection of the sperm head alone will produce a poor outcome, and a recent study proves this point (Moomjy *et al.*, 1999).

Once immobile, the spermatozoon may be aspirated into the injection pipette tail first by slowly turning the injector anticlockwise (see Figure 8.5c). It is essential at this point to emphasize the care needed in operating the injector screw control knob. Turning the control too far anticlockwise will cause a sudden in-rush of medium into the pipette. The sperm will be

(a)

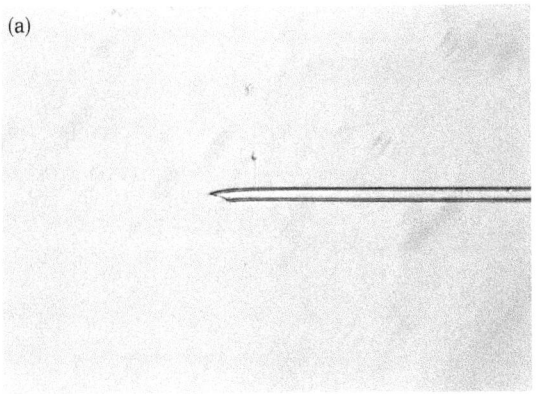

(b)

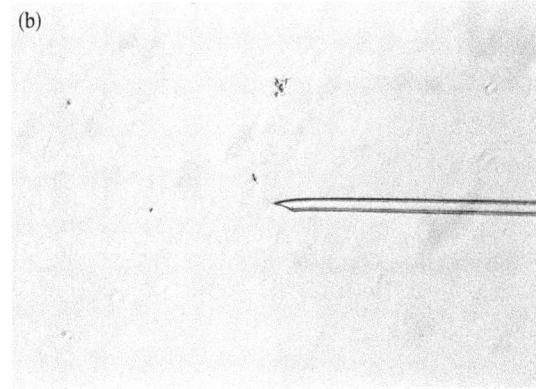

(c)

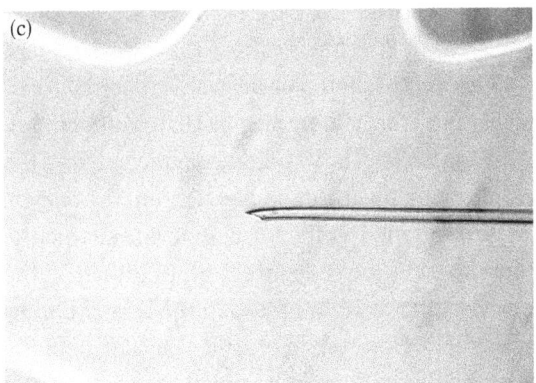

Figure 8.5 (a) The injection pipette is placed over the spermatozoon at right angles to its tail, with its tip in contact with the bottom of the ICSI dish. (b) The injection pipette is drawn rapidly across the tail of the spermatozoon, so that its tip, which is in contact with the bottom of the ICSI dish, damages the plasmalemma, leaving a permanent kink. (c) The spermatozoon is aspirated into the injection pipette, tail first.

lost and it will take a period of time for the pressure difference between the inside and the outside of the pipette to equalize. During this equalization process, it is impossible to aspirate or inject successfully. Hence, it is good practice to ensure that the movement of the spermatozoon along the injection pipette is completely under control before proceeding to manipulate the oocyte. This can be confirmed by stabilizing the position of the spermatozoon within the injection pipette using the injector.

8.4 MANIPULATION OF OOCYTES

The two most important considerations when manipulating the oocyte are to avoid the use of overly strong aspiration and to align the first PB at right angles to the line of the micropipettes. If excessive negative pressure is applied to the oocyte, the oolemma becomes sucked towards the holding pipette and deforms. Consequently, there is a risk of damage to the cytoskeleton of the oocyte. Furthermore, this deformation becomes exacerbated at injection because any resistance otherwise conferred by an intact oolemma is then compromised. Therefore, the use of slight negative

(a)

(b)

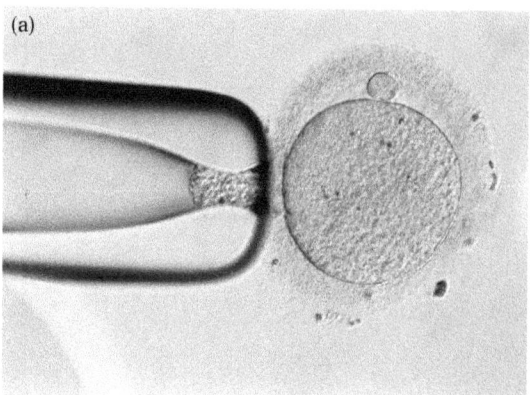
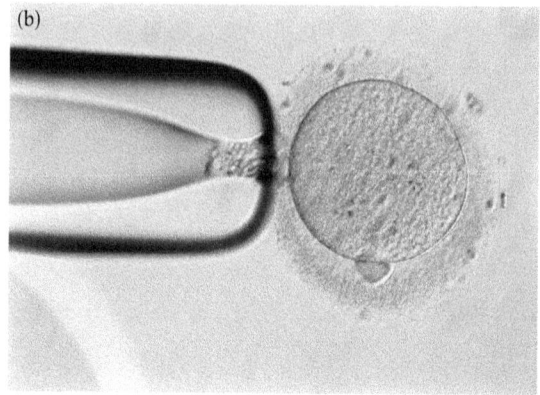

Figure 8.6 (a) The oocyte is aspirated on to the holding pipette with the first polar body lying in the 12 o'clock position. (b) The oocyte is aspirated on to the holding pipette with the first polar body lying in the 6 o'clock position.

pressure or even just capillary action should be all that is required to attach the oocyte gently but firmly to the holding pipette. On the other hand, the oocyte should not be held so loosely that it becomes detached from the holding pipette when withdrawing the injection pipette from the oocyte. Ideally, the oocyte should be positioned on the holding pipette so that the first PB lies at or near 6 or 12 o'clock (see Figure 8.6). In principle, the PB could be placed at any position at right angles to the line of the injection, the oocyte being a sphere. However, in practice, placement of the PB at 6 or 12 o'clock ensures that the injection pipette does not penetrate the oocyte closer to where the spindle is presumed to lie. It has been suggested that better-quality embryos result if ICSI is performed with the PB at the 6 o'clock position (Nagy *et al.*, 1995b). However, the difference observed was small (83% versus 79% embryos of transferable quality), and no differences in fertilization or survival rates were observed. Besides, logic dictates that it is irrelevant whether the PB is at 6 or 12 o'clock if injecting a sphere, and there does not seem to be any differential effect on pregnancy outcome providing ICSI is performed competently (Stoddart and Fleming, 2000).

Whenever manipulating oocytes, it is important to place the microinjection dish on to a heated stage. These are supplied with an aperture and there are pros and cons to using stages with different size apertures. Essentially, the larger the aperture, the greater the field of view; the smaller the aperture, the more efficient the heating of the dish. There are a number of ways in which the oocyte can be manipulated to lie attached to the holding pipette with its PB at 6 or 12 o'clock. One of these is to use the fine manipulator joystick and injector concurrently to position the holding pipette and aspirate the oocyte on to it. However, to position the oocyte with its PB at 6 or 12 o'clock using this technique, it is often necessary to

Figure 8.7 The holding pipette may be positioned to either side of the oocyte, either above or below its equator and either to the left or right of centre. Aspiration or expulsion of media into or out of the pipette, respectively, will cause the oocyte to spin towards or away from the pipette aperture, enabling the polar body to be brought into either the 6 o'clock position or the 12 o'clock position.

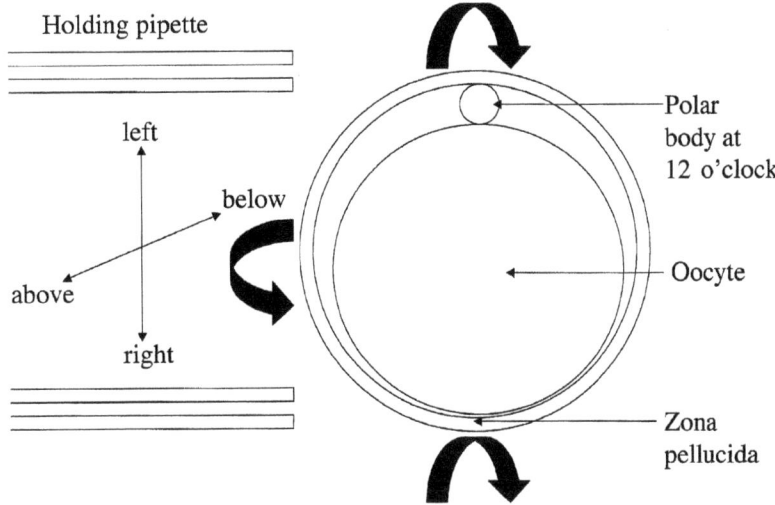

spin the oocyte in the appropriate direction as it approaches the holding pipette. Essentially, this is achieved by positioning the holding pipette, in two dimensions, in one of four different positions, depending upon which direction the oocyte needs to be rotated (see Figure 8.7). Similarly, the oocyte can be blown in the opposite direction to that when aspirated. Once perfected, this technique is very quick to apply. Another way that the oocyte may be manipulated such that its PB lies at 6 or 12 o'clock is to rotate it with the injection pipette while holding it gently on to the holding pipette. To do this, first aspirate the oocyte very gently on to the holding pipette regardless of the position of the PB. Then, using the sharp tip of the injection pipette, push against the appropriate area of the ZP to rotate the oocyte in the desired direction. If coronal cells remain attached to the oocyte, these too can be used as a means of indirectly attaching the oocyte to the holding pipette, but only if they can be made to lie in the same plane and at right angles to the PB. The advantage of using coronal cells for attachment of the oocyte to the holding pipette is that greater aspiration may be applied, with less risk of distorting the oolemma. Once the oocyte has been aligned on the holding pipette in the desired position, the oocyte may be injected.

8.5   INJECTION OF OOCYTES

Successful injection of oocytes is dependent upon a number of variables, including oocyte quality, technique, and the quality of the injection pipette. All oocytes for injection should be at MII, having extruded the first PB. This ensures that they contain a haploid set of chromosomes, so that a normal

Table 8.1 *Results of six different ICSI practitioners from the same centre*

ICSI practitioner	No. of eggs[a]	Fertilization rate (%)[b]	Cleavage rate (%)[c]	Embryo quality[d]	Pregnancy rate (%)[e]	Implantation rate (%)
A	1689	68	93	73% (1 + 2)	31	15
B	502	60	98	77% (1 + 2)	35	18
C	551	62	92	68% (1 + 2)	19	10
D	254	68	95	73% (1 + 2)	22	10
E	904	67	94	67% (1 + 2)	34	15
F	1012	66	94	72% (1 + 2)	23	13

[a] The number of eggs is the number of MII oocytes injected.
[b] The fertilization rate is the number of 2PN zygotes divided by the number of MII oocytes.
[c] The cleavage rate is per 2PN zygote.
[d] Embryo quality is graded on a standard scale, from 1 to 4, only grade 1 and 2 embryos also being considered suitable for cryopreservation.
[e] The pregnancy and implantation rates are calculated from the fresh transfer of one to three embryos on day 2 following oocyte retrieval.

diploid karyotype should be carried by the zygote following injection of another haploid set of chromosomes from the spermatozoon. Attempts have been made in the past to inject oocytes that are at MI (Hamberger *et al.*, 1995), but the fertilization rates achieved are much lower and there is always a greater risk of producing an aneuploid embryo. Arguably, a better approach would be to in vitro mature MI oocytes to MII before injection. Also, oocytes that have failed to fertilize following conventional IVF have been injected 24 hours following their aspiration as a form of rescue ICSI (Hamberger *et al.*, 1995). With this approach, the fertilization rates are almost as good as those normally achieved with routine ICSI, but only if freshly prepared spermatozoa from new ejaculates are injected. However, some authorities have expressed concern over this practice, as it may be possible that there was no sign of fertilization following IVF despite the entry of a spermatozoon. In such circumstances, a triploid embryo could be created following rescue ICSI. Germinal vesical stage oocytes should not be injected as a form of clinical treatment.

There is no single, correct way in which an oocyte should be injected. Rather, there are a number of different ways to achieve the same result, at least in terms of fertilization and oocyte survival. However, it is interesting to compare results between colleagues known to employ different methods for injecting the oocyte (see Table 8.1). It becomes immediately apparent that although different practitioners may achieve similar fertilization rates, the number of pregnancies resulting from the embryos created can vary wildly. The explanation for this may be that this is due simply to the many variables involved or a reflection of statistical variation, and pregnancy rates would even out providing enough data are analysed. However, the fact that there appears to be a variation in cleavage rate and embryo quality that correlates with the pregnancy data argues against this. It appears, therefore, that the injection technique needs to incorporate more than simply a method that ensures fertilization. Most probably, the technique used needs to minimize trauma to the oocyte that could cause damage to the cytoskeleton with subsequent impairment of cleavage. One way to minimize damage to the oocyte is to use a narrow and sharp injection pipette, preferably one that has been forged with a spike at its tip. Another way is to minimize the aspiration of ooplasm during the injection. Injection can be performed using a $20\times$ or $40\times$ objective lens. Although a higher magnification provides a closer view of what is happening, the field of view is restricted. This is an important point, considering the fact that it is necessary to be able to monitor the movement of the spermatozoon and ooplasm along the injection pipette. Therefore, injection using a $20\times$ objective lens is generally the better approach.

It is extremely important to use a fresh sterile injection pipette for each patient's oocytes, as it has been shown that foreign DNA may otherwise be carried over from one patient's oocytes and injected into another's (Chan *et al.*, 2000). Also, PVP has been suggested to be a toxin and putative carcinogen. However, it clearly facilitates control of the spermatozoon and may even potentiate oocyte activation. Although the world literature on ICSI has not yet identified any congenital problems with the use of PVP, it would nevertheless seem prudent to avoid injecting any more than 1–2 pl of medium along with the sperm. It is also important to keep a tally of which oocytes have been injected, so as to avoid accidentally injecting the same oocyte twice. This is a real possibility because the injection furrow seals within minutes following ICSI, making it very difficult to determine whether the oocyte has been injected previously. It is also important to wash the oocytes through several changes of bicarbonate-buffered medium to rapidly restore physiological temperature and pH following the ICSI procedure.

8.5.1 Microinjection of oocytes with mature spermatozoa

Assuming that the spermatozoon has been immobilized and aspirated into the injection pipette, and that the oocyte has been attached to the holding pipette with the PB at either 6 or 12 o'clock, injection of the spermatozoon may be proceeded with. Firstly, raise the oocyte just clear of the bottom of

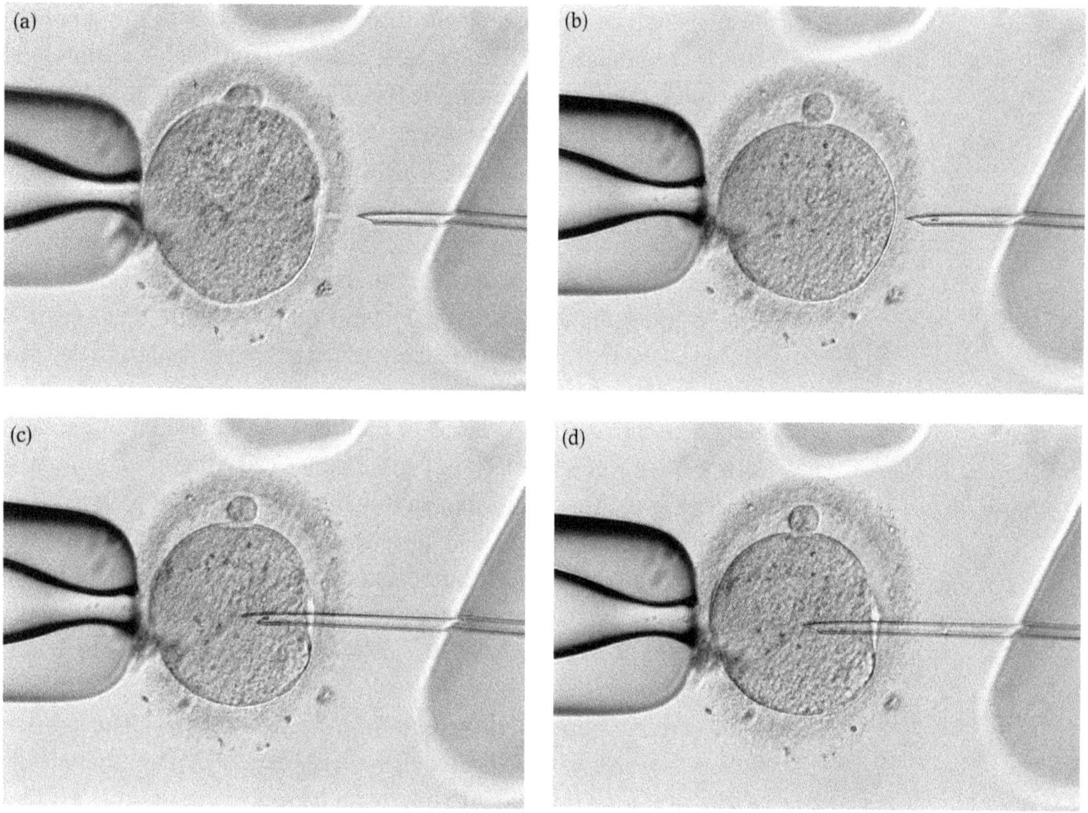

(a)

(b)

(c)

(d)

(e)

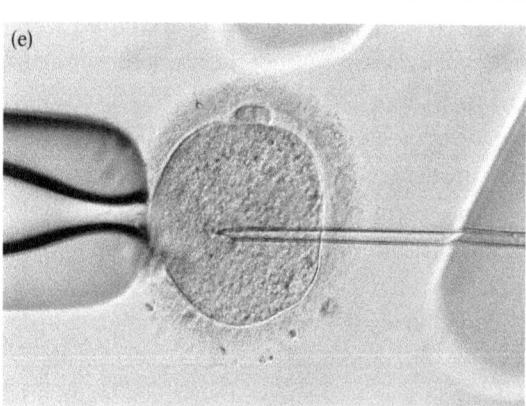

Figure 8.8 (a) The tip of the injection pipette is placed adjacent to the ZP of the oocyte, both being concurrently in focus. (b) The spermatozoon is moved along the injection pipette and brought to rest at its very tip. (c) The injection pipette is pushed through the ZP of the oocyte, causing an indentation of the oolemma. (d) The injection pipette is advanced halfway into the ooplasm of the oocyte, and ooplasm is aspirated into the injection pipette. (e) The aspirated ooplasm plus the spermatozoon is deposited well towards the centre of the oocyte.

the dish and focus on the oolemma. This ensures that the focal plane runs through the geometrical centre of the oocyte. Taking care not to disturb the oocyte, position the injection pipette almost adjacent to the ZP at the midline of the oocyte and raise or lower it until its very tip comes into sharp focus (see Figure 8.8a). At this stage, both oolemma and injection pipette tip should be in focus concurrently. This ensures that the injection pipette will initially pierce the oocyte at its midline.

Now, slowly turn the injector screw clockwise to move the spermatozoon towards the tip of the injection pipette – it will be necessary to eventually counteract this to avoid losing the spermatozoon out of the end of the injection pipette. To do this, turn the injector screw slowly anticlockwise as the spermatozoon approaches the tip of the injection pipette. Using fine control, it should be possible to stabilize the movement of the spermatozoon at the tip of the injection pipette (see Figure 8.8b).

The injection pipette may then be advanced carefully in a straight line towards the oocyte to penetrate the ZP. Confirm that the injection pipette will enter the oocyte at its midline by observing the pattern of indentation that it creates. It should be possible to see the point of indentation of the oolemma as well as those areas of the oolemma either side of it (see Figure 8.8c). In the vertical plane, the circumference of the oolemma either above or below the point of indentation may be visible (see Figure 8.8c). If this is the case, then the point of indentation lies either above or below the midline of the oocyte. To find and maintain the midline during the injection, it is necessary to raise or lower the injection pipette until the circumference of the oolemma above and below the point of indentation are coincident (see Figure 8.8c). This ensures that the injection pipette follows a path to the geometric centre of the oocyte. Be careful not to push the injection pipette much more than halfway into the oocyte, so as to avoid piercing the oolemma on the far side (see Figure 8.8d). Concurrent damage to the oolemma at both sides of the oocyte usually results in its rapid degeneration due to lysis. Occasionally, the oolemma will rupture in response to the passage of the injection pipette, as evident by its movement back over the tip of the pipette. Usually, however, the oolemma remains intact due to its inherent strength and elasticity. This will be apparent by the fact that the oolemma remains invaginated around the micropipette (see Figure 8.8c and d). Also, this will be confirmed when aspirating ooplasm during the next step of the procedure.

Once the injection pipette has penetrated the ZP, the pipette may be withdrawn slightly, but it is important to ensure that ooplasm remains around its opening (see Figure 8.8d). Withdrawing the injection pipette provides more space into which it can be thrust in the event that the oolemma proves difficult to penetrate. Ooplasm may now be aspirated into the injection pipette by slowly turning the injector screw in an anticlockwise direction (see Figure 8.8d). Initially, the flow of ooplasm into the injection pipette will be slow as it is impeded by the intact oolemma. Eventually, however, the oolemma will rupture to allow a sudden free flow of ooplasm. At this juncture, it is important to rapidly halt the influx of ooplasm into the injection pipette by quickly reversing the negative pressure applied by the injector. If an air injector is used for injection of the spermatozoon, the negative pressure may be equalized immediately with atmospheric pressure by transiently 'opening' the line. Should the oolemma fail to rupture despite aspiration of a fairly long column of ooplasm into the injection pipette, it is not advisable to continue the aspiration, as excessive aspiration may result in degeneration of the oocyte. In this circumstance, it is usually better to attempt to penetrate the oolemma by employing a very rapid jabbing movement of the injection pipette into the oocyte. This requires excellent control as the jabbing action has to be rapid enough to penetrate the elastic oolemma, but contact with the far side of the oolemma must be avoided. If the oolemma cannot be penetrated despite such efforts, it is usually better to compromise by depositing the spermatozoon into the oocyte rather than subjecting it to more excessive manipulation, which might well result in its demise. At least with the former approach there remains some likelihood of fertilization occurring, whereas an oocyte that has degenerated is no good to anybody.

Once the oolemma has been penetrated and there is free flow of ooplasm, all that remains is to carefully deposit the ooplasm that has been aspirated, along with the spermatozoon, into the oocyte (see Figure 8.8e). This is achieved by slowly turning the injector screw in a clockwise direction. Once the spermatozoon has exited the injection pipette, it is important to withdraw the pipette from the oocyte so as to prevent delivery of an excess volume of medium containing PVP. In this respect, it is good practice to slow down the outflow of ooplasm as the spermatozoon approaches the opening of the injection pipette, and to begin withdrawing the pipette as soon as the head of the spermatozoon has exited it. Also, it is advisable to deposit the spermatozoon well towards the centre of the oocyte in order to minimize the risk of it being expelled either during removal of the injection pipette or as the injection furrow closes up to repair the oolemma. Having successfully delivered the spermatozoon into the oocyte, the oocyte may be released from the holding pipette by turning the injector screw clockwise. If there are other oocytes remaining in the microinjection dish, these may be injected in similar fashion, one by one, before washing them all through into bicarbonate-buffered medium for culture. If difficulty is encountered with any one of a batch of oocytes being injected, it is better to wash the others through into bicarbonate-buffered culture medium and leave them in a CO_2 incubator until the problem has been resolved. In this way, only a single oocyte is subjected to prolonged exposure to the adverse conditions outside of an incubator.

8.5.2 Microinjection of oocytes with immature spermatozoa

It cannot be stated too strongly that the microinjection of human oocytes with immature spermatozoa is still an experimental procedure. We still have much to learn about the reproductive potential and long-term safety of using immature spermatozoa in ICSI, and success rates remain pitifully low. Therefore, this procedure cannot yet be considered suitable for routine clinical application. Consequently, ethical approval should be sought before treating patients with this procedure, having first obtained their fully informed consent. Likewise, screening of the patients for genetic diseases before treatment and follow-up of any resultant pregnancies or births is mandatory, as congenital malformations following ELSI have been reported (Zech *et al.*, 2000).

Injection of just the nucleus of a round spermatid (round spermatid nucleus injection; ROSNI) has been achieved in human oocytes (Yamanaka *et al.*, 1997), although this approach is applied less commonly. The standard technique required for the injection of immature sperm into oocytes does not differ markedly from that employed with mature spermatozoa (Tesarik and Mendoza, 1996). However, there are clearly differences in the manipulation that is possible with round and elongating spermatids. Also, subtle manipulations of the oocyte have been suggested to improve fertilization outcome. Elongated and mature spermatids may be manipulated and injected into the oocyte using precisely the same technique as that for mature spermatozoa (Fishel *et al.*, 1995a). On the other hand, manipulation with an injection pipette having an internal diameter of 6–7 μm is necessary for round and elongating spermatids. Use of an injection pipette with these dimensions not only aids the successful identification of round spermatids but also facilitates their deformation, which may be important for successful activation of the oocyte. Penetration of the oocyte with the injection pipette is achieved in the same way as with mature spermatozoa.

Although round spermatids have been found to have sufficient oocyte-activating factor to induce oscillations of intracellular calcium within oocytes (Sousa *et al.*, 1996; Yamanaka *et al.*, 1997), it has been suggested that vigorous aspiration of the ooplasm be effected before injecting them (Tesarik and Mendoza, 1996). This is recommended particularly when injecting round or elongating spermatids, as these do not appear to have the same ability as elongated and mature spermatids to activate the oocyte, particularly when recovered from patients with complete failure of spermiogenesis. Furthermore, it has been suggested that any deficiency in the ability of spermatids to activate oocytes may

Table 8.2 *Oocyte/zygote appearance following ICSI*

Appearance	Definition	Expected rate (%) (Stoddart and Fleming, 2000)	Ploidy
0PN + 1PB	MII (unfertilized)	15–20	Haploid
1PN + 2PBs	Monopronucleate	1–5	Haploid
2PN + 2PBs	Fertilized	65–70	Diploid
3PN + 1PB	Digyny	1–5	Triploid
3PN + 2PBs	Dispermy	1–5	Triploid
Necrotic	Degenerate	5–10	Unknown

PN, pronucleus/pronuclei.

be compensated for by using electrical or biochemical means. Following spermatid microinjection, human oocytes have been activated artificially using the calcium ionophore A23187 (Vanderzwalmen *et al.*, 1997). Such treatment would appear to enhance both fertilization and pregnancy rates, although the data to support this are minimal at present. Even so, the vast majority of zygotes and cleaved embryos produced with the injection of round spermatids never result in an ongoing pregnancy (Urman *et al.*, 2002), let alone a live birth. Hence, we must remain highly sceptical about the reproductive potential of immature gametes.

8.6   ASSESSMENT OF FERTILIZATION AND QUALITY CONTROL/ASSURANCE

Oocytes are assessed for evidence of fertilization 16–18 hours later, on the morning following the ICSI procedure. Various results will be seen, depending upon multiple factors, including the ICSI technique employed, oocyte quality, and the type of sperm cell injected (see Table 8.2 and Figure 8.9).

If ICSI fails to result in fertilization, then there will be no evidence of any pronuclei and the oocyte will remain arrested at MII (see Table 8.2 and Figure 8.9). There may be various reasons for such fertilization failure, including lack of damage to the sperm plasmalemma, lack of penetration of the oolemma, and an inability of the oocyte to respond to the activating stimulus of the spermatozoon injected. Normal fertilization is defined as the presence of two pronuclei (2PN) and two PBs (see Table 8.2 and Figure 8.9). However, it is not that unusual to see zygotes containing three or more PBs, presumably due to division or fragmentation of the first PB. In

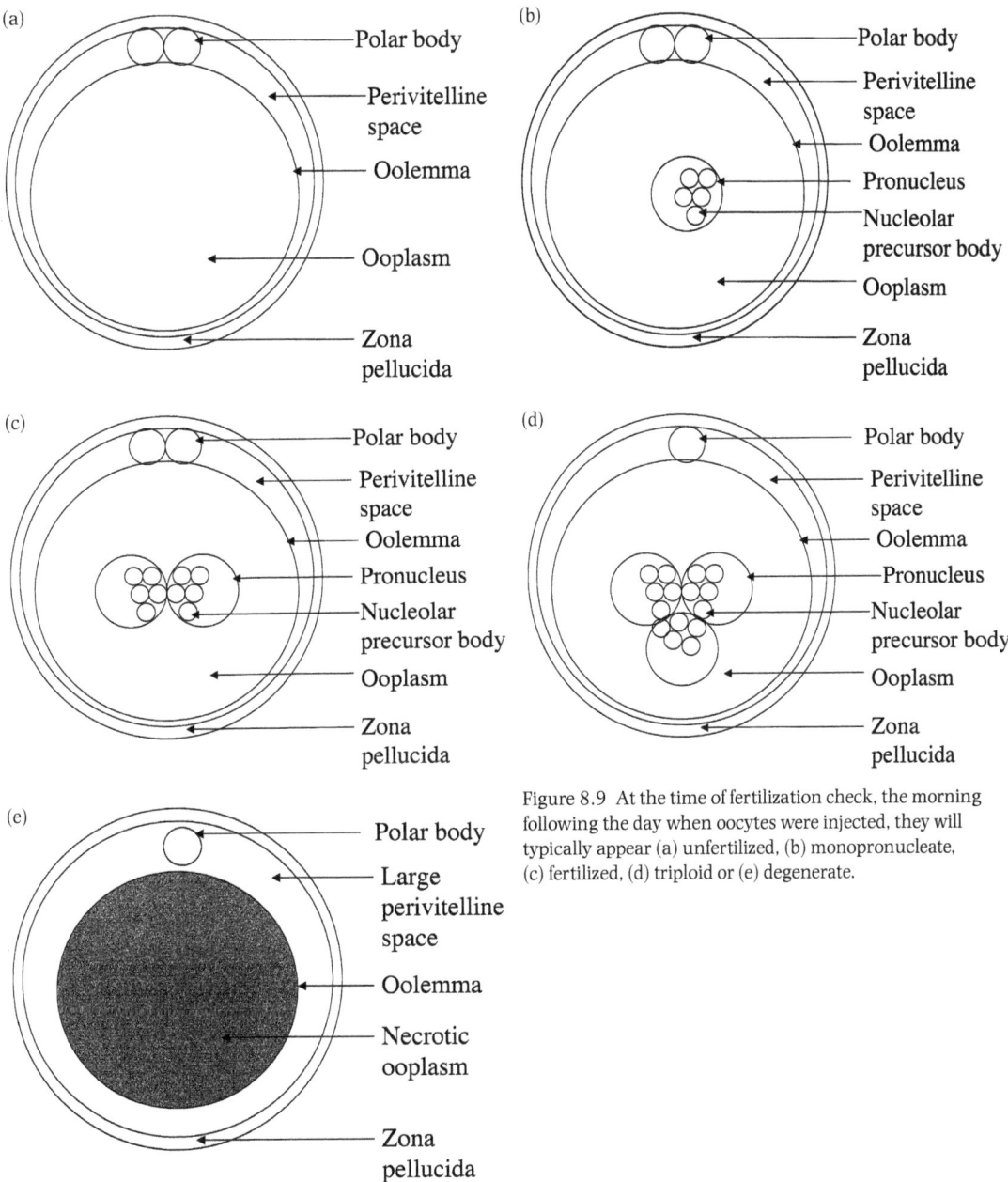

Figure 8.9 At the time of fertilization check, the morning following the day when oocytes were injected, they will typically appear (a) unfertilized, (b) monopronucleate, (c) fertilized, (d) triploid or (e) degenerate.

this event, the presence of two pronuclei despite the number of PBs may be taken alone as evidence of normal fertilization. Occasionally, oocytes with only a single pronucleus (1PN) will be seen (see Table 8.2 and Figure 8.9b). The most likely explanation for this is failure of sperm decondensation and male pronucleus formation, especially if the second PB is present.

Sometimes, the reason for such failure is evident from the presence of the spermatozoon within the PVS rather than in the ooplasm, it having been ejected from the oocyte. This typically results following failure to penetrate adequately the oolemma during the ICSI procedure. Otherwise, the similar size of the male and female pronuclei makes it very difficult to determine whether failure to complete fertilization is due to a lack of oocyte activation or sperm decondensation. Nevertheless, such 1PN oocytes should be checked again four hours later just in case the formation of the second pronucleus has been delayed for some reason. However, it is important that these should not be transferred if they should fail to exhibit a second pronucleus, as cytogenetic analysis of 1PN oocytes following ICSI shows more than 90% of them to be haploid, any subsequent cleavage being the result of parthenogenetic activation (Sultan *et al.*, 1995). Alternatively, oocytes containing three pronuclei (3PN) are observed occasionally (see Table 8.2 and Figure 8.9d). The possible reasons for this include failure of the oocyte to extrude the second PB and inadvertent injection of more than one spermatozoon into the oocyte. However, it is important not to confuse a vacuole for a pronucleus when examining apparently triploid zygotes. Pronuclei can be differentiated from vacuoles easily by the presence of nucleolar precursor bodies (usually three to five) (see Figure 8.9). Finally, a few oocytes may appear necrotic as they are undergoing degeneration (see Table 8.2 and Figure 8.9e). Oocytes may degenerate following injection for various reasons, including poor ICSI technique, poor injection pipettes, and inherent fragility of the oocytes (fragile oocyte syndrome). However, if the oocytes that were injected appeared to be of good quality but the rate of degeneration is above 10%, it will be necessary to troubleshoot the entire ICSI procedure. In summary, only normally fertilized zygotes (2PN) are suitable for transfer to the uterus.

Attention to all consumables, equipment and techniques utilized during the ICSI procedure should form the basis for ongoing quality control. Quality assurance is provided by the response of the oocytes to injection as well as the outcome following transfer of any embryos so created. The number of oocytes suitable for injection (MII) should reflect a maturation rate of more than 75%. Of those oocytes injected, more than 90% should survive injection and more than 60% should become fertilized normally (2PN). Pregnancy rates following transfer of embryos derived from ICSI should be comparable to those derived from routine IVF. Similarly, there should be no difference in the survival rate of embryos cryopreserved following either procedure.

8.7 TROUBLESHOOTING

8.7.1 Micropipette fitting, alignment and equilibration

8.7.1.1 *Problem – oil fails to exit the tool holder when the injector screw is turned clockwise*
Probable cause: There may be a block in the tool holder or the injector line. Occasionally, a novice may not appreciate that the tool holder in question is actually attached to an air injector, or that the oil injector has not been filled with oil.

Suggested remedy: Check the patency of the tool holder and injector line by using a replacement and ascertaining whether oil still fails to exit. If possible, remove any obvious cause of the blockage and, if necessary, replace any part that cannot be unblocked.

8.7.1.2 *Problem – the micropipette cannot be inserted past the sealing ring of the tool holder*
Probable cause: There may be the remnants of a broken micropipette inside the sealing ring, or the ferrule may still be tightened down.

Suggested remedy: Check that the ferrule is loosened off a couple of turns and, if necessary, remove it altogether to inspect the condition of the sealing ring inside the tool holder.

8.7.1.3 *Problem – the tool-holder cannot be attached to the retaining clip of the universal joint*
Probable cause: The retaining clip locking screw is not loosened off sufficiently.

Suggested remedy: Loosen off the retaining clip locking screw until the tool holder can be inserted easily.

8.7.1.4 *Problem – the tool holder cannot be rotated about its long axis whilst held by the retaining clip of the universal joint*
Probable cause: The retaining clip locking screw is not loosened off sufficiently.

Suggested remedy: Loosen off the retaining clip locking screw until the tool holder can be rotated easily.

8.7.1.5   *Problem – the range of the coarse manipulator is insufficient to position the micropipette directly over the objective lens of the inverted microscope*

Probable cause: The micropipette has been pushed too far into the tool holder and/or the tool holder has been placed into the retaining clip of the universal joint too far away from the centre of the microscope stage.

Suggested remedy: Loosen the ferrule of the tool holder and/or the locking screw of the retaining clip so that the micropipette can be brought closer to the centre of the microscope stage.

8.7.1.6   *Problem – the holding pipette cannot be seen down the microscope after having been positioned directly above the objective lens and adjusting the focus*

Probable cause: The micropipette has not been moved sufficiently far forward over the objective lens, or an objective lens of too high a magnification is being used.

Suggested remedy: Check that an objective lens with a magnification lower than 20× is in place and move the holding pipette forward so that it is clearly lying across its field of view. Then use the micromanipulator to move the micropipette backwards and forwards (over the objective lens) along the y-axis, at right angles to its long axis, while adjusting the coarse focus up and down until it comes into view.

8.7.1.7   *Problem – the injection pipette cannot be seen down the microscope after having been positioned close to the holding pipette and adjusting the focus*

Probable cause: The injection pipette has not been placed close enough to the holding pipette, or it is being missed because the focus is being adjusted too rapidly.

Suggested remedy: Looking down the microscope, move the injection pipette even further forward towards the holding pipette. Then, use the micromanipulator to move it backwards and forwards (over the objective lens) along the y-axis, at right angles to its long axis, while adjusting the coarse focus up and down very slowly until it comes into view.

8.7.1.8   *Problem – the tip of the injection pipette cannot be brought into focus on the bottom of the microinjection dish*

Probable cause: The point of contact between the injection pipette and the bottom of the microinjection dish is towards its heel, away from its tip.

Suggested remedy: Raise the injection pipette, increase the depth of the angle at which the tool holder points towards the microscope stage, remove the microinjection dish, and relocate the injection pipette down the microscope using the holding pipette as a landmark. The microinjection dish can then be replaced to test whether the tip of the injection pipette may now be brought into focus. If necessary, repeat this procedure until the tip of the injection pipette can be brought into focus on the bottom of the microinjection dish.

8.7.2 Gamete manipulation

8.7.2.1 *Problem – no spermatozoa can be seen after loading the PVP drop with an aliquot of the sperm preparation*
Probable cause: Either the spermatozoa have not yet had time to swim to the bottom of the PVP drop or too few spermatozoa have been added.

Suggested remedy: Allow the spermatozoa sufficient time (5–10 min) to swim to the bottom of the PVP drop and then scan the entire drop using the $10\times$ objective lens to locate them. If spermatozoa can still not be seen, load the PVP drop with another aliquot of the sperm preparation. Sometimes, the density or longevity of the spermatozoa is such that it will be necessary to add a much larger volume of the sperm preparation to the sperm drop. In this event, it will then prove necessary to aspirate spermatozoa from the sperm drop and transfer them to the PVP drop before manipulation.

8.7.2.2 *Problem – it is not possible to make contact with the sperm tail using the tip of the injection pipette.*
Probable cause: Either the angle of the tool holder relative to the microinjection dish is not steep enough, or the injection pipette has been pushed down too far, causing its tip to reflect away from bottom.

Suggested remedy: Adjust the angle of the tool holder or raise the injection pipette as necessary.

8.7.2.3 *Problem – spermatozoa stick to the tip of the injection pipette while attempting to immobilize them*
Probable cause: The spermatozoa or the injection pipette itself may be sticky.

Suggested remedy: Remove the spermatozoa attached to the injection pipette by rapidly moving the tip of the pipette against the bottom of the microinjection dish. If the spermatozoa remain attached, they will usually fall off if the injection pipette is moved rapidly in and out of the PVP drop, either up and down using the coarse manipulator or from side to side using the microscope stage control. Sometimes, replacing the injection pipette with a clean one will solve this problem, whereas occasionally this is simply the nature of the spermatozoa being manipulated. In the latter event, all that can be done is to persevere while minimizing the extent of manipulation to that required for sperm immobilization alone.

8.7.2.4 *Problem – the heads of the spermatozoa become detached from their tails during attempted immobilization*
Probable cause: The spermatozoa are unusually fragile.

Suggested remedy: All that can be done is to persevere while minimizing the extent of manipulation to that required for sperm immobilization alone. It is important to be aware of the fact that dissected spermatozoa should not be injected, as lack of sperm integrity can compromise normal mitotic division of the embryo, resulting in chromosomal mosaicism.

8.7.2.5 *Problem – spermatozoa stick to the bottom of the microinjection dish by their tails following immobilization, making it difficult to aspirate them into the injection pipette*
Probable cause: The spermatozoa are unusually sticky.

Suggested remedy: Aspirate the sperm head into the microinjection pipette and then move the micropipette forwards rapidly to dislodge the sperm tail from the bottom of the microinjection dish.

8.7.2.6 *Problem – it proves difficult to aspirate immobilized spermatozoa by their tails from the bottom of the PVP drop*
Probable cause: Either the opening of the injection pipette is not in the same focal plane as the sperm tail, or the injection pipette is blocked.

Suggested remedy: Adjust the height of the injection pipette to bring it into the same focal plane as the sperm tail or replace it, as necessary.

8.7.2.7 *Problem – spermatozoa rush into the injection pipette uncontrollably while attempting to aspirate them*
Probable cause: Either the injector screw has been turned too rapidly or excessive negative pressure resides within the injection pipette.

Suggested remedy: Use finer control of the injector or equalize the pressure inside and outside the injection pipette, as necessary.

8.7.2.8   *Problem – the spermatozoon does not fit into the injection pipette*
Probable cause: Either the injection pipette is too small or the sperm head is abnormally large.

Suggested remedy: Replace the injection pipette. If the problem persists, use an injection pipette with a slightly larger internal diameter, such as those supplied by some manufacturers for spermatid injection.

8.7.2.9   *Problem – spermatozoa drift within the injection pipette despite*
repeated attempts at stabilization
Probable cause: The oil or medium in the injection pipette has become mixed with air bubbles, compromising hydraulic control.

Suggested remedy: Replace the pipette. If this fails to resolve the problem, check for any source of temperature fluctuation. This can be a cause of the problem if using oil-driven injectors in an enclosed heated cage. In such cases, preferably replace the heated cage with a heated stage or, alternatively, replace the oil-driven injectors with injectors driven by air.

8.7.2.10   *Problem – the tip of the holding pipette cannot be brought into the same*
focal plane as the oocyte
Probable cause: The holding pipette is tilted upwards at its tip, initial contact between its heel and the bottom of the microinjection dish preventing its tip from moving into the same focal plane as the oocyte.

Suggested remedy: Adjust the angle of the tool holder.

8.7.2.11   *Problem – the oocyte either keeps falling off the holding pipette or*
becomes increasingly and excessively aspirated on to it
Probable cause: The oil or medium in the holding pipette has become mixed with air bubbles, compromising hydraulic control.

Suggested remedy: Replace the holding pipette.

8.7.2.12   *Problem – the oocyte becomes stuck to the holding pipette*
Probable cause: The oocyte is sticky, usually because some coronal cells remain attached.

Suggested remedy: The oocyte will usually fall off if the microscope stage control is used to move the holding pipette out of the injection drop of ICSI medium. Alternatively, the injection pipette may be used to knock the oocyte from the holding pipette.

8.7.3 Oocyte injection

8.7.3.1   *Problem – the spermatozoon cannot be seen in the injection pipette*
following orientation of the PB of the oocyte
Probable cause: The spermatozoon has drifted up or out of the injection pipette.

Suggested remedy: If the spermatozoon has drifted up into the injection pipette, it can often be recovered by turning the injector screw slowly clockwise. However, if no spermatozoon can be seen, then it will be necessary to prepare another for injection.

8.7.3.2   *Problem – the spermatozoon falls out of the injection pipette tip before*
injection of the oocyte
Probable cause: There is poor control of the spermatozoon within the injection pipette.

Suggested remedy: Blocking the opening of the injection pipette by pushing it up against the ZP will prevent the spermatozoon from falling out. However, this is only a temporary solution to the problem and appropriate steps should be taken to ensure that there is not a recurrence when attempting to inject other oocytes. Check that sufficient 'clean' medium is aspirated from the PVP drop before aspirating the spermatozoon, or, if necessary, replace the injection pipette. Do not be tempted to try and recover a spermatozoon that has fallen outside the injection pipette for the purpose of injection, as the resultant dilution of PVP will make control even more difficult.

8.7.3.3   *Problem – the ZP proves difficult to penetrate with the injection pipette*
Probable cause: The injection pipette is relatively blunt or the ZP is extremely elastic and tough.

Suggested remedy: If the injection pipette does not appear to be typically fine and sharp, then replace it rather than risk damage to the oocyte. If the ZP is truly tough and elastic, then a faster approach with the injection pipette will usually succeed in penetrating it.

8.7.3.4   *Problem – the oolemma fails to rupture following its aspiration into the*
injection pipette
Probable cause: The oolemma is unusually tough and elastic.

Suggested remedy: Attempt a few rapid jabbing movements of the injection pipette, taking great care not to hit the far side of the oolemma. If this still fails to cause the oolemma to rupture, rather than risk damaging the oocyte with a more aggressive approach advance the injection pipette two-thirds of the way into the ooplasm and deposit the spermatozoon. In this way, there is still some chance of a positive outcome.

8.7.3.5   *Problem – there is excessive aspiration of ooplasm following rupture of the oolemma and/or excessive outflow of medium following sperm deposition*
Probable cause: Either the injection pipette is partly blocked, or the oil/medium within it has become mixed with air bubbles, compromising hydraulic control.

Suggested remedy: Replace the injection pipette.

8.7.3.6   *Problem – the oocyte and/or ooplasm sticks to the injection pipette when withdrawing it following sperm deposition*
Probable cause: The ooplasm or injection pipette is unusually sticky.

Suggested remedy: Successive, short, rapid movements of the injection pipette while withdrawing it from the oocyte usually avoids this. However, this is only a temporary solution to the problem, and appropriate steps should be taken to ensure that there is not a recurrence when attempting to inject other oocytes. Essentially, the micropipette should be changed before proceeding with further injections.

8.7.3.7   *Problem – the oocytes appear shrunken following injection*
Probable cause: The oil overlay is not covering completely the drops of media, resulting in evaporation and increased osmolarity, or the oil is toxic.

Suggested remedy: Top up or replace the oil with a fresh batch.

9 Zona manipulation and embryo biopsy

'Zona drilling' was the term used originally to denote the technique of creating a hole in the ZP surrounding the oocyte (Gordon and Talansky, 1986). The first intuitive application of this procedure in human infertility was to provide a conduit via which spermatozoa could pass through the ZP (Cohen et al., 1988; Gordon et al., 1988). This approach to alleviating male-factor forms of infertility that were related to the inability of spermatozoa to bind to or penetrate the ZP was termed partial zona dissection (PZD). This involved physically cutting a hole or slit in the ZP using micropipettes. However, this approach was considered to be inefficient because it was suspected that partial or complete closure of the slit created might compromise sperm motility or even prevent access to the oocyte altogether. Therefore, the next logical step was to use ZD as a means of introducing spermatozoa directly into the PVS with the aid of a large microinjection pipette that could be passed through the hole thus created (Laws-King et al., 1987; Ng et al., 1988). This technique, originally termed 'microinjection sperm transfer' later became known as 'subzonal insemination'. With the introduction of very fine and sharp microinjection pipettes, ZD soon became unnecessary for the SUZI technique, as it became possible to pierce the ZP directly. Osmotic manipulation of the oocyte prior to SUZI was usually applied to enlarge the PVS, so as to avoid damage to the oolemma. Allegedly, precisely this type of inadvertent damage was responsible for the serendipitous development of the ICSI technique (Lanzendorf et al., 1988; Palermo et al., 1992). Consequently, ZD for the purposes of PZD and SUZI has become all but redundant due to the much greater efficiency of ICSI in procuring fertilization of the oocyte in male-factor infertility. Interestingly, it has been suggested that despite the use of fine and sharp injection pipettes, even ICSI might benefit from ZD, at least in those oocytes where the ZP proves difficult to penetrate (Abdelmassih et al., 2002).

ZD has also been applied to the embryo for a variety of purposes. One of these applications is known as 'assisted hatching' and relies upon the assumption that the blastocyst will 'hatch' more easily from the ZP if a hole or slit has been placed in it at an earlier stage of pre-implantation development. This technique was originally applied as a means of overcoming recurrent implantation failure, presumed to be due to a variety of factors, including those of excessive zona thickness and zona hardening (Cohen *et al.*, 1990). AH has not been applied universally, as it would appear that it is of benefit primarily only to those patients with a predisposition to producing poor-quality oocytes with unusually tough zonae. Another major application of ZD is in the PGD of embryos via blastomere biopsy. This technique was pioneered at around the same time as that of AH (Handyside *et al.*, 1990). A similar technique has been applied to mature oocytes to remove the PB as a source of material for PGD, but this is a less definitive test of the normality of any embryo that subsequently develops. Consequently, blastomere biopsy is the preferred approach in most centres that test embryos for sex-linked diseases and other genetic mutations. More recently, ZD has also been applied in the removal of fragments of cytoplasm from poor-quality embryos in an attempt to enhance their viability and implantation potential.

The method typically employed for ZD relies upon the use of acidified culture media, such as Dulbecco's, Earle's and Tyrode's, to 'burn' a hole in the ZP. Similarly, digestion of the ZP with enzymes such as chymotrypsin and pronase has also been utilized. Other measures to introduce a slit into the ZP have included the physical use of the micropipettes themselves. More sophisticated and more expensive methods have since been applied for the same purpose, including the use of contact and non-contact lasers. The choice of method is usually based upon cost considerations, since although the use of lasers is arguably quicker and easier, all of the different techniques employed for AH appear to yield comparable results (Balaban *et al.*, 2002). However, there have been concerns over the exposure of embryos to lasers in the past and, in some states and countries, AH and PGD are regulated strictly or even restricted completely. Nevertheless, in all likelihood, the twenty-first century will see increased and more widespread application of PGD for the identification of normal and viable pre-implantation embryos. In view of the evolution of the application of zona cutting and ZD, only those techniques currently in more widespread use will be discussed in this chapter. These are AH and blastomere biopsy.

9.1 ASSISTED HATCHING

Essentially, three different methods are typically utilized for the purpose of drilling a hole or cutting a slit into the ZP. These are ZD using acid Tyrode's, the use of holding and injection micropipettes for cutting a slit, and AH by laser. Lasers can be used to drill either holes or slits in the ZP and are easier and quicker to apply, although they are considerably more expensive to incorporate into an assisted conception programme. Interestingly, it has been suggested that partial AH or thinning of the ZP may produce better results than drilling a hole through it entirely (Mantoudis *et al.*, 2002). Embryos may be suitable for AH regardless of whether they result from IVF or ICSI and of whether they have been cryopreserved. Most often, four- to eight-cell embryos are selected for AH just prior to transfer to the uterus. However, with the advent of extended culture of pre-implantation embryos for blastocyst transfer, even blastocysts may be subjected to AH.

9.1.1 Patient selection

In view of the prevailing literature, which suggests that AH is of benefit only to certain groups of patients, it is desirable to utilize an objective set of selection criteria. This is helpful both in counselling those patients that arbitrarily request the technique and in identifying those that might actually benefit from it. Those criteria cited most commonly include the following:

- Patients that have experienced a failed implantation after the transfer of two or three good-quality embryos on two or more occasions, for no obvious reason.
- Patients that have an unusually thick ZP (greater than 15 μm) as measured with a graticule under the inverted microscope.
- Patients that have a high FSH level (greater than 14 mIU/ml) prior to ovarian stimulation.
- Patients over the age of 38 years.

It should be apparent that these criteria relate mostly to oocyte quality, either directly or indirectly. It is also important to appreciate that any single factor is not necessarily an absolute indication for AH. Therefore, the number of criteria that a patient meets is probably the best way to identify those most likely to benefit from AH.

9.1.2 Zona drilling with acid Tyrode's

Acid Tyrode's (pH 2.3–2.5) may be prepared in-house or obtained commercially (see Table 2.13). Likewise, micropipettes for ZD may be forged in the laboratory or purchased from a number of different manufacturers (see Table 2.10). Alternatively, a very basic but usable drilling pipette may be fashioned easily from an ICSI pipette simply by breaking off its tip with a holding pipette while observing the diameter of the point of breakage under high magnification on an inverted microscope. The most important requirement for a pipette to be used for ZD is that it should be fire-polished to an inner diameter of around 5–10 μm, which is much smaller than that of a holding pipette. The reason for this is that the flow of acid Tyrode's must be controlled precisely. This is necessary to avoid potential damage to any blastomeres that lie within the immediate vicinity of the point of rupture of the ZP. If the internal diameter of the drilling pipette is too large, then the flow of acid Tyrode's is controlled less easily. Essentially, the procedure is relatively simple, as follows:

1 Prepare a microinjection dish containing 50 μl droplets of Hepes-buffered culture medium, one for priming the holding pipette and one for each embryo to be subjected to AH. The dish must also contain a large droplet (100–200 μl) of acid Tyrode's. The droplets must be overlaid with light paraffin oil and should be incubated at 37 °C before use. Mount a holding pipette to one side of the micromanipulation system and a drilling pipette to the other.

2 Place the microinjection dish on to the heated stage of the inverted microscope, and prime the holding pipette with Hepes-buffered culture medium. Back-fill the drilling pipette with acid Tyrode's from the large droplet using negative pressure. Ensure that sufficient acid Tyrode's is aspirated, as it is annoying to have to interrupt the procedure in order to refill the drilling pipette. This should take only 30 seconds to one minute. Remember to reverse the negative pressure or equalize the pressure inside the drilling pipette with that of atmospheric pressure once the acid Tyrode's has been loaded.

3 Place the embryos for AH into the microinjection dish, one per droplet of Hepes-buffered culture medium.

4 Using the holding pipette, orientate the embryo so that the point of contact between the drilling pipette and ZP will be between adjacent blastomeres (see Figure 9.1). This is an important step to avoid blastomere damage immediately following rupture of the ZP.

5 Advance the drilling pipette so that it lies firmly against the opposing ZP and slowly release the acid Tyrode's solution under positive pressure until a breach is formed in the ZP (see Figure 9.1). It is important to monitor this process very closely, as initially it will seem as if the acid Tyrode's is having no effect, but suddenly the ZP will be seen to 'pop'. This is because some medium may be aspirated into the drilling pipette, diluting the initial flow of acid Tyrode's. However, once the ZP begins to thin, rupture follows within seconds.

Figure 9.1 The embryo is positioned on to the holding pipette such that the drilling pipette containing acid Tyrode's can be pushed up against the ZP at a point between two adjacent blastomeres. (a) Acid Tyrode's is expelled slowly from the drilling pipette adjacent to the ZP. (b) The drilling pipette is pushed up against the ZP while expelling acid Tyrode's. (c) The ZP is eventually breached.

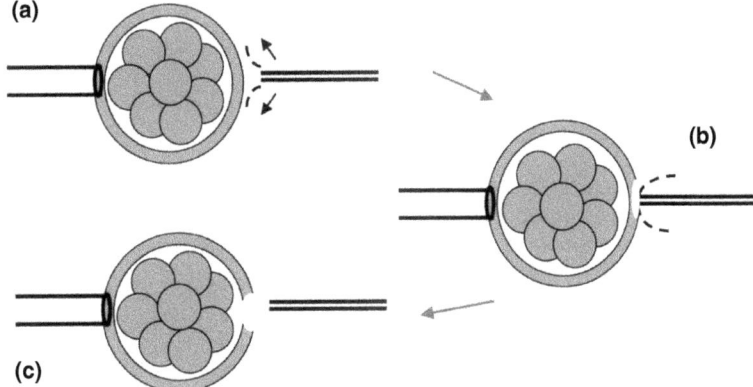

6   The drilling pipette must be withdrawn immediately from the ZP and the flow of acid Tyrode's ceased once the ZP has been ruptured, otherwise damage to the nearest blastomeres may result.

7   Immediately remove the embryo from the droplet where the AH has been performed and wash it through bicarbonate-buffered culture medium before proceeding to drill the next embryo.

Transfer of the embryos that have undergone AH may be performed immediately once the procedure is completed.

9.1.3   Zona dissection with micropipettes

This procedure, also known as zona tearing, involves the use of micropipettes to pierce the ZP while holding the embryo firmly on to a holding pipette, as follows:

1   Prepare a microinjection dish containing 50 µl droplets of Hepes-buffered culture medium, one for priming the holding pipette and one for each embryo to be subjected to ZD. The droplets must be overlaid with light paraffin oil and should be incubated at 37 °C before use. Mount a holding pipette to one side of the micromanipulation system and an injection pipette to the other.

2   Place the embryos for ZD into the microinjection dish, one per droplet of Hepes-buffered culture medium, and place the microinjection dish on to the heated stage of the inverted microscope. Prime the holding pipette with Hepes-buffered culture medium.

3   Using the holding pipette, orientate the embryo so that there is a clear area of PVS between the ZP and nearby blastomeres at one or other pole, so as to avoid blastomere damage during insertion of the injection pipette.

Figure 9.2 (a) The embryo is aligned on the holding pipette such that there is sufficient PVS between the blastomeres and the ZP at one pole. (b) The injection pipette is pushed through the ZP at one point and out again at another point, taking care to avoid any blastomeres. (c) The embryo is pushed along to a thicker section of the injection pipette, against which the holding pipette can be rubbed in order to tear a slit in the zona pellucida. (d) The ZP is eventually breached.

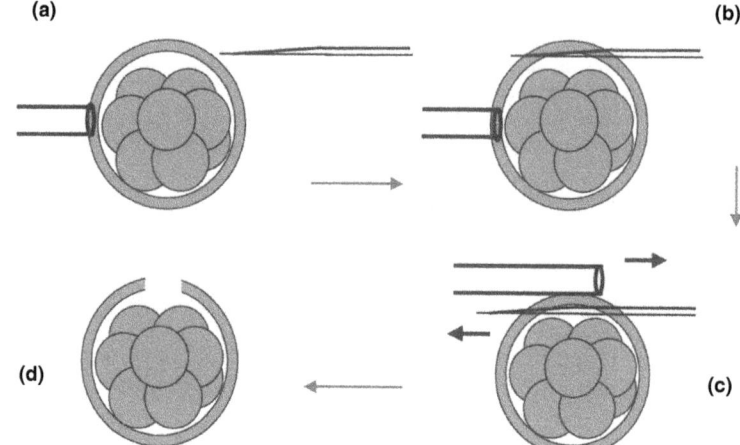

4 Pass the injection pipette through the ZP on one side of the embryo and again through the ZP on the opposing side of the embryo (see Figure 9.2b).

5 Using the holding pipette, move the embryo along the injection pipette to where it is wider and stronger, and rub the ZP between the injection and holding pipettes until it tears (see Figure 9.2).

6 Using the holding pipette, release the embryo from the injection pipette and orientate the embryo on to the holding pipette so that the injection pipette can be reinserted through the ZP at a different site, but exiting the embryo at one end of the first tear.

7 Repeat step 5 in order to create a fresh tear that will join up with the original one, so forming a V-shaped flap of zona.

Steps 6 and 7 are not obligatory for AH, but they are necessary to create a large enough hole for blastomere biopsy. Transfer of the embryos that have undergone ZD may be performed immediately once the procedure is completed and the embryos have been washed through bicarbonate-buffered culture medium.

9.1.4 Zona drilling by laser

Both contact and non-contact lasers may be used to puncture the ZP. There are a number of different systems available, some of which work in the ultraviolet spectrum and others of which work in the infrared spectrum (see Table 9.1). Non-contact lasers, especially those operating within the infrared spectrum, are considered to be safer as their potential for damaging surrounding tissue is far less.

The laser can be applied at a single point to create a hole or at several points adjacent to each other along the ZP to create a slit (see Figure 9.3). The size of the hole created is dependent upon the power of the laser and

Table 9.1 *Laser systems for ZD, AH and embryo biopsy*

Model	Supplier	Type	Wavelength
Fertilase	MTM Medical Technologies Montreux	Non-contact	Infrared
Saturn	Research Instruments Ltd	Non-contact	Infrared
ZLTS	Cell Robotics Inc	Non-contact	Infrared
Zona knife	SL Microtest GmbH	Non-contact	Infrared

Figure 9.3 A controlled short burst of a laser is fired at the ZP to burn a furrow through part of its circumference.

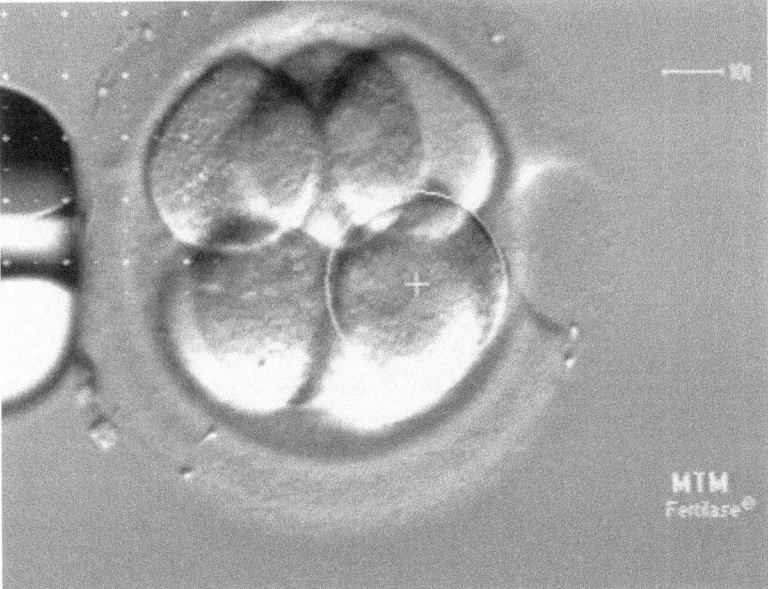

its firing duration and can be controlled precisely. With most systems, all that is usually required is to line up the part of the ZP to be drilled and fire the laser one or more times until a breach has been made. Naturally, the most important aspect of this technique is that once the laser has been fired, operator control is taken over by the machine. Therefore, it is crucial that the correct settings have been made so as to avoid creating too large a hole, which might otherwise damage the oocyte or blastomeres beneath the ZP. For this reason, it is often advisable to drill successive small holes to create a path through the ZP, rather than attempt to breach it with a single shot.

9.2 BLASTOMERE BIOPSY

The biopsy of blastomeres is usually performed on eight-cell embryos, since one or two blastomeres may be removed at this stage without

Table 9.2 *Commercial sources of calcium-/magnesium-free medium used for blastomere biopsy*

Medium	Supplier	Product no.
EM™-10	Vitrolife Fertility Systems	10020
QAH (Ca/Mg free)	SAGE BioPharma	ART-4100

compromising the viability of the embryo. Ideally, the embryo should have at least seven blastomeres if two are to be removed. Two blastomeres are often biopsied as a means of controlling for misdiagnosis. In this respect, it is advisable that patients requiring PGD have their oocytes totally denuded of cumulus cells and inseminated by ICSI rather than by routine IVF. This ensures that there are no supernumerary cells present that might otherwise interfere with the diagnosis, particularly if the nested PCR is to be used for PGD. Biopsy at this relatively early stage of pre-implantation development also allows sufficient time for the PGD to be made before ET. More recently, with the advent of extended culture of pre-implantation embryos for ET at the expanded blastocyst stage, early blastocysts have also been biopsied.

Biopsy is performed most easily using medium devoid of divalent cations (calcium- and magnesium-free; Dumoulin *et al.*, 1998). This media can either be prepared in-house or obtained commercially (see Table 9.2).

The rationale for the use of medium devoid of calcium and magnesium ions is that maintenance of cell–cell connections depends upon the presence of these ions. Therefore, blastomeres are held together less tightly in their absence, so facilitating the biopsy procedure. Micropipettes for blastomere biopsy may be forged in the laboratory or purchased from a number of different manufacturers (see Table 2.10). These should have an internal diameter of 40–50 μm. Ideally, the micromanipulation system should be fitted with a double tool holder so that the biopsy pipette may be interchanged rapidly and accurately with the drilling pipette. Otherwise, it is necessary to adopt the somewhat cumbersome procedure of replacing one pipette with another midway through the biopsy. Clearly, a double tool holder is not required if a laser system is employed for ZD.

9.2.1 Biopsy method

Naturally, blastomere biopsy relies upon first drilling a hole through the ZP that is large enough through which to introduce a biopsy pipette if necessary. Hence, either acid Tyrode's or a laser can be used for this purpose

Figure 9.4 The Petri dish used for blastomere biopsy contains droplets of Hepes-buffered media, Ca^{2+}-/Mg^{2+}-free media and acid Tyrode's.

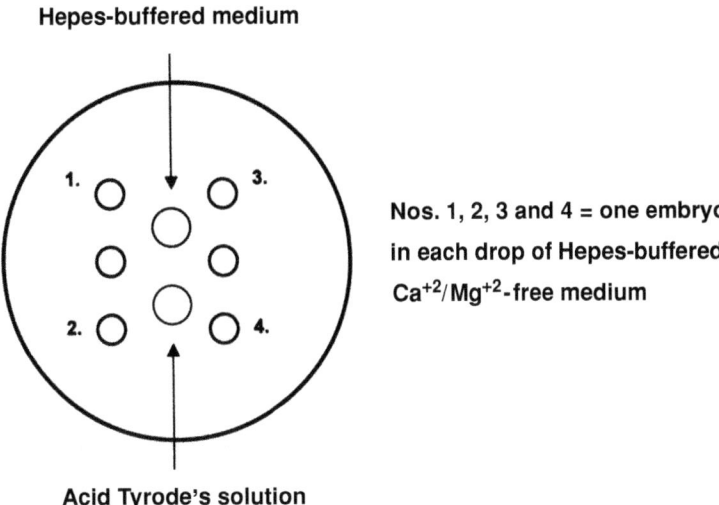

Hepes-buffered medium

Nos. 1, 2, 3 and 4 = one embryo in each drop of Hepes-buffered Ca^{+2}/Mg^{+2}-free medium

Acid Tyrode's solution

(see the relevant sections above). It is not very practical to attempt to tear a hole by mechanical means using an injection pipette. Besides, ideally, the hole created should not be too large, otherwise there is more opportunity for a number of blastomeres to be dragged outside the ZP along with the blastomere being biopsied. Consequently, the optimal size hole is one that is only just large enough through which to pass the biopsy pipette. If using acid Tyrode's for ZD during the biopsy procedure, then there are some extra steps to be followed, compared with the use of a laser. The procedure described below is for blastomere biopsy using acid Tyrode's:

1. Prepare a microinjection dish containing 10–20 µl droplets of Hepes-buffered Ca^{2+}/Mg^{2+}-free culture medium, one for each embryo to be subjected to biopsy, and a large droplet (20–50 µl) of acid Tyrode's (see Figure 9.4). The dish must also contain a large droplet (20–50 µl) of Hepes-buffered culture medium for priming the holding and biopsy pipettes (see Figure 9.4). All droplets must be overlaid with light paraffin oil and should be incubated at 37 °C before use.

2. Mount a holding pipette to one side of the micromanipulation system and mount drilling and biopsy pipettes to the other, using a double tool holder. The drilling and biopsy pipettes must be placed in the same plane, such that either can be visualized simply by moving one or the other into position. If a double tool holder is not available, then it will be necessary to mount the drilling pipette alone at this stage.

3. Place the microinjection dish for ZD on to the heated stage of the inverted microscope and prime the holding and biopsy pipettes with Hepes-buffered culture medium. Backfill the drilling pipette with acid Tyrode's from the

Figure 9.5 (a) The biopsy pipette is passed through the hole previously drilled through the ZP, and a blastomere is aspirated into it slowly and gently.

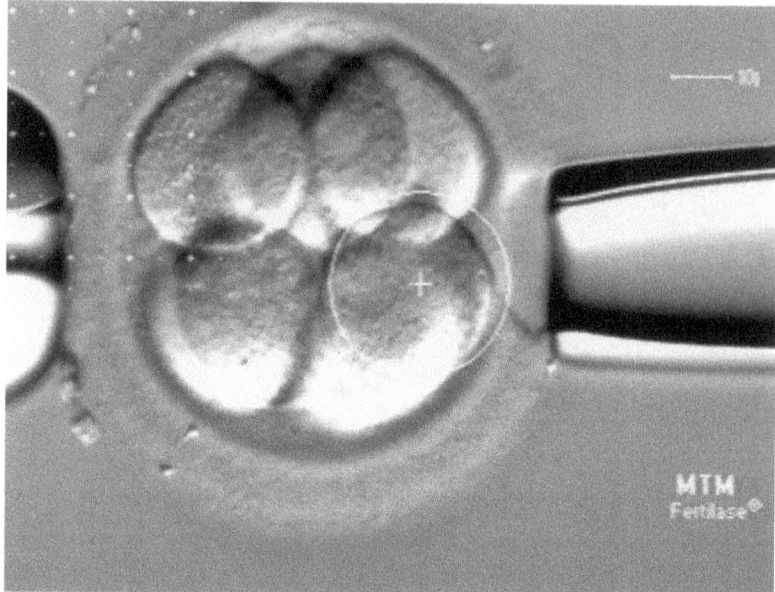

Figure 9.5 (b) The biopsied blastomere is expelled on to the bottom of the biopsy dish so that it can be collected and processed for PGD.

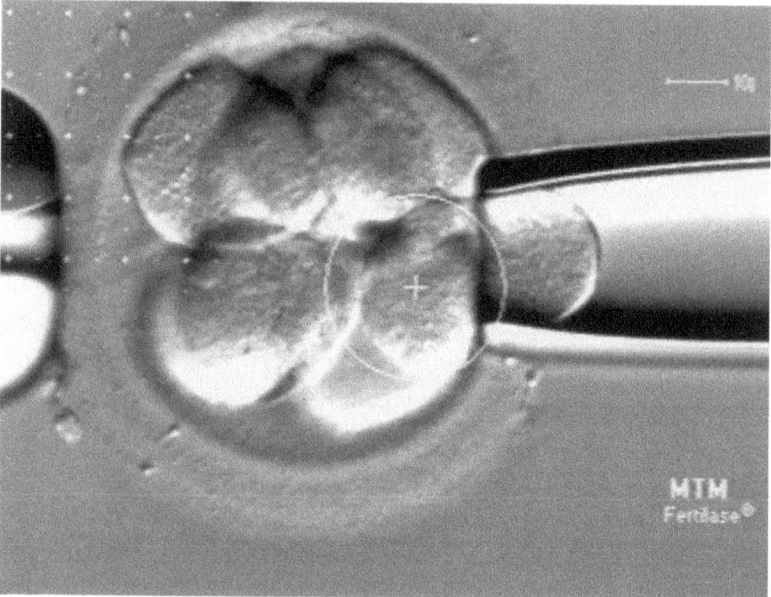

large droplet using negative pressure (as described in section 9.1.2). However, if using a double tool holder, take care to ensure that the biopsy pipette does not enter the droplet of acid Tyrode's, otherwise damage to the blastomeres may occur during the procedure.

4 Place the embryo for ZD into a droplet of Ca^{2+}-/Mg^{2+}-free Hepes-buffered culture medium in the microinjection dish. It is important to minimize the exposure of embryos to Ca^{2+}-/Mg^{2+}-free media; therefore, if more than one embryo is to be biopsied, then they should be subjected to this one at a time.

5 Using the holding pipette, orientate the embryo so that the point of contact between the drilling pipette and the ZP will be between adjacent blastomeres, one or both of which should appear normal (i.e. containing just a single nucleus).

6 Advance the drilling pipette and slowly release acid Tyrode's solution until a breach is formed in the ZP (as described in section 9.1.2).

7 Move the drilling pipette out of the field of view and replace it with the biopsy pipette, placing it near to the blastomere to be aspirated (both blastomere and pipette should be confocal at their equatorial planes).

8 Pass the biopsy pipette through the previously drilled hole in order to gain access to the blastomere to be aspirated. Using gentle aspiration, slowly draw the blastomere into the biopsy pipette (see Figure 9.5). This step should not be rushed and may take several minutes, depending upon the extent to which the embryo has become compacted. It is important to reduce the negative pressure exerted upon the biopsy pipette once the blastomere appears to become detached from its neighbours, so as to avoid its loss along the pipette.

9 Deposit the biopsied blastomere on to the bottom of the droplet so that it may be easily located, washed through into bicarbonate-buffered culture medium, and collected for PGD (see Figure 9.6).

10 Repeat the biopsy procedure for another blastomere if desired, or repeat the procedure on another embryo. Once each embryo has been biopsied, it should be immediately washed through into bicarbonate-buffered culture medium and incubated until the result of the PGD is known.

9.3 TROUBLESHOOTING

9.3.1 Assisted hatching

9.3.1.1 *Problem – backfilling the drilling pipette with acid Tyrode's is extremely slow or impossible*

Probable cause: There may be a block in the pipette or the injector line, or the drilling pipette may be too narrow.

Suggested remedy: Replace the drilling pipette with another one, and check the injector line while doing so. Ensure that the inner diameter of the drilling pipette used is not too narrow.

9.3.1.2   *Problem – the acid Tyrode's appears to have no effect on the ZP*
Probable cause: The acid Tyrode's may have been diluted to below its work-ing concentration due to the inadvertent influx of medium from the droplet containing the embryo.

Suggested remedy: Refill the drilling pipette with more acid Tyrode's, en-suring that the negative pressure exerted during the process has been reversed. If using an air injector, the simplest way to achieve this is to equalize the pressure inside the pipette with that of atmospheric pressure, by temporarily opening the closed line. If using an oil injector, opening the line is not a practical option, so instead it is necessary to exert an equal amount of positive pressure to stabilize the flow of acid Tyrode's. The acid Tyrode's is more efficient if it is at $37\,^{\circ}\mathrm{C}$, and rubbing the drilling pipette against the ZP while releasing the stream of acid may also help to rupture it.

9.3.1.3   *Problem – the embryo rolls off the holding pipette while attempting to pierce the ZP with an injection pipette*
Probable cause: This is more likely to happen if the holding pipette has a fairly narrow inner diameter, there being insufficient resistance to the shearing force applied while pushing the injection pipette against the ZP.

Suggested remedy: Use a holding pipette with a larger outside diameter. Alternatively, the shearing action of the injection pipette can be countered by performing the zona-tearing procedure with the embryo supported on the bottom of the droplet. This will present two opposing forces to the injection pipette: the holding pipette and the base of the microinjection dish.

9.3.1.4   *Problem – rubbing the ZP between the injection and holding pipettes fails to tear it*
Probable cause: The ZP may be particularly tough and elastic, and the contact between the pipettes may not be sufficient to tear the ZP.

Suggested remedy: Check that the embryo moves in response to the rubbing of the ZP between the pipettes to confirm that the contact between them is good. If the ZP still fails to rupture following further rubbing between the pipettes, move the embryo further along the injection pipette and try again. By doing this, a tear will eventually be effected since the increase in the diameter of the injection pipette as the embryo is moved along it causes the ZP to stretch and thereby become thinner.

9.3.2 Blastomere biopsy

9.3.2.1 *Problem – it is not possible to pass the biopsy pipette through the ZP following ZD*
Probable cause: The ZP has not been breached properly during ZD. Occasionally, it may appear that the ZD procedure has been successful, but in fact the ZP remains partly intact.

Suggested remedy: Replace the biopsy pipette with the drilling pipette and continue the ZD procedure until certain that the ZP has been ruptured. Since the ZP is probably thinned out by the initial attempt at ZD, it is necessary to expel the acid Tyrode's with extra care.

9.3.2.2 *Problem – when the drilling pipette is replaced with the biopsy pipette on the double tool holder, the biopsy pipette cannot be seen*
Probable cause: The drilling and biopsy pipettes are not in the same focal plane. This can be checked by observing that they touch the oil in the microinjection dish at the same time when lowered into it.

Suggested remedy: Adjust the biopsy pipette relative to the drilling pipette, such that both lie in the same focal plane.

9.3.2.3 *Problem – blastomeres remain attached to that being aspirated, and will exit the hole in the ZP if the procedure is continued*
Probable cause: The embryo being biopsied is relatively well compacted.

Suggested remedy: Check that the biopsy is being performed using Ca^{2+}-/Mg^{2+}-free culture medium. Aspirate the blastomere to be biopsied part of the way into the biopsy pipette and gently move the pipette up and down past the edges of the hole in the ZP. This will exert an additional shearing force between the aspirated blastomere and those remaining within the ZP. This approach should result in successful biopsy of the aspirated blastomere, although the procedure may take longer than usual.

9.3.2.4 *Problem – the embryo becomes dislodged from the holding pipette while attempting to aspirate a blastomere, and the hole in the ZP can no longer be seen*
Probable cause: Insufficient negative pressure may have been applied to the holding pipette, and the embryo may be particularly well compacted.

Suggested remedy: If the original hole in the ZP can no longer be seen, it will first be necessary to repeat the ZD procedure in order to create another hole. Try to identify a blastomere that appears attached more loosely to its neighbours than the others, and apply the ZD adjacent to it. Ensure that the embryo is held tightly to the holding pipette before aspirating this blastomere following ZD.

9.3.2.5   Problem – the biopsied blastomere lyses

Probable cause: The blastomere may have been damaged during the biopsy procedure, or it may be inherently fragile.

Suggested remedy: If the blastomere that has been biopsied lyses, then it will be extremely difficult, if not impossible, to identify it. Therefore, it will be necessary to biopsy another blastomere from the embryo. However this time, extra care should be taken to avoid subjecting the blastomere to excessive shearing forces during aspiration.

10 Microtool manufacture

Glass micropipettes are precisely constructed microtools forming the basis of a variety of investigative and clinically relevant techniques. They are used extensively in basic cellular research as channels into cells. Through these channels, substances can be injected or cellular contents extracted.

The fact that extremely high-quality microtools are available commercially should not necessarily discourage users from investigating the viability of making their own. The advantages are that the tools can be made on demand to one's own specifications, which can be far cheaper in the long run. In the early days of commercially available microtools, there were problems with continuity of supply and issues over quality. Nowadays, this does not seem to be such a problem (the market is becoming increasingly competitive), but lines of supply might still be intermittent in some parts of the world. Additionally, some more experienced and senior embryologists tend to consider microtool-making as a sort of rite of passage to which every newcomer to microinjection must be subjected. Certainly, while new techniques in micromanipulation continue to develop, new microtools need to be developed alongside, and manufacturers will usually start to mass-produce microtools only once it becomes clear that there is enough demand.

Whatever the reason for considering tool-making, it is still distinctly possible that embryologists will find themselves faced with such a task. While the techniques involved are not the easiest to master (many hours of practice may be necessary), they are not impossible if they are developed slowly and carefully, as outlined below. Remember that once the basic skills are mastered, many different sizes and shapes of microtool should be attainable.

Micropipettes are formed by heating glass capillary tubing to its softening point and then drawing it down to form a cone with an open-tip diameter ranging from a relatively large 50 μm to ultrafine tips of less

Figure 10.1 The typical
dimensions of an injection
pipette.

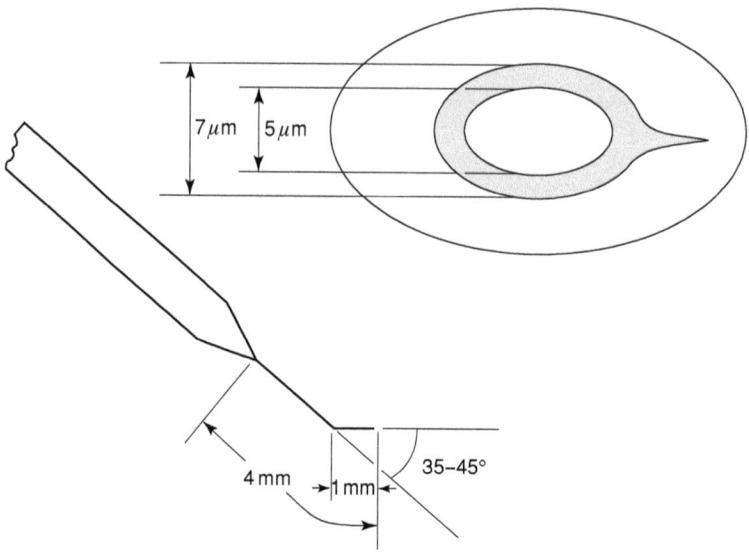

than 0.02 µm. The majority of microinjection techniques today utilize tip
diameters typically between 0.7 and 7 µm.

10.1 THE ICSI PIPETTE

While there is some difference of opinion as to what the ideal ICSI pipette
should look like (see Figure 10.1), certain characteristics seem to be essential:

- The inner diameter of the pipette tip should be 4–5 µm. Using thin-walled
  glass capillary tubes, this means that the outer diameter will be around
  7 µm. This is large enough to allow sperm to pass yet not so large as to
  allow the sperm to turn around inside the pipette or the pipette to damage
  irreparably the injected oocyte. The narrower the opening of the injection
  pipette tip, the greater the pressure that is required to push liquid out of
  the end.
- The 5 µm inner diameter/7 µm outer diameter should be consistent from
  the tip to around 4 mm along its length.
- There should be in the region of 5 mm of drawn pipette.
- The pipette should have a bend of between 35° and 45°. The bend should
  be placed about 1 mm from the tip.
- The pipette should be bevelled to an angle of about 35°.
- The holding pipette should be fashioned to hold an oocyte by gentle suction, preventing it from moving during the injection procedure but not
  damaging it.

Figure 10.2 The typical
dimensions of a holding pipette.

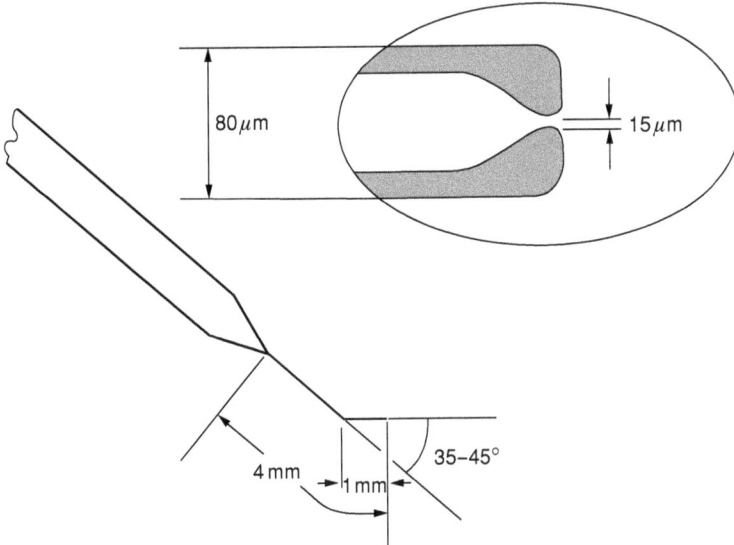

- The outer diameter should be about 80 μm with an inner diameter of
  15 μm once it is fire-polished (see Figure 10.2). This allows the oocyte to
  be held gently without the risk of it being sucked into the pipette.
- As with the injection pipette, the holding pipette should be bent to an
  angle of between 35° and 45°, the bend being placed about 1 mm from
  the tip.

10.2 HISTORICAL PERSPECTIVE

The simplicity of a piece of glass tubing belies the complexity of technique
required to produce, accurately and reproducibly, the micropipette characteristics that a researcher desires. Micropipettes were originally formed
manually by heating tubing over a flame and drawing it apart very rapidly.
While this technique yielded pipettes with very small-tip outer diameters,
it was difficult to make the tips reproducibly and sufficiently short and
straight to be useful. Timing is crucial in pulling micropipettes, and for
most humans it was not possible to achieve the requisite timing.

The breadth of functionality obtained from glass tubing comes from its
sensitivity to small changes in the heating and drawing process. Formation
of micropipettes is a function of the viscosity and the wall thickness of
the glass capillary. Viscosity is in turn dependent upon glass composition
and the temperature profile used to melt the glass. Given the number of
different pipette shapes required to satisfy the needs of the microinjection
specialist, it is important to have a great deal of control over the factors
that affect pipette formation.

Machines entered the micropipette pulling scene circa 1930. Early micropipette pullers provided features that have been incorporated in some form in all later instruments for pulling micropipettes. Those features include a heat source, a mechanical assembly to provide a means of support for the glass throughout the pulling process, an adjustable source of tension for pulling the micropipette, a sensing system used to detect the state of the glass, and a means for cooling the glass prior to tip formation.

Additional requirements for micropipettes dictate that the features be integrated in such a way as to provide an instrument capable of reproducibly pulling pipettes with a controllable configuration (shape and tip size). Controlled configuration means that the user is given the flexibility of producing pipettes with adjustable characteristics. Reproducibility means that there is a measure of dimensional stability between consecutive pulls.

10.3 CURRENT PIPETTE-PULLING TECHNOLOGY

Given the number of micropipette pullers on the market today, deciding which puller to purchase can be daunting. Selection requires choosing from vertical versus horizontal pullers; single-sided versus double-sided pullers; simplistic versus sophisticated; cheap versus expensive. The most basic pullers available on the market today are the vertical pullers. While they tend to be more simplistic and cheaper than the horizontal pullers available, their reliance on passive cooling of the glass naturally confers a steeper taper to the pipette geometry than a pipette produced with an actively cooled horizontal puller. This is quite the opposite of what is required for microinjection applications. Additionally, most of the technological advances in pipette pulling have been due to developments of horizontal pullers rather than vertical pullers. Except for the most undemanding of applications, vertical pullers have been superseded by horizontal pullers.

The current state-of-the-art puller for fabricating microinjection needles is Sutter Instrument Company's P-97 horizontal puller fitted with a box-shaped platinum heating element (see Figure 10.3). This microprocessor-controlled puller allows the user to store a multiple number of programs designed specifically to pull different types of pipette morphologies. The puller utilizes a patented velocity-sensing system for detecting the state of the glass. This scheme has resulted in a greater degree of puller reproducibility compared with pullers utilizing other detection methods. The instrument also features a solid-state air-delivery system, to provide for cooling of the glass, and an environmental chamber, to minimize the affects of humidity variation on the pulling process. The active cooling technique allows the user to shape pipettes in ways that are not possible with passively cooled systems.

Figure 10.3 The Sutter
Instrument Company P-97
horizontal puller is fitted with a
box-shaped platinum heating
element.

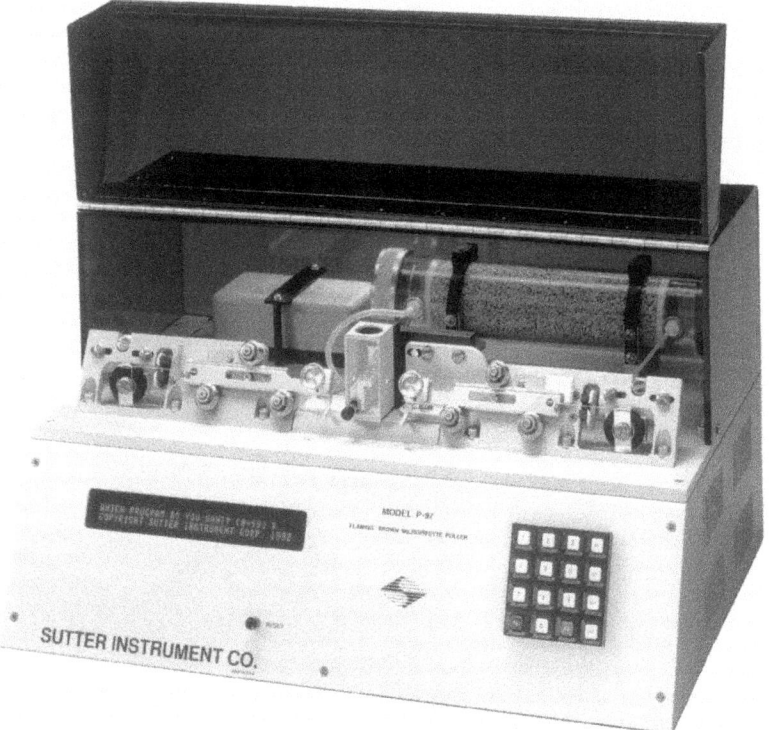

A typical program for the P-97 involves a dataset consisting of heat, velocity, pull, time and pressure. The heat reflects the heating current to the filament. The velocity determines the state of the glass, and serves as the system trip (which signals the pulling). The pull is the value of a hard pull activated once the velocity is reached. The time is the duration of the active cooling puff, which rapidly cools the glass. The pressure is the pressure of the cooling puff. Adjusting any one of these parameters can affect the morphology of the pipette. Generally speaking, the higher the heat, pull and velocity, the longer the pipette, the smaller the tip, and the more gradual the taper. The higher the time and pressure, the shorter the pipette and the more rapid the taper. For most microinjection applications, a heat value close to the calibration heat value is sufficient. Relatively modest pull values and high velocity values help to stretch out the glass into the long but gradual taper required for ICSI microtools.

Because of the number of degrees of programming freedom available with the Sutter puller, it can take a fair bit of time to derive a program suitable for pulling the pipette necessary for a specific application. Direct contact with the company can help reduce this burden. This brings up

Figure 10.4 The Narishige EG-400 microgrinder is fitted with a multispeed motor, a whetstone wheel, a micromanipulator, a light source, a monocular microscope, and a water-drip mechanism.

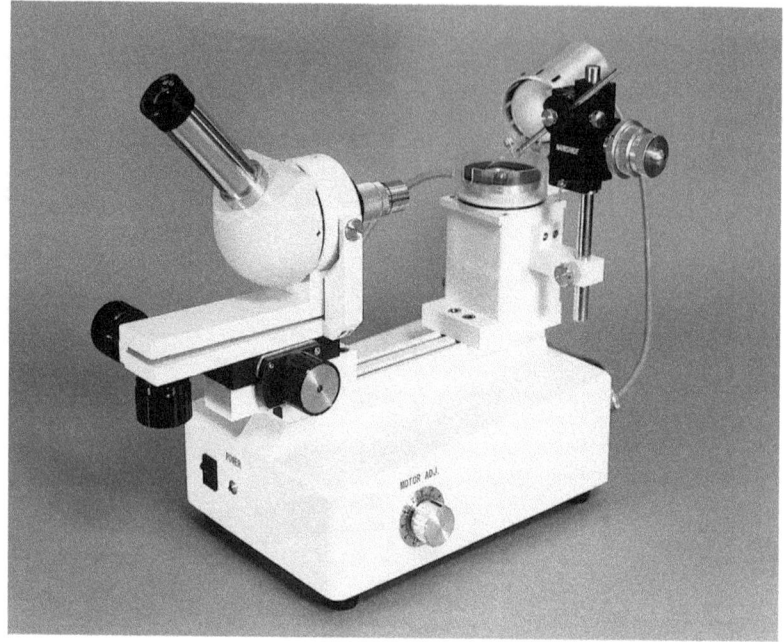

a final point in considering which pipette puller to purchase, and indeed should be a consideration for any laboratory equipment purchased. That is the often underrated but certainly important factor of the degree of technical support provided by the instrument manufacturer. This is perhaps best determined by discussing with peers who have experience with various manufacturers.

10.4 BEVELLING

Once a needle of the appropriate dimensions has been attained, the next stage in injection pipette preparation is that of grinding the pipette tip to produce a bevelled edge – rather like that of a hypodermic needle. This will enhance the ease with which the pipette can be pushed through the ZP and oolemma during the ICSI process.

The Narishige EG-400 and the Sutter BV-10 are both fitted with a multispeed motor driving a whetstone wheel, a micromanipulator, allowing the pipette tip to be placed on the whetstone at any angle, a light source, a microscope for visualizing the pipette tip, and a mechanism for keeping the grinding surface wet (see Figures 10.4 and 10.5). Of these two instruments, the Sutter is capable of a greater degree of grinding precision, having a grinding surface that is optically flat to an extremely high tolerance and a wobble-free motor drive. More details of bevelling techniques can be found in Brown and Flaming (1974).

Figure 10.5 The Sutter BV-10
grinder.

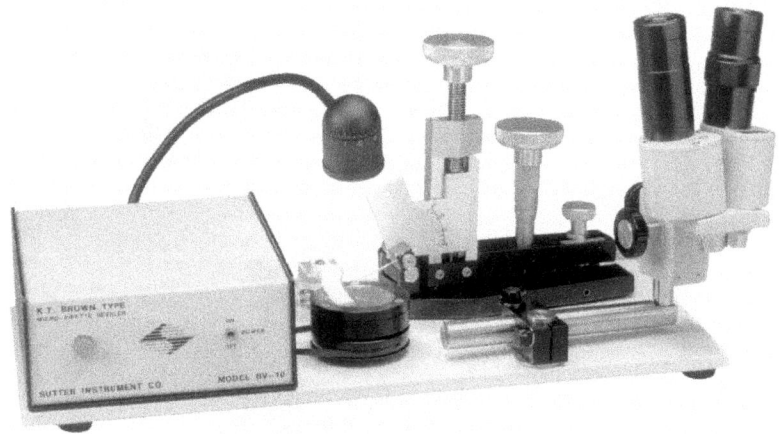

The recommended angle of bevel is approximately 35° for an ICSI
pipette. This can be set precisely by reading off the required angle on the
pipette holder on the manipulator before lowering the pipette on to the
grinding wheel. The pipette should be lowered on to the whetstone until
the tip just touches the surface and the pipette shank bends very slightly.

The pipette should usually be left in contact with the grinding surface
for approximately three minutes with the wheel speed set on maximum,
although these values may vary depending on the hardness of the glass
and the size of the unground tip. It will be necessary – as with pipette
pulling – to experiment with different settings to obtain the required result.
Once the grinding process is complete, place a pen mark on the upper face
of the blunt end of the pipette before removing it from the grinder. This
will help with the correct orientation when putting the pipette in the
microforge for subsequent processing.

During the grinding process, the whetstone should be humidified constantly with a slow water drip. This keeps the inside of the pipette free from
glass dust, as capillary action constantly washes water into and out of the
opening.

It is not necessary to grind the tip of the holding pipette.

10.5 THE MICROFORGE

10.5.1 Setting up

A microforge is required for the final steps in pipette preparation, including
breaking and fire-polishing the holding pipette, putting a spike on the injection pipette, and bending both. The Narishige microforges are supplied

Figure 10.6 The Narishige
microforge model MF-900.

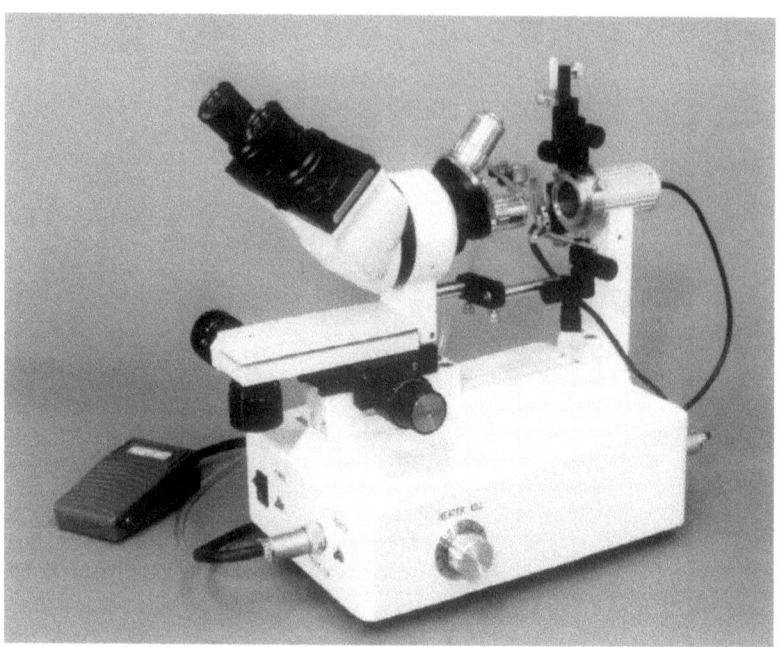

with $10\times$ eyepieces and $4\times$ and $10\times$ objective lenses. As an option, it is possible to order two $15\times$ eyepieces and one $33\times$ long-working-distance objective (Narishige code MF-OPT), giving a total magnification of $495\times$. There were two versions of the now-discontinued MF-90 microforge: the later one had the heating element mounted on a bar attached to the main body of the forge, and the older version had the heater attached directly to the objective lens. In both cases, the instrument was designed to allow the heater to remain in the field of view wherever the microscope was moved in relation to the pipette. The latest model from Narishige, the MF-900 (see Figure 10.6), retains this feature. Whichever microforge model is used, the heater block is normally adjusted so that the heating element enters the field of view horizontally, from the left. This is accomplished by experimenting with the heater block in different positions, and by adjusting the micromanipulator to which the heater block is attached. The orientation of the pipette holder can be adjusted by rotating it around the light source so that the tip enters the microscope field of view from above (see Figure 10.7) or from the right (see Figure 10.8). This gives the orientations needed for all forging processes.

There are two sets of controls for moving the pipette in relation to the microscope/heater assembly. One set moves the pipette itself and is found on top of the light source. The other set moves the microscope/heater assembly in relation to the pipette (giving the impression that the pipette is being moved when viewed through the microscope) and is found below

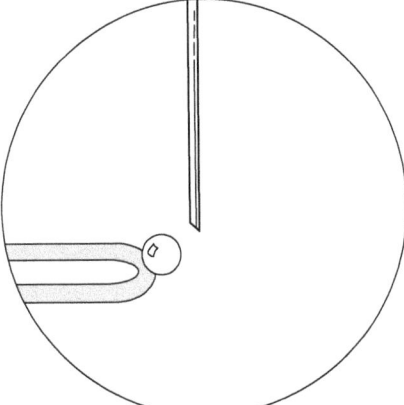

Figure 10.7 The pipette holder of the Narishige microforge has been orientated such that the pipette tip enters the field of view of the microscope from above.

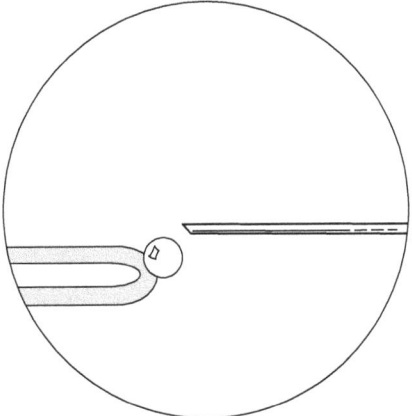

Figure 10.8 The pipette holder of the Narishige microforge has been orientated such that the pipette tip enters the field of view of the microscope from the right.

the eyepieces. It is a matter of personal preference which controls are used, but in general the adjustment on the pipette holder should be used initially to bring the pipette tip into the field of view, while the second set on the microscope should be used for fine adjustments while forging.

Before pipette processing can begin, it is necessary to place a small bead of glass on top of the heater element. This is then used to ensure that the element itself never comes into direct contact with the pipette, giving a greater degree of control over forging operations. With the heater control adjusted so that the element glows dull red, a pipette is lowered on to the hot element (see Figure 10.9). As the glass melts, the pipette should be lowered continuously until a bead of approximately 20–30 μm diameter has formed. Switch off the heat, break the pipette close to the bead with a pair of fine forceps, withdraw the broken pipette and discard it, and finally heat the bead gently until the jagged portion is absorbed (see Figure 10.10). The microforge is now ready to process holding and injection pipettes.

Figure 10.9 Lowering a pipette on to the hot element of the microforge melts the glass to form a glass bead.

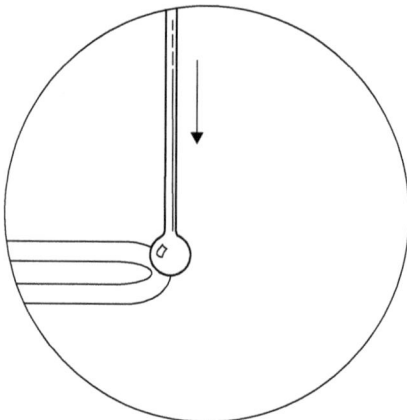

Figure 10.10 The glass bead on the heating element of the microforge is heated gently until the jagged portion is absorbed.

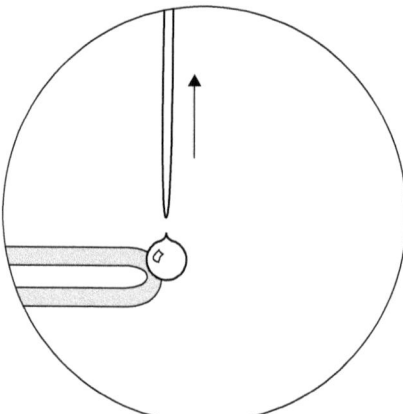

10.5.2 The holding pipette

The pipette should be placed in the holder and the holder rotated around the light source so that the pipette tip enters the field of view from the right:

- With the heat off, gently lower the pipette on to the glass bead at a point where the outer diameter of the pipette is approximately 80 µm (see Figure 10.11).
- Turn down the heat control to a minimum.
- Press and hold the heater footswitch control.
- While watching through the microscope, slowly turn up the heat until there is a thin film of molten glass between the glass bead and the pipette (see Figure 10.12).
- Turn off the heat by releasing the footswitch.

Figure 10.11 The holding pipette is lowered gently on to the glass bead at a point where the outer diameter of the pipette is approximately 80 μm.

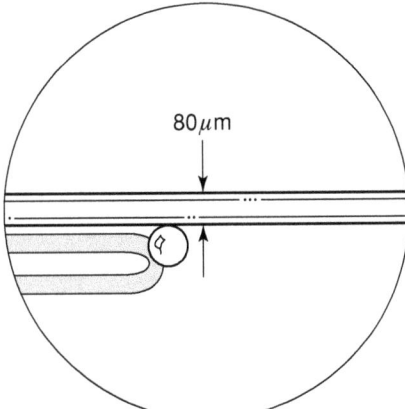

Figure 10.12 The heat is increased slowly until a thin film of glass forms between the glass bead and the holding pipette.

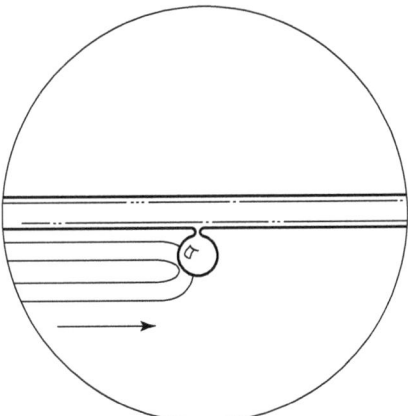

The heater element expands when it is heated, therefore as the element cools it will contract. Since the glass bead and the pipette are now welded together, the contracting element will pull the pipette and cut it, cleanly, at the point where the bead was attached (see Figure 10.13). The original pipette tip may still be attached to the glass bead; if so, manoeuvre the pipette to gently push the old tip off the bead (see Figure 10.14).

The pipette is now ready for fire polishing:

- Turn the heat control to minimum.
- Press and hold the footswitch to activate the heater.
- Bring the new tip of the pipette into close proximity with the heater element (see Figure 10.15).
- Remember that as the heat is turned up, the element will expand and move towards the pipette (see Figure 10.16).

Figure 10.13 As the heating element of the microforge cools, it contracts and snaps the holding pipette at the point where it was attached to the glass bead.

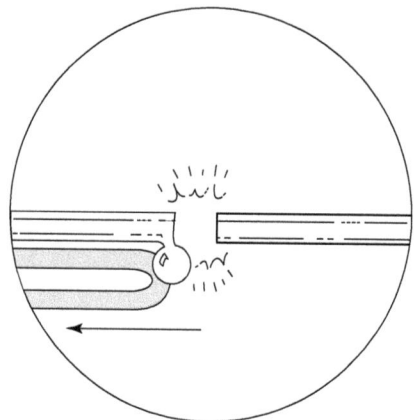

Figure 10.14 The holding pipette is manoeuvred in such a way as to sever its contact with the glass bead.

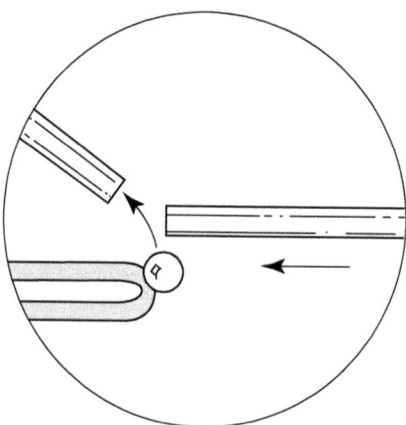

- Slowly turn up the heat watching the pipette tip until it is rounded, with an opening of approximately 15 μm (as in Figure 10.2).
- Release the footswitch control to deactivate the heater.

To put a bend in the pipette, rotate the holder so that the pipette is held vertically with the tip just out of the bottom of the field of view using the 10× objective (see Figure 10.17):

- Turn down the heat to minimum.
- Press and hold the footswitch and slowly turn up the heat so that it glows orange (approximately 35% power).
- Using the x-axis (left-to-right) control (on the Narishige MF-90 and MF-900 models, this control is below the eyepieces at about chin-height), slowly bring the heater element towards the pipette shank. As the element approaches the pipette shank, the pipette will begin to bend to the left (see Figure 10.18). If the heat is too high, or if the element is too close to the

Figure 10.15 The newly formed tip of the holding pipette is brought into close proximity with the heating element of the microforge.

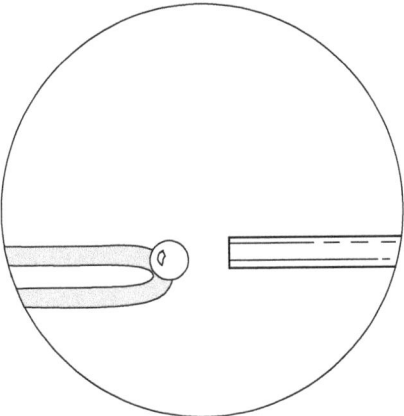

Figure 10.16 As the heat is increased, the heating element of the microforge expands and moves towards the holding pipette.

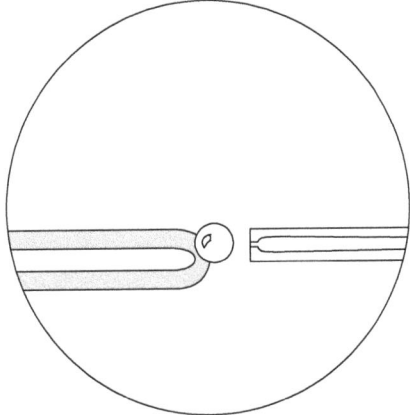

pipette, the glass may melt too quickly and the pipette will bend to the right.

- As soon as the bend is at the required angle (35–45°), release the footswitch to cut off the power. Once sterilized, the pipette will be ready to use.

10.5.3 The injection pipette

The spike on the tip of the injection pipette is a matter of personal preference. Some users believe that the freshly bevelled micropipette is sharp enough to penetrate the oocyte without the need for a spike. Indeed, some believe that the act of putting a spike on the pipette tip dulls the sharp bevelled edge, and so they miss out this step altogether. If a spike is required, however, the pipette should be placed in the microforge pipette holder so that it enters the field of view from above, directly over the glass bead,

Figure 10.17 The pipette holder is rotated such that the holding pipette is held vertically with its tip just out of the bottom of the field of view.

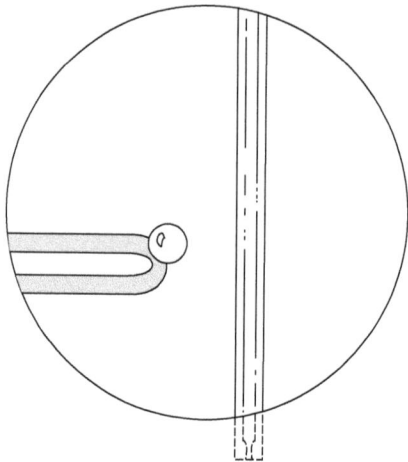

Figure 10.18 The heating element of the microforge is moved slowly towards the shank of the holding pipette until it begins to bend to the left.

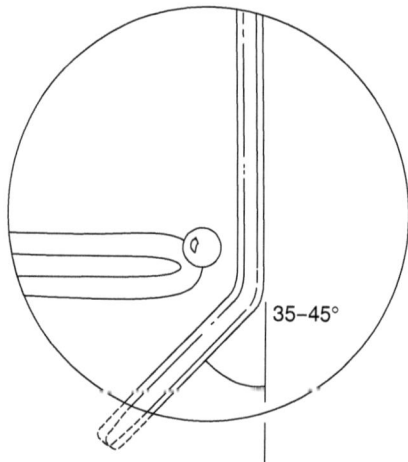

35–45°

with the hole facing directly forwards (use the pen mark made during the grinding process) (see Figure 10.19):

- Heat the glass bead with about 20% power or enough that the bead is just molten but the heating filament does not glow (this will require practice).
- Locate the Y-axis control (up–down) on the microscope. In one smooth movement, dip the pipette towards the glass bead, touch it lightly, and withdraw it immediately (see Figure 10.20).
- The very tip of the pipette should melt as it comes into contact with the glass bead and, as it is withdrawn, a sharp spike of glass should be drawn out on the pipette tip. This technique may take some practice to perfect.

Figure 10.19 The injection pipette is placed into the pipette holder of the microforge so that it enters the field of view from above, with the open face of the bevel facing forwards and directly over the glass bead.

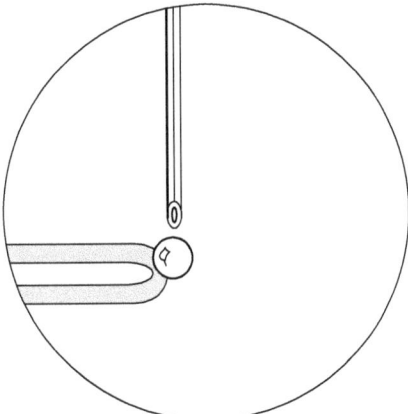

Figure 10.20 The tip of the injection pipette is lowered towards the heated glass bead until it makes contact with it, and then withdrawn immediately to draw out a sharp spike.

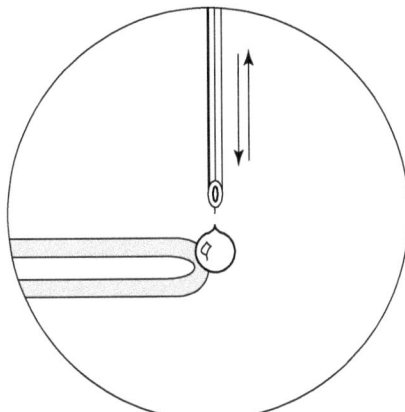

The injection pipette can now be bent in the same way as the holding pipette. Ensure that the pipette enters the field of view from above, with the hole of the bevel facing forward (use the pen mark again). This ensures that when it is mounted on the right-hand micromanipulator, the bevel points towards the bottom left of the microscope field of view. This is generally accepted to be the default set-up for the injecting pipette, and the direction of the bevel will influence the point of deposition of the sperm. See Nagy *et al.* (1995b), Blake *et al.* (2000), Hardarson *et al.* (2000) and Stoddart and Fleming (2000) for more research into the effects of sperm deposition site.

10.6 PIPETTE STERILIZATION AND STORAGE

While prefabricated microtools usually come prepackaged individually, home-made pipettes must be sterilized and stored appropriately. Once forged, it is vital that the micropipettes are sterilized and stored in a

Table 10.1 *Effects on the micropipette of altering pulling parameters*

Parameter	Increase	Decrease
Heat	Smaller opening	Larger opening
	Longer taper	Shorter taper
Pull	Smaller opening	Larger opening
	Longer taper	Shorter taper
Velocity	Smaller opening	Larger opening
Time	Shorter taper	Longer taper
Air flow	Shorter taper	Longer taper

dust-free environment. Metal boxes are ideal for this purpose, as they provide a dust-free environment and can be subjected to heat sterilization. Heat sterilization can be achieved by baking the metal box containing the micropipettes at $160\,°C$ for three hours. After allowing the box to cool, the lid should be opened only to remove a micropipette under aseptic conditions, such as those within a laminar flow hood.

10.7 TROUBLESHOOTING

10.7.1 Micropipette puller

10.7.1.1 *Problem – it is difficult to program parameters that produce the desired pipette shape*

Probable cause: This is often simply the selection of the wrong instrument. While many users are able to pull ICSI pipettes on a vertical-type puller, horizontal pullers are generally accepted to pull better, more gently tapering pipettes that are easier to grind and forge into good ICSI needles. Probably the most popular puller on the market is the Sutter, and the steps below refer to the Sutter horizontal puller range, although they may be applicable to other horizontal pullers (data reproduced courtesy of Sutter Instrument Company).

Suggested remedy: Use the changes in parameter shown in Table 10.1 to alter the shape of the pipette. Start with a clean filament and change one parameter by no more than five units at a time time.

10.7.1.2 *Problem – pipette shape is inconsistent from one pull to the next*

Once the program that produces the desired pipette shape has been achieved, maintaining consistency from one pull to the next can be a challenge. There are many reasons for inconsistency, some of which are explained below for the Sutter Instrument Company range of horizontal pullers. Again, the following account has been adapted from Sutter's own troubleshooting guide, which is located on the company's website.

Probable cause: Old or damaged filament. If the platinum filament (box or trough) is over two years old or the puller is in high use, the filament can be worn thin and will provide uneven heating to the glass. It may also be possible that the filament has survived a collision with a glass rod and is now bent or misshapen.

Suggested remedy: Replace the filament. Refer to the manual or contact Sutter for instructions. (Note that a new filament requires a new ramp test. If the filament has been replaced, then a new ramp test will need to be run. Sutter's filaments are hand-made, and the thickness and width of the platinum may vary slightly. This normal variation could represent 20–40 units of heat. If you are going from a trough to a box filament, then the new ramp value could increase two-fold. Run a ramp test and adjust the heat values accordingly.)

Probable cause: Distorted or misaligned filament.

Suggested remedy: If the filament has just been replaced and variability is still a problem, check the following: a trough filament should be shaped so the walls angle inward by 80–70°. A box or trough filament should be centred over the air jet, and the air jet should sit 2–3 mm below the base of the filament. The glass should run through the centre of a box filament and through the bottom third of a trough filament. To check the alignment of the filament relative to the air jet, pull a micropipette with a long taper and compare the right and left pipettes. If they are not identical in length, nudge the filament in the direction of the shorter pipette. Repeat this procedure until both pipettes are the same length. Refer to the manual or contact Sutter for further instructions about adjusting the alignment of the filament and the glass.

Probable cause: Moist Drierite granules. The rear right canister on the base plate contains a desiccant, Drierite, which should be light blue in colour. If the granules are lavender or pink, then they are saturated with moisture and the cooling of the glass will be variable.

Suggested remedy: Remove the Drierite and bake out the moisture. Refer to the Sutter manual or contact Sutter for instructions on how to do this.

Probable cause: Other mechanical problems, such as build-up of dirt and oils on the puller bars and bearings, restricted pulley or cable tension.

Suggested remedy: Check the bevelled edge of the puller bars and the groove in the bearings (where the puller bars reside) for dirt and grime. These can be wiped down and cleaned with 70% ethanol on a cotton bud or applicator. To check for obstructions, depress the spring stop and ensure that the puller bars slide smoothly from left to right. It should also be possible to rotate the bearings by holding the puller bar stable and rolling a thumb or finger over the bearing. Never oil the bearings!

The right and left pulleys (black or metal wheel that the cable is guided over) should both spin freely when both puller bars are pulled back in the locked position within the spring stops. If these do not spin freely, contact Sutter for parts and instructions.

To check the cable tension, hold both puller bars together and depress/tap the cable between the bumper and the pulley with a forefinger. The cables should have about 1–2 mm of slack and should not be taut. It should be possible to push down slightly on each cable and hear the pull solenoid plunger (within the puller cabinet) hit its stop. A knocking or clunking sound will be heard. If this is not the case, contact Sutter for further instructions.

It should be emphasized that there may be other factors affecting consistency that are not mentioned here. A good pipette puller manufacturer should have a customer support hotline or website, which should be able to explore any problems further. It may be worthwhile checking the effectiveness of a company's support network before buying their equipment.

10.7.2   Micropipette grinder

10.7.2.1   *Problem – once grinding is complete, small particles of dust can be seen inside the pipette*
Probable cause: These particles are probably glass dust from the grinding process, which stick to the inside of the pipette by static electricity.

Suggested remedy: The use of a humidifying system to keep the grinding surface moist is the most effective way of minimizing this. Many commercially available grinders (Sutter BV-10, Narishige EG-44 and EG-400) have their own humidifying mechanisms, but one can be fashioned relatively easily. There are two options here: either apply drops of water to the whetstone wheel directly from above (this is how most commercially available instruments work) or gently force water down the inside of the pipette as it is being ground. Either method works. For more information, see Brown and Flaming (1974).

10.7.2.2 *Problem – there is inconsistency in the size of the tip opening between pipettes*

Probable cause: There are a number of possibilities here, including pressing the pipette tip too hard on the grinding surface, leaving it in contact too long during grinding, and starting out with inconsistently pulled pipettes.

Suggested remedy: After ensuring that one starts out with consistently pulled pipettes, and leaving the tip in contact with the wheel for the same amount of time (this time will vary depending on the instrument used, hardness of glass, amount of water on the wheel, etc.), the next most obvious check is ensuring that the tip is placed on the grinding surface with the same force each time. Without complex sensing apparatus, this is impossible, which is why it is essential to monitor the placement of the tip using a microscope. Both the Sutter BV-10 and the Narishige EG-400 have microscopes (it is an option on the BV-10). Another problem to look out for is the movement of the grinding surface itself. The Narishige instruments are direct-drive units, based on an up-turned computer fan, and any motor vibrations are transmitted to the grinding surface. This can damage the tip. The Sutter BV-10 is coupled magnetically and so is virtually vibration-free. Sutter also guarantees an optically flat grinding surface (see section 10.4)

The micromanipulator used to position the pipette is important too. Ensure that it is not running down on its own (see section 3.5.1.1).

10.7.3 Microforge (Narishige MF-90/900)

10.7.3.1 *Problem – the heating element/glass bead is out of focus*

Probable cause: The heating element should remain in focus at all times, even if the pipette tip is out of focus. If the heating element appears blurred, then it needs to be readjusted.

Suggested remedy: Reposition the position of the heating block assembly with respect to the front of the microscope objective. This can be easy if the heater assembly is fixed to the frame of the microforge, but it will be harder if the heater assembly is fixed to the objective itself (as in earlier models). If the latter is the case, then the heater assembly must be moved every time the user changes objectives. Consider sending back the unit to Narishige and requesting an upgrade to the newer heater mounting – on the microforge body. Once the heater is correctly aligned, the glass bead should stay in focus no matter how much the microscope focus is adjusted, because the distance between the heater assembly and the objective remains constant (see also Section 10.9.3.2)

10.7.3.2 *Problem – it is difficult to focus clearly on the pipette and/or the heating element*

Probable cause: There are two possibilities here: the first is that the microscope focusing rack is damaged, in which case the unit will need to be returned to Narishige for repair. The second possibility is that the light source is too bright or not diffuse enough.

Suggested remedy: Some early models of MF-900 were distributed with clear plastic covers over the light source, making the light too concentrated to work well with the microscope. Using a white translucent cover (supplied as standard on later models) can help remedy this. Request a replacement cover from Narishige.

10.7.3.3 *Problem – the pipette holder will not rotate around the light source*

Probable cause: This was a design oversight on early models of the MF-900 (serial numbers beginning with 96).

Suggested remedy: The unit should be returned to be upgraded so that the pipette holder can rotate.

10.7.3.4 *Problem – the heater element will not glow, no matter how much power is supplied*

Probable cause: (1) The footswitch is not plugged in properly or there is a loose connection. (2) The heating element has burned out/broken. (3) The forge has developed a fault and needs to be returned for repair.

Suggested remedy:

(1) Plug in the footswitch properly.

(2) There is no protection in the Narishige microforge circuitry to prevent the user from supplying too much current to the heater and thus burning it out. If the heater is glowing fiercely bright, then too much current is flowing and the power should be cut (release the footswitch) and the setting dialled down. Also, the amount of current needed to make the element glow will depend on the resistance of the platinum wire dictated by its length.

(3) Contact the Narishige distributor.

10.7.3.5   *Problem – when adjusting the x- or y-axis movement of the microscope, the pipette seems to wobble off-axis*

Probable cause: The axis controls work by pushing a pointed screw against a flat plate pushing the whole microscope assembly with respect to the microforge body. This off-axis movement, or wobble, usually happens after the plate has been damaged, either in transit (the axes are usually tied with string when shipped from Narishige) or if the axis has been allowed to snap back against the spring force. The plate becomes dented.

Suggested remedy: This is something that can be tolerated depending upon the severity, but eventually the user should consider a repair by Narishige.

11 Transgenesis and the generation of knock-out mice

11.1 **TRANSGENESIS**

The word 'transgenic' refers to an animal or plant that has been transplanted with an exogenous gene. Unlike ICSI and other manipulation techniques on human oocytes and embryos, embryo manipulation in animals, particularly in mice, involves the introduction of a foreign gene to produce either overexpression or disruption of expression of the targeted gene. Transgenic animals are generated to study gene regulation in a tissue-specific (spatial) and developmental stage-specific (temporal) manner. In livestock production, transgenic technology can be applied to develop improved strains and increased disease resistance (Wheeler and Walters, 2001). Transgenic animals can also be utilized as models for various human diseases, wherein the probable causative gene mutation or deletion can be analysed fully throughout development (Campbell, 2002; Petters and Sommer, 2000) and possible therapies can be trialled to alleviate the human disease conditions. Applications of the transgenic mouse include fate mapping of cells during development and acting as markers for unknown regions in the chromosome (Jaenish, 1988). A commonly used technique developed by Gordon *et al.* (1980) is direct DNA microinjection into the pronuclei of fertilized mouse zygotes. This results in a stable chromosomal integration of the foreign DNA, usually in a head-to-tail array. Since the foreign DNA is present in every cell, including the germ cells, generally integration occurs at the one-cell stage before DNA replication, although later-stage integration can also occur, creating a mosaic mouse. The number of copies integrated varies, and the transgenes are usually integrated in a single chromosomal locus. Because the transgene can insert randomly into the mouse genome, one consequence of transgene production is the creation of insertional mutations with various phenotypic effects. This may be caused by either a gain of function mutation or production of negative mutants through the expression of some transgene. The transgene can act as a marker for the mutated gene, thus allowing the characterization of new genes, which may play a role in normal development (Jaenish, 1988; Meisler, 1992).

Another method is the indirect introduction of the transgene into the mouse genome by using DNA-transfected embryonic stem cells (ESCs) to produce chimaeric mice. This is useful in instances where the transgene may have a dominant lethal effect on the embryo.

Other ways of introducing genes into the germ line include retroviral infection of the embryos (Cabot *et al.*, 2001; Chan *et al.*, 2002; Harvey *et al.*, 2002; Haskell and Bowen, 1995; Mizuarai *et al.*, 2001; Robertson *et al.*, 1986; Schnieke *et al.*, 1983) and nuclear transplantation (Campbell, 2002; Latham and Solter, 1993; Prather *et al.*, 1999; Wilmut *et al.*, 2002; Wolf *et al.*, 1998). This chapter will briefly discuss pronuclear microinjection into a fertilized mouse egg (see Figure 11.1) and DNA-transfected ESC injection into a mouse blastocyst.

11.1.1 DNA preparation

The DNA for microinjection has to be purified from contaminants produced during DNA purification that may affect the viability of the injected zygotes. There are several factors that may affect the frequency of DNA integration into the mouse genome, such as the form of the DNA molecule, DNA concentration, and the composition of the injection buffer. Linearized DNA is five-fold more efficient than the circular form (Brinster *et al.*, 1985). The use of a lower DNA concentration (1–2 ng/μl) results in an increase in the number of zygotes that develop both in vitro and in-utero (Brinster *et al.*, 1985). A reduced amount of ethylene diamine tetra-acetic acid (EDTA) in the injection buffer also leads to an increase in the survival rate.

The protocol for DNA preparation is modified from Sambrook *et al.* (1989). Approximately 20 μg of DNA is digested with the appropriate restriction enzymes. The fragments are separated by electrophoresis through an agarose gel, and the band of interest is excised out with the use of a scalpel blade. This gel is then transferred into dialysis tubing that is sealed at one end with a dialysis clip and filled with 1 × Tris-acetate/EDTA (TAE) electrophoresis buffer (see Table 6.2 in Sambrook *et al.*, 1989). The dialysis bag is flattened to squeeze out most of the buffer, leaving about 200 μl. The other end is then sealed, avoiding air bubbles, and the bag is placed in an electrophoresis tank containing 1 × TAE. The DNA is electro-eluted from the gel into the dialysis bag by electrophoresis at about 100 V for two hours, and then the polarity of the current is reversed for about a minute to release the DNA from the wall of the bag. The buffer containing the DNA is collected into an Eppendorf tube. The bag is washed with fresh

Figure 11.1 Transgenic mice are produced following the transfer of embryos that have had DNA injected into one or more of their pronuclei.

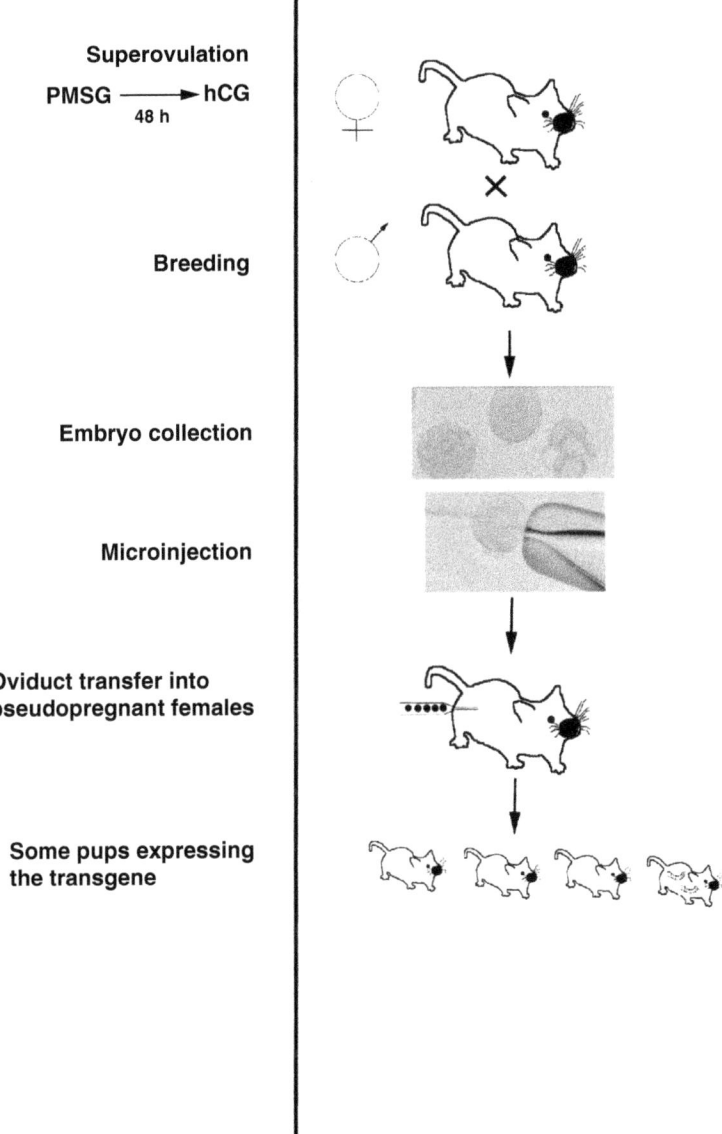

Superovulation

PMSG $\longrightarrow$ hCG
48 h

Breeding

Embryo collection

Microinjection

Oviduct transfer into pseudopregnant females

Some pups expressing the transgene

1× TAE (200 μl) and pooled with the first collection. The electroeluted DNA is extracted with buffered phenol, then with phenol/chloroform, and precipitated by adding one-tenth the volume of 3 M sodium acetate (pH 5.2) and 2.5 volumes of ethanol. This is then centrifuged and the DNA pellet resuspended in 50 μl of microinjection buffer (10 mM Tris, pH 7.6; 0.1 mM EDTA, pH 8.0). The DNA suspension is purified further by passing it through a sephacryl resin (e.g. MicroSpin™ S-200 HR column) following the manufacturer's protocol. The DNA is run on an agarose gel to determine the concentration and then diluted to a final concentration of 2 ng/μl.

11.1.2 Media preparation

The media used in mouse pronuclear microinjection are similar to those used in ICSI procedures: an incubation medium (M16) containing bicarbonate buffered by 5% CO_2 and a manipulation medium (M2) that is Hepes-buffered and so is stable outside the incubator (M2 and M16 preparation) (Gordon, 1993; Hogan *et al.*, 1994). The media are also available commercially (e.g. M2 medium, M7167, and M16 medium, M7292, Sigma). M16 droplets are placed in 35-mm or 60-mm tissue culture plastic Petri dishes and then overlaid with mineral oil (embryo-tested, M8410, Sigma). M16 has to be pre-equilibrated for at least an hour in 5% CO_2, 95 % air at 37 °C before use, while the M2 is kept at 37 °C during the manipulation procedures.

11.1.3 Mouse strain

The mouse strain used can affect the overall efficiency of microinjection, with the hybrid strains showing an eight-fold increase in efficiency over inbred strains (Brinster *et al.*, 1985). However, some experiments may require the use of a mouse strain with a defined genetic background, such as FVB/N (Taketo *et al.*, 1991), C57BL/6J, BALB/CJ and C3H mice. However, certain inbred strains of mice may have an inherent pathological phenotype. A good example is the FVB/N strain, which exhibits neurological pathology and retinal degeneration, which may have a major impact on transgenic research (Gimenez and Montoliu, 2001; Goelz *et al.*, 1998). Older FVB/N mice have a higher incidence of developing spontaneous lesions in the lungs (Mahler *et al.*, 1996).

11.1.4 Source of fertilized one-cell eggs/zygotes

To ensure the collection of a large number of fertilized eggs, donor mice are superovulated by intraperitoneal injection of PMSG, which mimics FSH, and 42–48 hours later injection with hCG, which mimics luteinizing hormone, to synchronize and promote ovulation before mating with the males. Younger females (three to four weeks old) are recommended for use, but older females (five to eight weeks old) can also be used. It is important that the hCG is given before the release of the endogenous hormone (48 hours post-PMSG injection). On the day of 'plugging' (checking for the deposition of semen and seminal fluid within the vagina), females are sacrificed and the oviduct collected in M2. The cumulus mass that contains the fertilized eggs is visible through the swollen ampulla

Figure 11.2 (a) A mouse oviduct collected on the day following mating is characterized by a dilated ampulla (Amp) towards one end and the anterior part of the uterus (Ut) at the other end. (b) Zygotes (Zyg) within the cumulus mass (Cum) are released into the media after tearing the ampulla (Amp). (Photographs provided by Dr Edna Hardeman, Muscle Development Unit, Children's Medical Research Institute, Westmead, Sydney, Australia.)

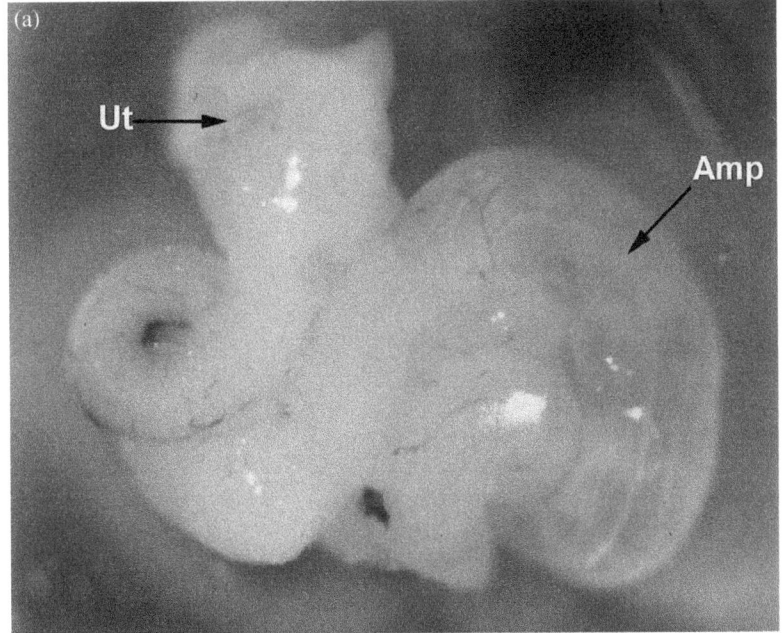

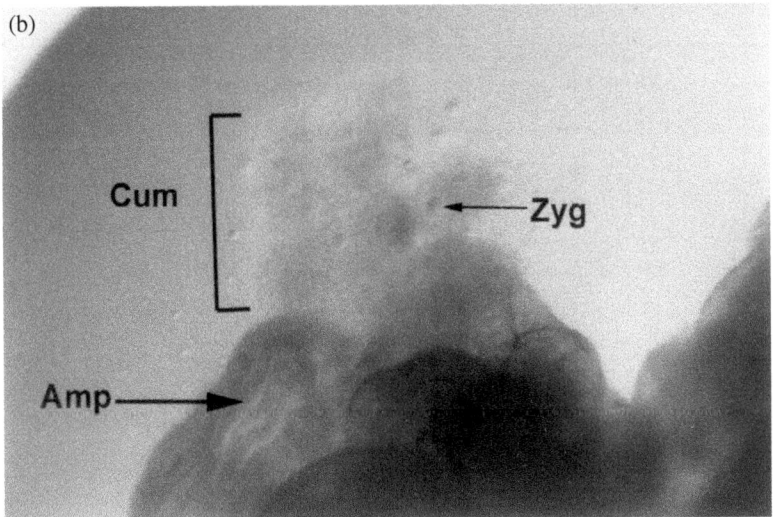

(if collection is done early in the morning; see Figure 11.2a) and is released into the media by tearing the wall of the oviduct (see Figure 11.2b). The eggs are released from the mass by using hyaluronidase diluted in M2 at a concentration of 300 µg/ml. Fertilized eggs are then washed several times in M2 before transferring to M16 for culture before microinjection. Zygotes with two pronuclei and two PBs are used for microinjection (see Figure 11.3a).

Figure 11.3 (a) A normal mouse zygote is characterized by having two polar bodies (PB) and two pronuclei (PN). (b) Microinjection into the pronucleus of a mouse zygote. Note the enlargement of the injected pronucleus (En PN) compared with the uninjected pronucleus (PN). (Photographs provided by Dr Edna Hardeman, Muscle Development Unit, Children's Medical Research Institute, Westmead, Sydney, Australia.) HP, holding pipette; IP, injection pipette.

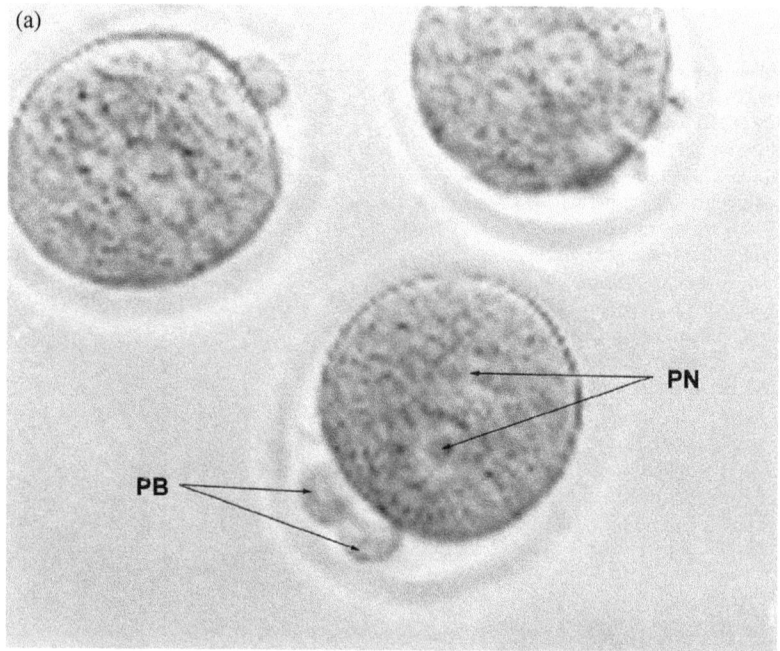

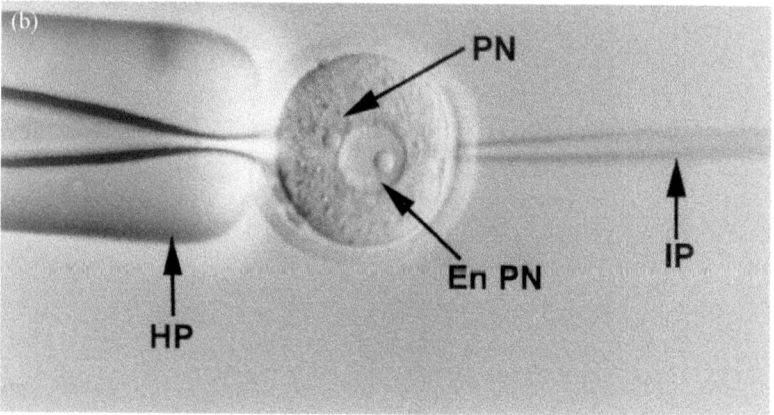

11.1.5 Pipettes

There are three kinds of pipettes used in the production of transgenic mice: transfer pipettes, holding pipettes and microinjection pipettes. The transfer pipettes are made from hand-drawn disposable glass Pasteur pipettes and are usually attached to rubber tubing connected to a mouthpiece to facilitate collection and transfer of zygotes during the manipulation procedures.

The holding pipettes can also be hand-drawn using a glass capillary (outer diameter 1 mm, inner diameter 0.8 mm, length 15 cm, Wild Leitz,

Table 11.1 *Commercially available holding pipettes for pronuclear microinjection*

Supplier	Product no.
Conception Technologies	HP-95-00
	HP 120-00
	HP120-XX
Eppendorf	5175-108-000
Humagen Fertility Diagnostics	10-MPH-95
	10-MPH-95-B
	10-MPH-120
	10-MPH-120-B
	10-MPH-150
	10-MPH-180

335-520119), polishing the tip with a deFonBrune-type microforge (see section 10.5.2). They are also available commercially (see Table 11.1) and can be used for both one-cell and blastocyst injection. The holding pipettes are utilized to fix the zygote in place during the microinjection.

The injection pipettes can be drawn mechanically using a Flaming/Brown micropipette puller (e.g. Model P-97, Sutter Instruments; see section 10.5.3). Thin-walled borosilicate glass capillaries with filament (1.0 mm outer diameter, 0.75 mm inner diameter; e.g. from World Precision Instruments, TW100F-4) are set on the puller with the middle of the capillary sitting over the heating element. The pipettes are usually drawn just before use. The use of commercially produced injection pipettes (e.g. FemtotipII from Eppendorf, 5242-957-000) is becoming more popular, although cost is the limiting factor. The pipette is loaded with the DNA immediately before microinjection, either by capillary action by dipping the blunt end of the pipette into the DNA solution (due to the presence of a filament inside the pipette) or by using a loading pipette tip (e.g. Microloader from Eppendorf, 5242-956-003). The tip of the injection pipette should be of optimum length and the diameter not too large to ensure a high survival of the injected zygotes.

11.1.6 Pronuclear microinjection

The microinjection protocol and equipment required are quite similar to those used in human ICSI, except that the injection pipette is loaded with DNA and injection is directly into one or both pronuclei. The zygotes are removed from M16 and washed through several droplets of M2 before transferring them into the injection dish (e.g. four-well glass slide from Nunc, 177399) containing about 10 μl microdrops of M2 covered with mineral oil. Groups of 10–20 zygotes are transferred into each M2 microdrop. Using the 10× objective, the holding pipette is slowly lowered into the injection chamber/dish and positioned near a zygote. The injection pipette is then lowered to a level wherein the holding and injection pipettes and the zygote are all on the same plane. Microinjection is performed using the 20× or 40× objective. The ZP is pierced gently with the injection pipette until it has been inserted into the pronucleus. The injected pronucleus will swell as positive pressure is applied (see Figure 11.3b). The pipette is then withdrawn and the injected zygote separated from the unmanipulated fertilized eggs. The injection pipette is replaced for each group of zygotes, or more frequently if the survival is low. Usually 60–80% of injected zygotes survive microinjection. They are then transferred into M16 and cultured for about 30 minutes or overnight before transfer into pseudopregnant females (non-superovulated females mated with vasectomized males).

11.1.7 Transfer of injected embryos into recipient females

11.1.7.1 *Oviduct transfer*

Zygotes that survive the injection are transferred into the oviduct of plugged pseudopregnant females through the infundibulum. Transfer can be done using one-cell zygotes (same-day transfer) or two-cell embryos after an overnight incubation in M16. The embryos are washed in several droplets of M2 prior to the transfer. The recipient female is anaesthetized (e.g. using ketamine 0.2 mg/g and xylazine 0.1 mg/g, i.p.) and placed on a dissecting microscope with the dorsal side up. A skin incision is made just below the ribcage (upper flank area) using a small pair of scissors (e.g. delicate scissors from B. Braun, BC65), exposing the abdominal muscles. With another pair of scissors, an opening is made into the peritoneum over the fat pad/ovary area. The oviduct is exposed by pulling the fat pad through the incision and held in place over the back of the mouse by a clamp (e.g. using bulldog clamps from B. Braun, BH020). The infundibulum (the most anterior part of which is the natural opening of the oviduct) is visible through the bursa covering the ovary and part of the oviduct. A tear is made on the bursa directly above the infundibulum, avoiding the capillaries. While keeping the tear open with fine-tipped forceps (e.g. jeweller's forceps from B. Braun, BD330), the transfer pipette containing the embryos is then inserted into the infundibulum and teased deeper into the oviduct. The embryos are transferred gently

Figure 11.4 A loaded transfer pipette, showing alternating columns of air bubbles (arrowheads) and media containing the zygotes (Zyg). (Photograph provided by Dr Edna Hardeman, Muscle Development Unit, Children's Medical Research Institute, Westmead, Sydney, Australia.)

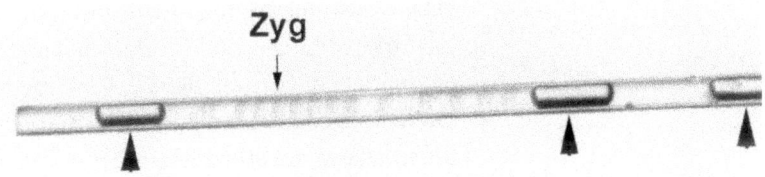

along with a minimum amount of M2. An air bubble drawn into the transfer pipette immediately after the embryos can function as an indicator that all embryos have been transferred successfully (see Figure 11.4). About 15–20 embryos are transferred into one or both oviducts. The fat pad is released from the clamp and grasped with a pair of forceps, then returned carefully into the peritoneal cavity without touching the oviduct. The muscle incision is closed with absorbable suture (e.g. Vicryl 5–0, ETHICON) and the skin incision is closed with non-absorbable suture (e.g. Ethilon 5–0, ETHICON). Around 5–50% of the pups born should carry the transgene.

11.1.7.2 *Uterine transfer*

Uterine transfers are generally performed for embryos at the blastocyst stage. The recipient females (day 2.5 pseudopregnant) are operated on exactly as for the oviduct transfer up until the point at which the reproductive tract is externalized. For uterine transfers, the first 5–10 mm of the uterus must be exposed and laid out so that it is relatively straight. A hole is then made at the top of the uterus using a 26G needle, avoiding blood vessels in the wall of the uterus. The transfer pipette containing the embryos is then inserted a few millimetres into the hole and the embryos are expelled. It is not possible to see through the wall of the uterus when the embryos have been expelled successfully, so it is common to use a system of air bubbles in the transfer pipette above the embryos to indicate when sufficient medium has been blown out to release them. About six to eight embryos should be transferred per uterus, and single-sided or double-sided transfers can be performed. After transfer of the embryos, the recipient is closed up exactly as for oviduct transfers.

11.2 GENERATION OF KNOCK-OUT AND TRANSGENIC MICE USING ESCs

Blastocyst injection is a technique used to return ESCs grown and manipulated in vitro to the in vivo environment. ESCs can be isolated from blastocyst-stage embryos – they make up the inner cell mass (ICM) of blastocysts and are totipotent, meaning they are undifferentiated and have the potential to differentiate into any cell type in the body. Under the appropriate in vitro conditions, ESCs can be grown and expanded indefinitely. They can be manipulated by the addition of exogenous genes, or by the specific removal or alteration of endogenous genes and then studied in vitro by driving the cells down various differentiation pathways. The real power of ESC work, however, can be realized when ESCs are returned to the in vivo environment by means of blastocyst injection (or alternately morula co-culture), generating complete organisms carrying the defined genetic manipulations generated in the ESCs. In this way, genetic changes as specific as a single base mutation can be studied with respect to their effect on normal growth, development and function of the entire organism or any of its component cells, tissues or organs.

The potential exists for genetic manipulation via ESCs in any organism for which ESCs can be derived and cultured successfully – this technology is applied most commonly to the mouse, but it is being developed further in rats, monkeys and humans, among others. There is also potential for future clinical applications of ESC technology in humans by driving manipulated ESCs down specific differentiation pathways and then returning resultant cell types to the specific target tissue/organ (e.g. brain cells for Alzheimer's disease patients, islet cells for diabetics, etc.).

11.2.1 Source of ESCs

ESCs have been isolated from a number of different mouse strains (see Table 11.2), facilitating the generation of gene-targeted mice in these strains. Where possible, it is preferable to use ESCs of the same strain as that in which you wish to generate the mouse model. The choice of ESC strains is still relatively limited compared with the huge number of mouse strains available, however, so for some mouse models there may be no option but to conduct studies in a mixed genetic background. If this is not suitable for a specific mouse model, then the alternative is to conduct extensive back-crossing to change the model from one strain to another. This cannot always be achieved successfully, however, as in some cases the targeted gene or genes lie within regions that determine the essential character of a particular strain. An example is the tumour necrosis factor (TNF) cytokine family of genes that lie within the major histocompatibility complex (MHC) region of the genome (Koerner *et al.*, 1997). For immunological models targeting any of this cytokine gene family, the strain of ESCs used will determine to a large extent the phenotype displayed by the resultant mouse line generated, as the MHC and TNF family genes are unlikely to be segregated by standard back-crossing protocols.

Table 11.2 *ESC lines*

ESC line	Mouse strain	Reference
CCE	129/Sv/Ev	Robertson *et al.* (1986)
D3	129/Sv	Doetschman *et al.* (1985)
J1	129/Sv	Li *et al.* (1992)
R1	129/Sv X 129/Sv-CP	Nagy *et al.* (1993a)
E14TG2a	129/O1a	Hooper *et al.* (1987)
BL/6 III	C57BL/6	Ledermann and Burki (1991)
Bruce 4	C56BL/6	Koentgen *et al.* (1993)

In all cases, it is important to understand the underlying characteristics of the strains chosen, as these may influence phenotypes displayed by the mice after introduction of the specific genetic manipulations.

11.2.2 Design of the targeting construct

The most common application of ESC technology has been in the generation of gene knock-out mice. This is where a specific gene or region of the genome has been targeted for a precise manipulation by homologous recombination, which renders the chosen gene inactive and thus a functional gene product is no longer produced. However, ESC manipulation also lends itself to transgenesis by either targeted or random integration. This has the advantage that, at least for some genes, the pattern of integration and expression of the transgene can be analysed in vitro prior to any in vivo experimentation (this may have ethical implications if it allows a reduction in the use of animals).

Random transgenesis makes use of a classic transgenic construct that is transfected into the ESCs (generally by electroporation, i.e. the application to the cells of a short electrical current that temporarily opens pores in the plasma membrane and allows the entry of DNA molecules) (Thomas and Capecchi, 1987). Consequently, the construct is incorporated in much the same manner as introduction to the cell via pronuclear injection.

Targeted transgenic and knock-out strategies require the use of homologous flanking regions of DNA around the construct that, on transfection, locate their homologous regions in the genome and replace the intervening sequence with that of the targeting construct (see Figure 11.5). In this manner, genetic modifications as precise as single base changes are possible.

For most gene knock-out constructs, it is necessary to include a selectable marker, such as the classic neomycin resistance cassette

Figure 11.5 The targeting construct replaces some or all of the coding region of the gene with a positive selectable marker, allowing cells incorporating the construct to survive selection. Outside the homologous flanking arms of the targeting construct, there may be a negative selectable marker that will be lost on homologous recombination. If the construct is integrated randomly, then the negative selectable marker will also be incorporated and under selective pressure will kill the cell.

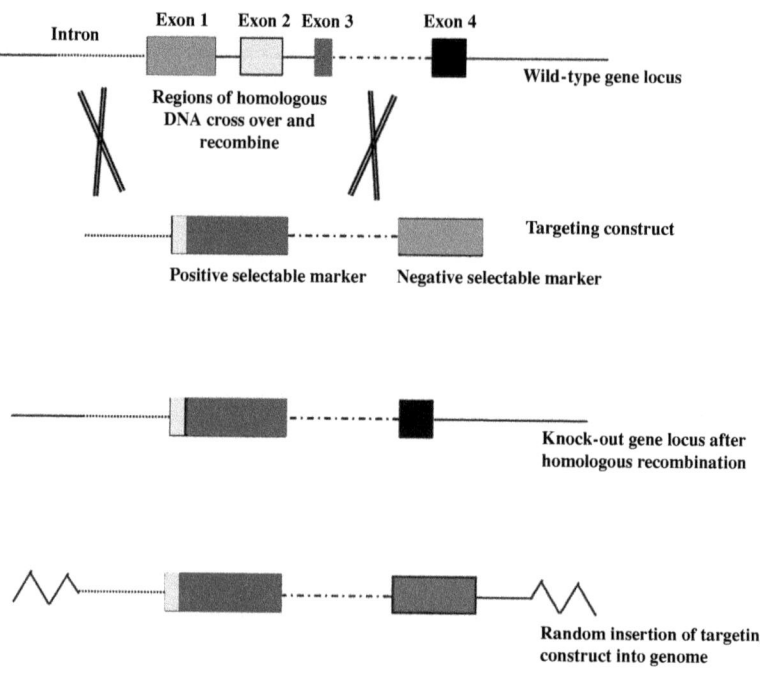

(an example of positive selection). This allows easy identification of cells in which construct integration has been successful (cells incorporating the targeting construct will express the neogene and will be able to grow in the presence of exogenous neomycin, which would otherwise kill them). It is also possible to combine positive selection with negative selection to discriminate between homologous recombination and random integration. For this, a selectable marker such as the Herpes simplex virus thymidine kinase gene can be added to the targeting construct outside the flanking arms of homology. If the construct is incorporated into the cell via homologous recombination, then this gene will be lost. If the construct is inserted randomly, however, the gene will also be incorporated, and in the presence of ganciclovir (a synthetic guanine analogue harmless to normal cells) toxic metabolites will be produced that ultimately kill the cell. As homologous recombination is generally a rare event (1–2% is a common rate of homologous recombinants to random integrants for many targeted genes), the use of a combined positive/negative selection strategy can enrich the identification of homologous recombinants by 2–2000 times (Galli-Taliadoros et al., 1995).

As ESCs are diploid and transfection normally targets only a single allele, screening for homologous integration of the targeting construct by a readout of the output from the targeted gene will not be useful in most cases due to the compensatory effects of the non-targeted wild-type allele.

11.2.3 ESC culture

The culture of ESCs requires some degree of care to ensure the cells remain totipotent and are able to contribute to all tissues of the developing mouse. Leukaemia inhibitory factor (LIF) was shown (Smith *et al.*, 1988; Williams *et al.*, 1988) to be the single ingredient able to maintain murine ESCs in an undifferentiated state. However, despite the addition of LIF to the culture medium, ESCs may tend to differentiate unless the other culture conditions are ideal. ESCs generally prefer to be slightly crowded rather than very sparse on the culture dish, and they benefit from frequent and regular passaging. This has the added benefit of removing differentiating cells as they do not tend to survive trypsinizing and replating well. Standard ESC culture medium is high-glucose DMEM containing 10–15% FCS (ESC qualified), 110 mg/l sodium pyruvate, 2 mM L-glutamine, antibiotics (50 U/ml penicillin and 50 µg/ml streptomycin), 0.1 mM non-essential amino acids, 100 µM 2-mercaptoethanol, nucleotides (30 µM A,C,G,U and 10 µM T) and 1000 U/ml LIF. Cells are passaged every two to three days and plated at approximately $2–5 \times 10^6$ cells/10 cm diameter culture dish. Comprehensive culture techniques for ESCs are available widely (see Abbondanzo *et al.*, 1993; Robertson, 1987).

The use of embryonic mouse fibroblasts as a feeder layer is relatively common, and most ESC lines appear to prefer growing in this manner. The feeder cells provide various growth factors (including LIF) as well as a more appropriate extracellular environment for the ESCs than the tissue culture surface alone. If not using feeders, it is essential to gelatinize the tissue culture surface (0.1% in distilled water, sufficient to cover the surface for 15–30 minutes, then aspirate off the remaining solution) to facilitate ESC adhesion and reduce differentiation. Embryonic fibroblasts can be isolated from the torsos (minus the liver) of day-13–14 embryos from virtually any mouse strain. However, for the feeders to remain alive during any selection procedures, it is helpful to isolate the fibroblasts from a mouse line carrying the same selectable markers as used in the targeting construct. To prevent the feeders overgrowing the ESCs, they are growth-arrested by either irradiation (25 Gray) or with mitomycin-C treatment (30 µM for four hours followed by extensive washing) and plated at approximately $1–2 \times 10^6$ cells/10 cm diameter culture dish.

11.2.4 Source of blastocysts

The source of embryos for blastocyst injection needs to be considered carefully. For easy recognition of chimaeric animals resulting from successful blastocyst injection, it is most common to use embryos from a strain with a markedly different coat colour to that of the ESC strain. However, various factors, including the developmental rate of the donor embryos, play a role in determining which combinations of ESC and donor embryo strains are compatible and will result in successful chimaerism and subsequent germ line transmission. As most of these factors are largely undetermined, most work tends to be done in tried- and-true combinations.

Depending on the donor strain of choice, superovulation may be an option to produce large numbers of embryos for injection. However, some strains of mice yield lower-quality embryos when superovulated, negating the gain in embryo quantity, and so for these strains natural mating may be preferred. For most donor strains, blastocysts can be harvested on the morning of day 3 (post-plugging) and injected either immediately or at some time later on the same day. Due to the different developmental rates of mouse strains, some may require earlier harvesting and overnight in vitro maturation to reach an appropriate stage for injection (Lemckert *et al.*, 1997). Embryos are generally harvested in a Hepes-buffered medium (e.g. M2) and cultured in microdrops of a bicarbonate-buffered medium (e.g. M16) under oil at $37\,°C$, 5% CO_2. Blastocysts are injectable from the early expanding stage right through to fully expanded blastocysts, although for the inexperienced injector the later stages may be easier due simply to a larger target (blastocoel) being available. Care must be taken not to allow the embryos to overdevelop, however, as the membranes become very rubbery and hard to penetrate, while the entire embryo becomes fragile and collapses easily when handled. Embryos tending toward this state can be slowed in their development by storage for a while at $4\,°C$, although this should be avoided for prolonged periods as there is a risk of the embryo halting development entirely.

11.2.5 Preparation of ESCs for blastocyst injection

ESCs for blastocyst injection are easiest to use if the feeder cells (if used) are first depleted from the cell preparation. Cells for injection should be growing vigorously (log phase) when taken for injection so it is usually best to passage the cells the day before injection.

The following items are required for the preparation of ESCs:

- Dish of ESCs in log phase growth
- PBS

- Trypsin/EDTA
- ESC medium
- Injection medium
- One or two gelatinized culture dishes
- Centrifuge tube

Injection medium comprises ESC medium with reduced FCS levels (5–10% FCS), 20 mM Hepes and 50 U/ml DNase (optional). This must be embryo tested before use. The level of FCS favours embryonic development over ESC growth and helps reduce the stickiness of the ESC membranes. The DNase, if used, can help digest any DNA released by damaged cells. Hepes maintains pH outside the CO_2 incubator. The ESCs are prepared as follows:

1 Wash cells well with PBS.
2 Trypsinize thoroughly (for 5–10 minutes at 37 °C) with a minimum volume of trypsin/EDTA.
3 Add ESC medium and pipette thoroughly to completely disrupt all cell clumps and yield a single cell suspension.
4 Plate the cell suspension on to a gelatinized culture dish and incubate for 20–30 minutes to allow the fibroblasts to adhere.
5 Draw up the supernatant containing non-adherent cells and repeat Step 4 if desired.
6 Place the supernatant into a centrifuge tube and pellet the cells at a low speed for about five minutes.
7 Discard the supernatant, resuspend the cells in injection medium, and store on ice until required.

Once the cells are prepared for injection, they should be used as soon as possible, because maintenance of ESCs on ice for extended periods will not facilitate chimaera production. If the injection session is expected to last for more than a couple of hours, it is recommended that a second plate of cells be prepared.

11.2.6 Blastocyst injection

ESCs are usually injected into blastocysts at the rate of about 10–15 cells per embryo. However, different combinations of ESC lines and donor embryo strains will behave differently, so some variation from this figure may be necessary.

When the embryos are ready to inject and the cells have been prepared, they should be transferred to the injection chamber. This can be a chamber slide containing injection medium and covered with a layer of oil, a

Petri dish full of injection medium, or any other vessel that offers good optical qualities for injection. The injection chamber design must prevent desiccation of the ESCs and embryos, and make it possible to keep track of where the embryos are at all times.

The injection chamber can then be placed on the microscope stage (use of a cooling stage set to approximately 12 °C is recommended where possible, as this helps stiffen the membranes of the blastocysts and facilitate injection), and the holding and injection pipettes can be introduced. One embryo at a time should be held firmly by suction with the holding pipette, ensuring the ICM is away from the line of injection, and then the ESCs drawn up into the injection pipette.

The injection pipette is adjusted so that it will enter the embryo close to its horizon and, where possible, at a junction between the trophecto-derm cells (see Figure 11.6a). The pipette should be introduced into the blastocoel in a short, sharp, controlled movement, and the ESCs expelled carefully (see Figure 11.6b). The injection pipette can then be withdrawn and the embryo released from the holding pipette.

After injection, embryos will collapse, but they will start to re-expand within a couple of hours. They can be transferred to the uterus of day 2.5 pseudopregnant mice (or alternatively to the oviduct of day 0.5 pseudo-pregnant mice) within four to six hours (see section 11.1.7), and pups will be born approximately 17–20 days later.

11.3 GENERATION OF KNOCK-OUT MICE THROUGH MORULA CO-CULTURE

Chimaeric mice can be produced by micromanipulation techniques other than blastocyst injection. Morula co-culture has some advantages over blastocyst injection in that it is a simpler technique. It requires far less specialized and expensive micromanipulation equipment, needs less training and expertise, and much greater numbers of embryos can be handled in a day's work. It utilizes outbred donor mouse strains (e.g. CD1) that can be superovulated successfully, significantly reducing costs. However, its benefits are limited somewhat by the fact that only a few ESC strains appear suitable for the technique, while blastocyst injection has far more flexibility in this regard. Also, blastocyst injection appears capable of producing germ-line-transmitting chimaeras even if the ESCs are somewhat marginal in their totipotency, whereas morula co-culture requires absolute totipotency to achieve this result (Wood et al., 1993).

Figure 11.6 (a) The trophectoderm is a layer of cells with a quilted appearance, lining the inside of the ZP. To facilitate penetration of the trophectoderm and reduce damage to the blastocyst, the injection pipette should be inserted at a junction between these cells. (b) Following penetration of the ZP and trophectoderm, ESCs are injected into the blastocoel.

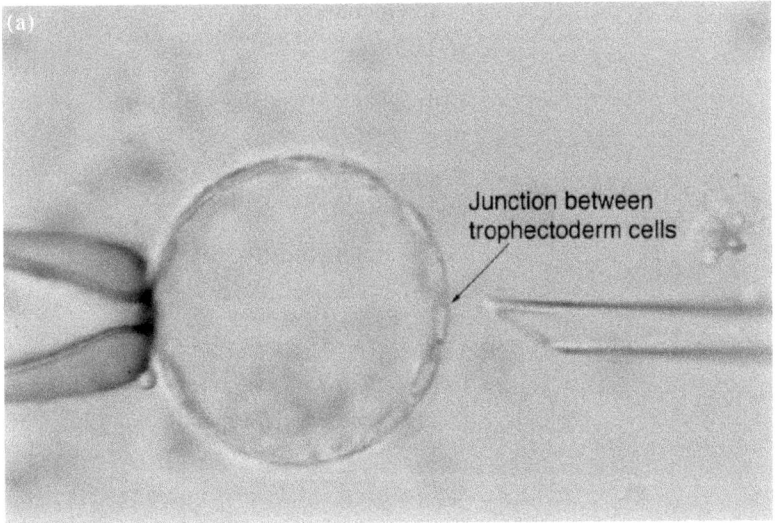

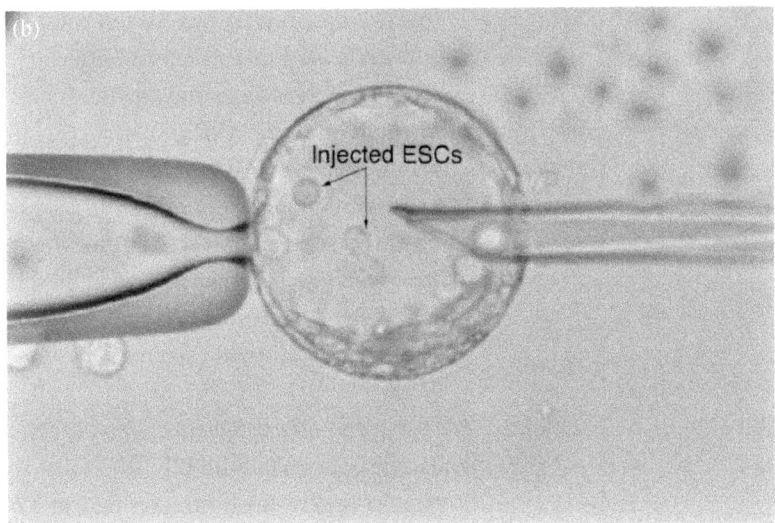

11.3.1 Preparation of ESCs for co-culture

Morula co-culture can be performed in two main ways: by culturing zona-stripped morulae on a lawn of single ESCs, or by culturing zona-stripped morulae in microwells with a small clump of ESCs. The ESCs are efficiently internalized by the developing embryo and can contribute significantly to the ICM of the resultant blastocyst (Wood *et al.*, 1993). As is the case for blastocyst injection, ESCs perform best if growing in log phase when prepared for co-culture.

The following items are required for the preparation of ESCs for morula co-culture:

- Dish of ESCs in log phase growth
- PBS
- Trypsin/EDTA
- ESC medium
- Co-culture medium
- Acid Tyrode's solution

Co-culture medium comprises ESC medium with 5–10% FCS, 20 mM Hepes and 23 mM lactate. This must be embryo-tested before use. The ESCs are prepared for morula co-culture as follows:

11.3.1.1 *For the preparation of a single cell suspension*
1. Wash the ESCs well with PBS.
2. Trypsinize thoroughly (five to ten minutes at $37\,°C$) with a minimum volume (at least 1 ml) of trypsin/EDTA.
3. Add 10 ml ESC medium and pipette thoroughly to completely disrupt all cell clumps and yield a single cell suspension.
4. Place the cell suspension into a centrifuge tube and pellet the cells at a low speed for about five minutes.
5. Discard the supernatant, resuspend the cells in a small volume of co-culture medium, and take a small aliquot for counting.
6. Adjust the cell concentration to $0.5–1 \times 10^6$ cells/ml and plate out 15 μl drops on to co-culture dishes.

11.3.1.2 *For the preparation of small clumps of cells*
1. Wash the cells well with PBS.
2. Trypsinize briefly (a few minutes only at $37\,°C$, monitoring the cells) with a minimum volume (at least 1 ml) of trypsin/EDTA.
3. Add 10 ml ESC medium and pipette gently to lightly disrupt the colonies and yield small ESC clumps of about five to ten cells each.
4. Under a good dissecting microscope, select suitably sized cell clumps for co-culture and gather them together in a small culture dish or similar until required.

11.3.2 Morula co-culture
Morulae for co-culture need to be at the compacting stage, which occurs at approximately 8–16 cells. Earlier embryos risk disintegration into individual blastomeres once the ZP is removed because the individual cells do not attach to one another as strongly as those in compacted embryos

(Wood *et al.*, 1993). ESCs also appear to adhere more tightly to compacting/compacted embryos, and thus the co-culture is more likely to result in their successful internalization.

These embryos can generally be harvested from day 2.5 donor mice. Once harvested, the embryos need to be stripped of their ZPs using acid Tyrode's solution (Sigma, T1788, embryo tested) as follows:

1 Place drops of Tyrode's solution on to culture dishes.
2 Collect a small number of embryos in as small a volume of medium as possible, and add to the drop of Tyrode's solution, mixing gently to ensure the embryos are bathed in the solution rather than culture medium that has been carried over.
3 Monitor the embryos constantly to check when the ZP has been dissolved.
4 As soon as the ZP has been dissolved flood the drop of Tyrode's solution with medium to inactivate the Tyrode's and prevent the embryos sticking to the culture dish.
5 Gather the embryos and wash them through a number of drops of medium, then transfer them back to microdrops until ready to use.

Once stripped, the embryos are sticky and will adhere easily to the surface of culture dishes. They are also very fragile as they lack the physical protection of the ZP, and so great care needs to be taken when handling them.

For co-culture on a lawn of ESCs, five to ten stripped embryos can then be added to each of the preplated ESC microdrops and cultured for two to three hours until a number of ESCs can be seen adhering to the embryo. The embryos are then removed from the ESC lawn and returned to microdrop culture in embryo medium overnight until they have developed through to blastocysts.

For co-culture with clumps of ESCs, microwells can be made in the base of culture dishes using the Hungarian darning needle technique (see Figure 11.7). Each well should be sufficiently large to accommodate only a single embryo. The zona-stripped embryos are placed into the microwells; then a clump of ESCs is placed on top of the embryo in the microwell (if possible, nestled into a junction of the blastomeres so as to maximize contact with the embryo). The embryos are then cultured overnight to the blastocyst stage.

After the co-culture period, the embryos can be transferred to the uterus of day 2.5 or the oviducts of day 0.5 pseudopregnant mice (see section 11.1.7). Pups can be expected approximately 17–20 days after embryo transfer.

Figure 11.7 The darning needle is pressed on to the surface of the embryo culture dish (I) and rotated slightly, whilst pressing downwards (II), to create a small depression in the base of the dish (III). The optimal size for a microwell created in this fashion is marginally larger than the diameter of a zona-stripped morula (IV). N.B. The culture dish must contain microdrops of media before the microwells are created to prevent air bubbles becoming trapped within them.

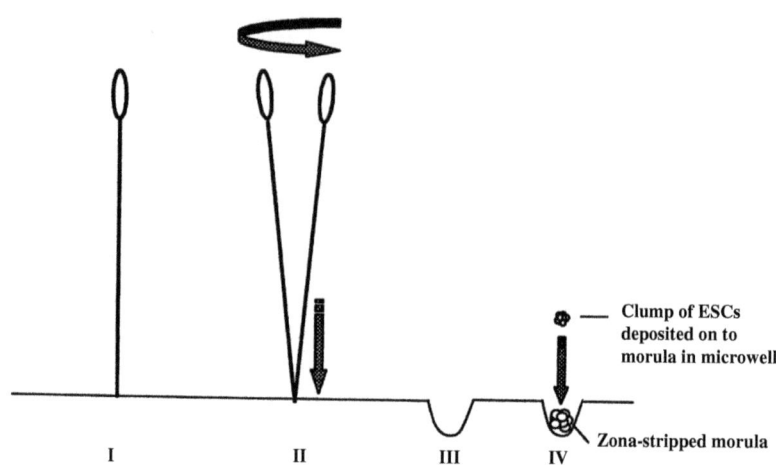

11.4 TROUBLESHOOTING

11.4.1 Problem – neither pronucleus is visible during microinjection

Probable cause: Fertilized eggs are not yet ready for microinjection.

Suggested remedy: There is a 'window of microinjection' for a period of about three to five hours where both pronuclei are at their maximum size. The mouse strain used and the time of hCG administration determine the optimum time for microinjection. Generally, if the hCG is administered at 1 p.m., then the optimum time for injection is between 1 p.m. and 6 p.m. the following day.

11.4.2 Problem – pronuclei do not enlarge during microinjection of DNA

Probable cause: Blocked injection pipette. A self-pulled pipette is usually not patent or is still sealed at the tip after pulling with the pipette puller.

Suggested remedy: Tap the injection pipette gently against the holding pipette to break off the tip and allow the flow of the DNA.

11.4.3 Problem – microinjection DNA becomes diluted with M2

Probable cause: Backflow of media into the microinjection pipette.

Suggested remedy: Use a microinjector that provides positive pressure to ensure continuous flow of the DNA, thus preventing backflow of the media.

11.4.4 **Problem – the embryo rotates when sucked on to the holding pipette, causing the ICM to change position**

Probable cause: The diameter of the holding pipette is greater than that of the embryo, and the embryo is jumping up off the base of the injection chamber to reach the holding pipette opening.

Suggested remedy: Make or buy holding pipettes with an outer diameter that is smaller than, or at most equal to, that of the embryos.

11.4.5 **Problem – the embryo moves around when it is being injected and is not held sufficiently steady by the holding pipette**

Probable cause: The holding pipette is angled so that the tip is not perpendicular to the base of the injection chamber.

Suggested remedy: (1) Adjust the angle of the holding pipette so that the last few millimetres of the holding pipette are parallel to the floor of the injection chamber and the tip is perpendicular. In this way, the embryo can be held firmly by the holding pipette flat to the floor of the injection chamber. (2) Ensure the embryo is being injected exactly at the hemisphere (as viewed from the side). In this way, the forward pressure from the injection pipette will be against the region of maximum support from the holding pipette, preventing movement of the embryo.

11.4.6 **Problem – it is hard to control the flow of ESCs into or out of the injection pipette**

Probable cause: The internal diameter of the injection pipette is too large.

Suggested remedy: Try making/buying injection pipettes where the internal diameter is only fractionally larger than the ESCs.

11.4.7 **Problem – It Is hard to penetrate the blastocyst with the injection pipette – the embryos collapse first**

Probable cause: The timing of injection is incorrect.

Suggested remedy: Adjust the timing of the injection so that most of the embryos are at an expanded blastocyst stage.

Probable cause: The membranes of the embryos are rubbery.

Suggested remedy: Use a cooling stage if possible (set to 10–15 °C), or precool the embryos and injection medium in the fridge or on ice for about ten minutes before injection. This helps stiffen the membranes and makes injection easier. If precooling the embryos and medium, inject only small batches of embryos at a time and replace the embryos and injection medium frequently.

Probable cause: The injection pipette is blunt.

Suggested remedy: The micropipette can easily become dulled by cell debris, or the point can be broken if knocked against the base of the injection chamber or the holding pipette. Check the point on the micropipette and be prepared to change it frequently if it is not performing as expected.

Probable cause: The injection technique is suboptimal.

Suggested remedy: Target the junction between two trophectoderm cells and be sure to use a short, sharp, jabbing action to pierce through the cell layer into the blastocoel.

11.4.8 Problem – the ESCs rush out of the embryo when the injection pipette is withdrawn

Probable cause: Injection has increased the pressure in the blastocoel.

Suggested remedy: Allow time after the ESCs have been expelled into the blastocoel for the pressure to equilibrate, or actively draw back some fluid from the blastocoel cavity (carefully avoiding the ESCs) before withdrawing the micropipette – you can even afford to reduce the pressure to the extent that the embryo collapses very slightly.

11.4.9 Problem – it is not possible to keep the injected separate from non-injected embryos

Probable cause: Using a depression injection chamber causes aggregation of the embryos in the chamber as the embryos converge at the bottom of the well.

Suggested remedy: Use a flat four- or eight-well tissue culture glass slide. The media chamber is detached, leaving the glass slide with the gasket separating the wells. This gasket also prevents the oil from spreading over a large area of the slide, thus ensuring that the M2 droplet is always covered.

11.4.10 Problem – the oviduct wall is punctured during transfer

Probable cause: The glass transfer pipette has a jagged tip.

Suggested remedy: After cutting the pulled pipette with a diamond pen, expose the tip for a few seconds near a naked flame to bevel the end. This will also allow deeper penetration of the pipette into the oviduct, as it will be easier to thread the oviduct over the pipette.

11.4.11   Problem – backflow of media/bursal fluid/blood into the transfer pipette

Probable cause: Not enough media or oil in the pipette.

Suggested remedy: Aspirate enough media or oil into the pipette until the capillary action stops. However, oil droplets can line the inside of the pipette and hamper the smooth flow of the embryos during the transfer procedure. M2 can be used as an alternative liquid to prevent this backflow. Generally, M2 is aspirated until capillary action stops, then an air bubble is sucked in, then a series of small amounts of M2 and air bubbles are sucked in, with the last column of M2 containing the injected embryos (see Figure 11.4).

11.4.12   Problem – bleeding in the infundibulum/oviduct area

Probable cause: Rupture of blood vessels/capillaries when tearing the bursa to access the infundibulum during oviduct transfer of injected embryos.

Suggested remedy: Flush the area with sterile saline solution to wash away the blood. Then dry the area using sterile Whatmann paper cut into small pieces. Replace the soaked paper as the need arises.

11.4.13   Problem – unable to determine whether DNA is toxic to the embryo without waiting until recipient females give birth

Probable cause: Contaminants such as phenol or ethanol may have come through during DNA preparation, which is toxic to the injected embryos.

Suggested remedy: Culturing a number of injected embryos until the blastocyst stage will generally reflect the quality of the microinjection DNA. Around 90% of non-injected one-cell embryos develop to the blastocyst stage in culture. The number will be lower in the injected embryos, but at least 50% should develop to the blastocyst stage. This will also assess the quality of the media.

11.4.14   Problem – unable to assess the pregnancy status of recipient females

Probable cause: The transferred embryos may not be developing in utero and are being reabsorbed. This may be due to a lethal effect of the injected DNA on normal mouse development. Embryos that are high transgene expressors may also die in utero.

Suggested remedy: A simple way of determining whether the females are getting pregnant is by weighing them after oviduct transfer. They should gain weight by about 3–5 g a few days after the procedure. Weighing the females on a regular basis (every three to five days) until about two weeks post-transfer is a simple way of gauging pregnancy status.

11.4.15 Problem – lack of pups born to recipient females (uninjected blastocysts/unmanipulated morulae give plenty of pups)

Probable cause: ESCs grow and divide rapidly and are capable of overgrowing the blastocyst/morula rather than coming under its control and growing in a regulated manner.

Suggested remedy: (1) Try using fewer ESCs per embryo so that any chemical or contact signals provided by the blastocyst/morula are not diluted amongst too many ESCs to be effective. Good chimaeras can be produced with very few ESCs. (2) Try altering the injection or co-culture medium so that it favours embryo development over ESC growth. This may be sufficient to shift the balance in favour of chimaerism rather than ESC growth overtaking the embryo.

11.4.16 Problem – chimaeras have low ESC-derived coat colour/are unable to transmit targeted allele to F1 pups

Probable cause: Too few ESCs have been used to generate chimaeras.

Suggested remedy: Try generating chimaeras using more ESCs per embryo (bearing in mind the possible problems raised in section 11.4.15).

Probable cause: ESCs have undergone some crisis during culture that has caused them to differentiate to some degree.

Suggested remedy: (1) Try generating chimaeras with another cell line carrying the same genetic manipulation. (2) Review tissue culture conditions to ensure that the best possible reagents/conditions are being used and, if necessary, begin transfection of ESCs from the start.

12 New and advanced techniques

The successful development of micromanipulation techniques for ICSI and PGD has stimulated research into further potential clinical applications. Putative beneficial uses of this technology have included the use of empty ZPs for the cryopreservation of spermatozoa (Cohen *et al.*, 1997a), the transfer of ooplasm from one oocyte to another (Cohen *et al.*, 1997b), the transfer of a GV from one oocyte to an enucleated oocyte (Zhang *et al.*, 1999), ploidy reduction by removal of pronuclei from polyploid zygotes (Rawlins *et al.*, 1988), and the removal of fragments of cytoplasm from fragmented embryos (Alikani *et al.*, 1999). Almost all of these techniques are still at an early research stage and have yet to be proven unequivocally to have beneficial clinical application. Indeed, some of these techniques have become controversial due to concern over their safety, such as the possible inheritance of defective mitochondrial DNA, which could lead to disease in later life. It is not within the scope of this book to review exhaustively all of the new applications currently being researched. However, some of these techniques merit further description by virtue of their perceived benefit to the enhancement of reproductive and therapeutic potential. Consequently, these will be discussed briefly in this chapter.

12.1 CRYOPRESERVATION OF SPERMATOZOA WITHIN THE ZP

Some patients have sparingly few spermatozoa, such as those presenting with cryptozoospermia and those requiring surgical sperm recovery, particularly patients with non-obstructive azoospermia. In these instances, conventional methods for cryopreserving spermatozoa are relatively ineffective because of the extreme difficulty, following thawing, in locating and identifying the few motile spermatozoa that were originally frozen. Nevertheless, it may be important to cryopreserve whatever can be retrieved from the ejaculate or a biopsy taken from either the epididymis or testis, particularly where there is no guarantee of retrieving anything on a subsequent occasion. Therefore, there is a need to develop techniques whereby a few or even single spermatozoa may be recovered successfully following cryopreservation. Jacques Cohen and colleagues (1997a) designed one solution to this problem: their approach utilizes empty ZP prepared from mammalian oocytes. Following removal of the entire contents of the oocyte by aspiration into a micropipette, motile human spermatozoa can be transferred into the empty ZP using a standard ICSI injection pipette. ZP bearing human spermatozoa can then be equilibrated with cryoprotectant containing glycerol, loaded into embryo freezing straws, and frozen using a fast protocol. Upon thawing prior to use in a treatment cycle, the spermatozoa within the ZP can be located and aspirated using an ICSI micropipette. This approach benefits from the knowledge that any spermatozoa recovered from the ZP are likely to be effective in achieving fertilization providing that they were viable at the time of freezing. However, there may be some concern over the use of biological material from another species, although the ZP is a relatively inert tissue. In such instances, a modified approach might be to use empty ZP prepared from donated human oocytes or embryos.

12.2 FRAGMENT REMOVAL

Fragmentation of human embryos is often seen, especially in patients of advanced maternal age. The degree and pattern of fragmentation is generally related to the likelihood of pregnancy occurring following embryo transfer, with highly fragmented embryos usually resulting in implantation failure (Alikani *et al.*, 1999). The cause of fragmentation and its effect upon embryogenesis remain to be established. However, it is likely to be related in some way to apoptosis (Jurisicova *et al.*, 1996). It has been suggested that such fragments might induce apoptosis of neighbouring blastomeres through toxin release during degeneration. Fragmented embryos can be genetically normal, so it may benefit their development if fragments are removed. Fragments can be removed from embryos following ZD (see sections 9.1.2–9.1.4). Typically, a micropipette with an outer diameter of 10–12 μm is passed through the hole drilled in the ZP and fragments are removed carefully by gentle aspiration (Alikani *et al.*, 1999). This technique shows promise for the rescue of embryos that might otherwise fail to develop normally and implant.

12.3 VISUALIZATION OF THE MEIOTIC SPINDLE FOR ICSI

Embryos generated from sperm microinjection generally have lower morphology scores than embryos generated from standard IVF techniques (Hsu *et al.*, 1999). This may be due in part to the physical insertion of a pipette into the oocyte and the mechanical aspiration of the ooplasm, or in part by the ability to disrupt the meiotic spindle during preparation for microinjection or during ICSI (Eichenlaub-Ritter *et al.*, 2002). The routine process of aligning the PB of the oocyte at a position away from the microinjection pipette is one method of reducing the risk of disrupting the spindle. However, this relies on the assumption that the PB and spindle are still in close proximity following removal of the cumulus cells and denudation of the oocyte via the mechanical removal of the coronal cells.

Determining the location of the meiotic spindle in a live oocyte being used for microinjection has been a difficult technique in the past. In mammals that have a large, obvious meiotic spindle, the spindle can be detected easily using optics such as Nomarski DIC; however, in human oocytes, it is somewhat more difficult. Whilst a small (15–20 μm in length) translucent oval can often be seen either perpendicular or close to the oolemma (using $800\times$ magnification), positively identifying this structure as a spindle instead of other cytoplasmic inclusions such as microvacuoles is a difficult task. The use of fluorochromes to positively locate the spindle is effective in oocytes used in research, but this approach is useless in oocytes being used for live microinjection. These problems can be overcome by the use of polarized light (PolScope and LC-SpindleView, Cell Robotics International). Modifications to the bright field light pathway and the use of attachments to the inverted microscope allow birefringence (the splitting of one beam of light into two) to be detected and the degree of divergence of light around the spindle can be measured. The use of complex algorithms within software programs allows this information to be displayed as a digital image for storage, or the spindle location can even be seen down the eyepieces of the inverted microscope. This ingenious process allows the spindle to be visualized relatively simply and non-invasively.

Recently, polarized light has been used to determine the presence, absence or location of the meiotic spindle in human oocytes. This non-invasive process has already shown that oocytes with visible spindles display a higher fertilization and development rate (Wang *et al.*, 2001a; Wang *et al.*, 2001b) and that the spindle is highly thermosensitive (Wang *et al.*, 2001c; Wang *et al.*, 2001d). Previous research indicates that the first polar body (PB1) is a poor indicator of the location of the meiotic spindle (Silva *et al.*, 1999; Hardarson *et al.*, 2000). Furthermore, oocytes aligned for ICSI relative to the spindle instead of the PB1 develop embryos of better morphology and have less fragmentation (Cooke *et al.*, 2003). Indeed, it may be possible to control the polarity and subsequent development of

Figure 12.1 The locations of the PB1 and the meiotic spindle vary within different MII oocytes. The PB1 is in the 12 o'clock position in the two oocytes at the top of the figure but the spindle location can be far from (a) or near to (b) it. The PB1 in the two oocytes at the bottom of the figure is at 2 o'clock (c) and at 11 o'clock (d), but the spindle is not located nearby. Injection of the oocytes with the spindle located at 3 o'clock (a) or 9 o'clock (d) could have resulted in damage to it.

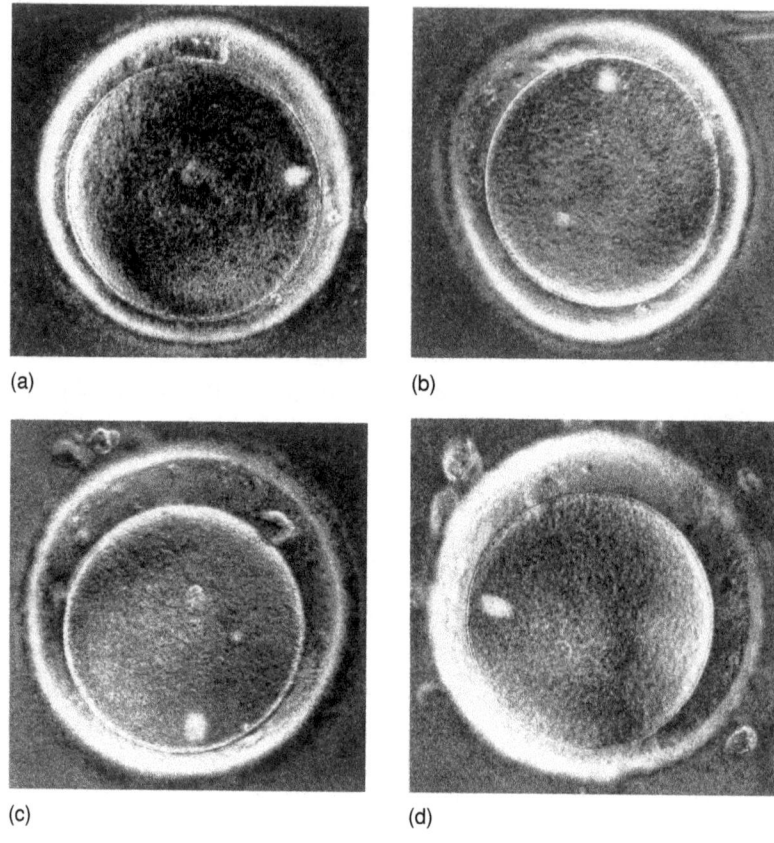

(a)

(b)

(c)

(d)

microinjected oocytes using visualization of the meiotic spindle (Cooke *et al.*, 2003).

The four oocytes in Figure 12.1 show the meiotic spindle as a bright white area within the ooplasm when viewed using the PolScope. The meiotic spindle can be seen at many locations around the oocyte and even in the opposite hemisphere of the oocyte to that of the PB1. Whilst the PB1 may have had a relationship with the spindle at the time of its extrusion into the PVS, the subsequent movement of the PB now means that it is really not a reliable marker of the location of the meiotic spindle.

The use of a PolScope to identify the meiotic spindle and align oocytes and embryos has not been used in any great numbers or indeed in a large number of IVF units. However, it demonstrates the current limitations of laboratory-based manipulation and alignment of oocytes. These new and more in-depth techniques associated with microinjected oocytes may become necessary to consistently avoid the maternal spindle and aid in the control of polarity and the subsequent improvement in development of human embryos.

12.4 OOPLASMIC TRANSFER AND GV TRANSFER

Some patients may experience infertility due to an inherent defect within the oocyte itself, such as insufficient cytoplasmic mitochondria or incomplete cytoplasmic maturation. Whilst the use of donor oocytes in place of a patient's own oocytes constitutes an obvious solution to this problem, most patients would prefer an approach that enables them to remain the genetic parent of their children. In an attempt to resolve these issues, various concepts have been formulated and developed by Cohen and colleagues (1997b). In theory, it is conceivable that such problems might be remedied by supplementing the patient's oocytes with ooplasm from donor oocytes, so restoring their reproductive potential. There are several ways in which ooplasmic transfer may be achieved, including electrofusion. However, the simplest method is to aspirate a small volume of ooplasm from a donor oocyte along with a spermatozoon, injecting both into the patient's oocyte during an ICSI procedure. Another, technically more demanding, approach is to remove the GV from immature donor oocytes and replace them with the GV from the patient's own immature oocytes (Zhang *et al.*, 1999). The oocytes reconstructed in this way can then be matured in vitro prior to ICSI. Both ooplasmic transfer and GV transfer maintain the genetic parentage of the patient. However, concern has been expressed over the transfer of mitochondrial DNA, present within the ooplasm, from the donor oocyte to the patient's oocyte and the possible consequences this might have on subsequent health in later life (Hawes *et al.*, 2002). Indeed, the Food and Drug Administration (FDA) of the USA effectively banned such treatment in 2001, amid concern over the unknown safety of any treatment that genetically alters oocytes or embryos.

12.5 SOMATIC CELL NUCLEAR TRANSFER

Human embryos derived by somatic cell nuclear transfer (SCNT) offer a means of therapeutic cloning that has the potential to overcome the major problem of histocompatibility. The SCNT procedure involves the enucleation of a mature oocyte followed by microinjection of a somatic cell nucleus into its ooplasm, and oocyte activation to initiate embryogenesis. Using such an approach, embryo development up to the six-cell stage has been reported recently (Cibelli *et al.*, 2001). The technique employed by these authors included the aspiration of the oocyte's chromosomes and adjacent cytosol using a 10-μm internal diameter, blunt micropipette and piezoelectric device following their visualization with the fluorescent dye bisbenzimide. Adult cumulus cells were used as the source of somatic cell nuclei, the nuclei being isolated by aspirating the cells in and out of a 5-μm internal diameter micropipette. The isolated nuclei were then injected into the ooplasm of the enucleated oocytes and the reconstructed oocytes were activated one to three hours later by exposing them to 5 μM ionomycin for four minutes followed by 2 mM 6-dimethylaminopurine for three hours (Nakagawa *et al.*, 2001). The fact that SCNT in the human oocyte has resulted in only limited embryonic development suggests that many technical problems inherent in the technique have yet to be overcome, including enucleation, nuclear transfer, oocyte activation, and reprogramming of the somatic cell nucleus. However, the putative therapeutic potential of ESCs derived through SCNT demands that these problems be overcome. Furthermore, modification of somatic cell nuclei before nuclear transfer offers the potential for gene therapy via the generation of genetically modified ESCs.

12.6 HAPLOIDIZATION

Haploidization is a theoretical method that has been forwarded as a potential means of allowing women without their own oocytes to become the genetic and biological mothers of their offspring (Tsai *et al.*, 2000). This technique relies upon oocyte reconstruction from artificially haploidized somatic cells and enucleated oocytes and, therefore, represents a form of semi-reproductive cloning. Theoretically, at least, there are several ways in which this might be achieved. It appears that the ooplasm of the mature human oocyte has the capacity to force a somatic cell nucleus to undergo a premature M phase (without the S phase) of mitosis, resulting in the extrusion of one set of single-chromatid chromosomes within a pseudo-PB2 (Tesarik *et al.*, 2001). Alternatively, the diploid somatic cell nucleus can be transformed into a haploid nucleus following meiosis and extrusion of the PB1, effectively yielding a reconstructed oocyte. This technique involves the enucleation of a GV oocyte (see section 12.4) followed by subzonal injection of a somatic cell and electrofusion to initiate embryogenesis. Haploidization has been shown recently to have potential for oocyte reconstruction using the mouse as an animal model (Palermo *et al.*, 2002). The technique employed by these authors initially required the production of ooplasts through the aspiration of the GV from mouse oocytes using a 20-μm internal diameter blunt micropipette. Adult human endometrial stromal cells were used as the source of somatic cell nuclei, the cells being isolated, injected into the PVS of the ooplasts, and then subjected to electrofusion. The oocytes reconstructed in this way were cultured until they extruded the PB1, most of those undergoing this transformation subsequently being shown to have a haploid complement of chromosomes. Oocytes reconstructed in this way can be fertilized by ICSI and therefore may provide a means of producing embryos containing both maternal and paternal genomes. Another modification of this technique has been to use haploidized cumulus cells to fertilize mouse oocytes, suggesting a possible avenue for azoospermic men to become the biological and genetic parents of their own offspring (Lacham-Kaplan *et al.*, 2001).

Naturally, the therapeutic promise of these techniques of SCNT and haploidization must be tempered by full consideration of inadvertent aneuploidies, inadequate somatic cell nuclear reprogramming, and abnormal genomic imprinting, to name but a few of the possible risks. Therefore, it would be scientifically and ethically irresponsible to apply these techniques clinically without their full validation in animal models. Indeed, micromanipulation has proven to be a technique that has enabled us to realize fully our reproductive potential and yet at the same time has challenged the ethics of our society in ways previously unimaginable.

Appendix
Suppliers and manufacturers of equipment and consumables

Baxter Healthcare Corp.
1 Baxter Parkway, Deerfield, IL 60015, USA
Tel:+1 847 948 2000; fax:+1 847 948 4489
http://www.baxter.com

B. Braun Medical Ltd
Thorncliffe Park, Sheffield S35 2PW, UK
Tel:+44 114 225 9000; fax:+44 114 225 9111;
email: info.bbmuk@bbraun.com
http://www.bbraun.co.uk

BDH Laboratory Supplies
Merck House, Poole, Dorset BH15 1TD, UK
Tel:+44 1202 660 444; fax:+44 1202 666 856; email: export@bdh.com
http://www.bdh.com

Becton Dickinson & Company Ltd
1 Becton Drive, Franklin Lakes, NJ 07417–1886, USA
Tel:+1 888 237 2762; fax:+1 800 847 2220; email: labware@bd.com
http://www.bd.com

Cambridge Research & Instrumentation (CRI), Inc.
35-B Cabot Road, Woburn, MA 01801, USA
Tel:+1 781 935 9099; fax:+1 781 935 3388; email: sales@cri-inc.com
http://www.cri-inc.com

Campden Instruments Ltd
4 Park Road, Sileby, Loughborough, Leicestershire LE12 7TJ, UK
Tel:+44 870 240 3702; email: mail@campden-inst.com
http://www.campden-inst.com

Carl Zeiss
Königsallee 9–21, 37081 Göttingen, Germany
Tel:+49 551 5060 660; fax:+49 551 5060 480;
email: mikro.verkauf@zeiss.de
http://www.zeiss.de

Cell Robotics International, Inc.
2715 Broadbent Parkway NE, Albuquerque, NM 87107, USA
Tel:+1 505 343 1131; fax:+1 505 344 8112; email: crii@cellrobotics.com
http://www.cellrobotics.com

Conception Technologies
6835 Flanders Drive, Suite 500, San Diego, CA 92121, USA
Tel:+1 858 824 0888; fax:+1 858 824 0891;
email: info@conceptiontechnologies.com
http://www.conceptiontechnologies.com

COOK IVF
12 Electronics Street, Brisbane Technology Park, Eight Mile Plains, QLD 4113, Australia
Tel:+61 7 3841 1188; fax:+61 7 3841 1288;
email: custserv@cookaust.com.au
http://www.cookivf.com

Eppendorf AG
Barkhausenweg 1, 22339 Hamburg, Germany
Tel:+49 40 53 8010; fax: 49 40 538 01556;
email: eppendorf@eppendorf.com
http://www.eppendorf.com

ETHICON Inc.
PO box 151, Somerville, NJ 088760151, USA
Tel:+1 800 255 2500; fax:+1 732 562 2212;
email: customersupport@eesus.jnj.com
http://www.ethiconinc.com

Falcon
See Becton Dickinson & Company Limited

GIBCO BRL
Invitrogen Ltd, 3 Fountain Drive, Inchinnan Business Park, Paisley PA4 9RF, UK
Tel:+44 141 814 6100; fax:+44 141 814 6287; email: mail@invitrogen.com
http://www.invitrogen.com

GlaxoSmithKline
Glaxo Wellcome UK Ltd, Stockley Park West, Uxbridge, Middlesex UB11 1BT, UK
Tel:+44 20 8990 9000; fax:+44 20 8990 4321
http://www.gsk.com

Graticules Limited
Pyser-SGI Ltd, Fircroft Way, Edenbridge, Kent TN8 6HA, UK
Tel:+44 1732 864 111; fax:+44 1732 865 544; email: sales@pyser-sgi.com
http://www.pyser-sgi.com

Greiner GmbH
Maybachstrasse 2, D-72636 Frickenhausen, Germany
Tel:+49 70 229 480; fax:+49 70 2294 8514
http://www.greiner-lab.com

Gynetics Medical Products
St Odilialaan 125, 3930 Hamont-Achel, Belgium
Tel:+32 11 645 872; fax:+32 11 640 677; email: info@gynetics.be
http://www.gynetics.be

Hamilton Company
PO Box 10030, Reno, NV 895200012, USA
Tel:+1 775 858 3000; fax:+1775 856 7259;
email: sales@hamiltoncompany.com
http://www.hamiltoncompany.com

Hobson Tracking Systems Ltd
697 Abbey Lane, Sheffield, South Yorkshire S11 9ND, UK
Tel/fax:+44 114 235 0076

Hoescht AG
Aventis S.A., F-67917, Strasbourg, France
Tel:+49 69 30 51 40 72; fax:+49 69 30 53 67 87; email: info@hoechst.com
http://www.hoechst.com

Hoffman Optics
Modulation Optics Inc., 100 Forest Drive at East Hills, Greenvale, NY 11548, USA
Tel:+1 516 484 8882; fax:+1 516 621 4768; email: modopt@aol.com
http://www.modulationoptics.com

Humagen Fertility Diagnostics Inc.
2400 Hunter's Way, Charlottesville, VA 22911, USA
Tel:+1 434 979 4000; fax:+1 434 295 5912; email: humagen@earthlink.net
http://www.humagenivf.com

Hunter Scientific Ltd
Unit 1, Priors Hall Barn, Widdington, Saffron Walden, Essex CB11 3SB, UK
Tel:+44 1799 541 688; fax:+44 1799 541 703;
email: sales@hunterscientific.com
http:// www.hunterscientific.com

Irvine Scientific
2511 Daimler Street, Santa Ana, CA 92705-5588, USA
Tel:+1 949 261 7800; fax:+1 949 261 6522; email: nucleus@irvinesci.com
http://irvinesci.com

Leica Microsystems AG
Ernst-Leitz-Strasse 17-37, 35578 Wetzlar, Germany
Tel:+49 6441 290; fax:+49 6441 292 590
http://www.leica-microsystems.com

Lindsey Optical Ltd
2a Walden Road, Sewards End, Saffron Walden CB10 2LE, UK
Tel:+44 1799 513 613; fax:+44 870 163 4672;
email: sales@lindseyoptical.co.uk
http://www.lindseyoptical.co.uk

Linkam Scientific Instruments
8 Epsom Downs Metro Centre, Waterfield, Tadworth, Surrey KT20 5HT, UK
Tel:+44 1737 363 476; fax:+44 1737 363 480; email: info@linkam.co.uk
http://www.linkam.co.uk

LIP (Equipment & Services) Ltd
Bibby Sterilin Ltd, Tilling Drive, Stone, Staffordshire ST15 0SA, UK
Tel:+44 1785 812 121; fax:+44 1785 813 748;
email: export.enquiry@lip.org.uk
http://www.lip.org.uk

MediCult Imperial Laboratories Ltd
Møllehaven 12, DK-4040 Jyllinge, Denmark
Tel:+45 46 79 0200; fax:+45 4 679 0300;
email: medi-cult@medi-cult.dk
www.medi-cult.com

MicroData Instrument Inc.
1207 Hogan Drive, South Plainfield, NJ 07080, USA
Tel:+1 908 222 1717; fax:+1 908 222 1365; email: info@microdatamdi.com
http://www.microdatamdi.com

MidAtlantic Diagnostics Inc.
438 North Elmwood Road, Marlton, NJ 08053, USA
Tel:+1 856 762 2000; fax:+1 856 762 2009;
email: info@midatlanticdiagnostics.com
http://www.midatlanticdiagnostics.com

Millipore Corp.
80 Ashby Road, Bedford, MA 01730, USA
Tel:+1 617 275 9200; fax:+1 781 533 3110
http://www.millipore.com

MTM Medical Technologies Montreux SA
PO Box 431, Rue du Collège 26, CH-1815 Clarens/Montreux, Switzerland
Tel:+41 21 989 8787; fax:+41 21 989 8789; email: mtm@mtmsa.ch

Narishige Scientific Instrument Laboratory
27-9 Minamikarasuyama 4-chome, Setagaya-ku, Tokyo 157-0062, Japan
Tel:+81 3 3308 8233; fax:+81 3 3308 2005; email: sales@narishige.co.jp
http://www.narishige.co.jp

NidaCon International AB
Mölndalsvägen 22, S-412 63 Gothenburg, Sweden
Tel:+46 31 405 440; fax:+46 31 405 415; email: contact@nidacon.com
http://www.nidacon.com

Nikon Instech Company Ltd
Parale Mitsui Building, 8 Higashida-cho, Kawasaki-ku, Kanagawa 2100005, Japan
Tel:+81 44 223 2167; fax:+81 44 223 2182;
email: bio_micr@nikongw.nikon.co.jp
http://www.ave.nikon.co.jp/inst

Nunc A/S
Kamstrupvej 90, Postbox 280, DK-4000 Roskilde, Denmark
Tel:+45 4631 2000; fax:+45 4631 2175; email: infociety@nunc.dk
http://www.nuncbrand.com

Olympus Optical Company Ltd
43–2, 2-chome, Hatagaya, Shibuya-Ku, Tokyo, Japan
Tel:+81 3 3377 2286; fax:+81 3 3375 6550; email: pr_dept@olympus.co.jp
http://www.olympus.co.jp/indexE.html

Pharmacia Corp.
100 Route 206 North, Peapack, NJ 07977, USA
Tel:+1 908 901 8000; fax:+1 908 901 8379;
email: webmaster.int@am.pnu.com
http://www.pharmacia.com

Research Instruments Ltd
Kernick Road, Penryn, Cornwall TR10 9DQ, UK
Tel:+44 1326 372 753; fax:+44 1326 378 783;
email: support@research-instruments.com
http://research-instruments.com

Rocket Medical plc
Imperial Way, Watford, Hertfordshire WD24 4XX, UK
Tel:+44 1923 651 404; fax:+44 1923 240 334;
email: exportsales@rocketmedical.com
http://www.rocketmedical.com

SAGE BioPharma
Bedminster One, 135 Route 202/206, Bedminster, NJ 07921, USA
Tel:+1 908 306 5790
http://www.sagebiopharma.com

Sarstedt
Postfach 12 20, D-51582 Nümbrecht, Germany
Tel:+49 22 933 050; fax:+49 22 9330 5122; email: info@sarstedt.com
http://www.sarstedt.com

Sefi Medical Instruments Ltd
50 Disraeli Street, Haifa 34334, Israel
Tel:+972 4 825 1651; fax:+972 4 825 8903; email: makler@netvision.net.il
http://sefimedical.com

Sigma-Aldrich Corp.
30350 Spurse Street, St Louis, MO 63103, USA
Tel:+1 314 771 5765; fax:+1 314 771 5757; email: custserv@sial.com
http://www.sigmaaldrich.com

SL Microtest GmbH
MMI AG, Flughofstrasse 37, 8152 Zürich-Glattbrugg, Switzerland
Tel:+41 1 809 1010; fax:+41 1 809 1011;
email: postmaster@sl-microtest.com
http://www.sl-microtest.com

Sutter Instrument Company
51 Digital Drive, Novato, Ca 94949, USA
Tel:+1 415 883 0128; fax:+1 415 883 0572; email: info@sutter.com
http://www.sutter.com

The Pipette Company Pty Limited
3032 Stirling Street, Thebarton, SA 5031, Australia
Tel:+61 8 8152 0266; fax:+61 8 8152 0277; email: tpc@pipetteco.com
http://www.pipette.com

Vitrolife Sweden AB Fertility Systems
Mölndalsvägen 30, SE-412 63 Göteborg, Sweden
Tel:+46 21 721 8000; fax:+46 31 721 8090; email: fertility@vitrolife.com
http://www.vitrolife.com

Wallace Women's Healthcare
Portex Limited, Hythe CT21 5BN, UK
Tel:+44 1303 260 551; fax:+44 1303 266 761; email: info@wallaceivf.com
http://www.smiths-medical.com

Wild Leitz

See Leica Microsystems AG

Wilkes Iris Diaphragm Co. Ltd

Widco Works, London Road, Bexhill-on-Sea, East Sussex TN39 3LE, UK

Tel:+44 1424 217 630; fax:+44 1424 215 406; email: ashley@wilkes-iris.com

http://www.wilkes-iris.com

WillCo Wells B.V.

WG-Plein 287, 1054 SE Amsterdam, the Netherlands

Tel:+31 20 685 0171; fax:+31 20 685 0333; email: info@willcowells.com

http://www.willcowells.com

World Precision Instruments Inc.

175 Sarasota Center Boulevard, Sarasota, Fl 34240, USA

Tel:+1 941 371 1003; fax:+1 941 377 5428;

email: microinjection@wpiinc.com

http://www.wpiinc.com

References

Abbondanzo, S., Gadi, I. and Stewart, C. (1993). Derivation of embryonic stem cell lines. In *Methods in Enzymology*, ed. P.M. Wassarman and M.L. De Pamphilis. p. 803. New York: Academic Press.

Abdelmassih, S., Cardoso, J., Abdelmassih, V., Dias, J., Abdelmassih, R. and Nagy, Z. (2002). Laser-assisted ICSI: a novel approach to obtain higher oocyte survival and embryo quality rates. *Hum. Reprod.* **17**, 2694–9.

Al-Hasani, S., Bauer, O., Ludwig, M., *et al.* (1999). Results of intracytoplasmic sperm injection using the microprocessor controlled TransferMan Eppendorf manipulator system. *Middle East Fertil. Soc. J.* **1**, 41–4.

Alikani, M., Cohen, J., Tomkin, G., Garrisi, G., Mack, C. and Scott, R. (1999). Human embryo fragmentation in vitro and its implications for pregnancy and implantation. *Fertil. Steril.* **71**, 836–42.

Aslam, I. and Fishel, S. (1998). Short-term in-vitro culture and cryopreservation of spermatogenic cells used for human in-vitro conception. *Hum. Reprod.* **13**, 634–8.

Aslam, I., Robins, A., Dowell, K. and Fishel, S. (1998). Isolation, purification and assessment of viability of spermatogenic cells from testicular biopsies of azoospermic men. *Hum. Reprod.* **13**, 639–45.

Balaban, B., Urman, B., Alatas, C., Mercan, R., Mumcu, A. and Isiklar, A. (2002). A comparison of four different techniques of assisted hatching. *Hum. Reprod.* **17**, 1239–43.

Balakier, H., Bouman, D., Sojecki, A., Librach, C. and Squire, J. (2002). Morphological and cytogenetic analysis of human giant oocytes and giant embryos. *Hum. Reprod.* **17**, 2394–401.

Barnes, F., Crombie, A., Gardner, D., *et al.* (1995). Blastocyst development and birth after in-vitro maturation of human primary oocytes, intracytoplasmic sperm injection and assisted hatching. *Hum. Reprod.* **10**, 3243–7.

Bellve, R. (1993). Purification, culture and fractionation of spermatogenic cells. *Methods Enzymol.* **225**, 84–113.

Blake, M., Garrisi, J., Tomkin, G. and Cohen, J. (2000). Sperm deposition site during ICSI affects fertilization and development. *Fertil. Steril.* **73**, 31–7.

Blanchard, Y., Lavault, M., Quernee, D., Le Lannou, D., Lobel, B. and Lescoat, D. (1991). Preparation of spermatogenic cell populations at specific stages of differentiation in the human. *Mol. Reprod. Dev.* **30**, 275–82.

Bongso, T., Sathananthan, A., Wong, P., *et al.* (1989). Human fertilization by micro-injection of immotile spermatozoa. *Hum. Reprod.* **4**, 175–9.

Bras, M., Dumoulin, J., Pieters, M., Michiels, A., Geraedts, J. and Evers, J. (1994). The use of a mouse zygote quality control system for training purposes and toxicity determination in an ICSI programme. *Hum. Reprod.* **9** (Suppl. 4), 23.

Brinster, R., Chen, H., Trumbauer, M., Yagle, M. and Palmiter, R. (1985). Factors affecting the efficiency of introducing foreign DNA into mice by microinjecting eggs. *Proc. Natl. Acad. Sci. USA* **82**, 4438–42.

Brown, K. and Flaming, D. (1974). Beveling of fine micropipette electrodes by a rapid precision method. *Science* **185**, 693–5.

Cabot, R., Kuhholzer, B., Chan, A., *et al.* (2001). Transgenic pigs produced using in vitro matured oocytes infected with a retroviral vector. *Anim. Biotechnol.* **12**, 205–14

Campbell, K. (2002). A background to nuclear transfer and its applications in agriculture and human therapeutic medicine. *J. Anat.* **200**, 267–75.

Cha, K. and Chian, R. (1998). Maturation in vitro of immature human oocytes for clinical use. *Hum. Reprod. Update* **4**, 103–20.

Cha, K., Koo, J., Ko, J., Choi, D., Han, S. and Yoon, T. (1991). Pregnancy after in vitro fertilization of human follicular oocytes collected from nonstimulated cycles, their culture in vitro and their transfer in a donor oocyte program. *Fertil. Steril.* **55**, 109–13.

Chan, A., Chong, K., Martinovich, C., Simerly, C. and Schatten, G. (2002). Transgenic monkeys produced by retroviral gene transfer into mature oocytes. *Science* **291**, 309–12.

Chan, A., Luetjens, C., Dominko, T., *et al.* (2000). Foreign DNA transmission by ICSI: injection of spermatozoa bound with exogenous DNA results in embryonic GFP expression and live Rhesus monkey births. *Mol. Hum. Reprod.* **6**, 26–33.

Cibelli, J., Kiessling, A., Cunniff, K., Richards, C., Lanza, R. and West, M. (2001). Somatic cell nuclear transfer in humans: pronuclear and early embryonic development. *J. Regenerative Med.* **2**, 25–31.

Cohen, J., Malter, H., Fehilly, C., *et al.* (1988). Implantation of embryos after partial opening of oocyte zona pellucida to facilitate sperm penetration. *Lancet* **2**, 162.

Cohen, J., Elsner, C., Kort, H., *et al.* (1990). Impairment of the hatching process following in vitro fertilization in the human and improvement of implantation by assisting hatching using micromanipulation. *Hum. Reprod.* **5**, 7–13.

Cohen, J., Malter, H., Talansky, B. and Grifo, J. (1992). *Micromanipulation of Human Gametes and Embryos.* New York: Raven Press.

Cohen, J., Garrisi, G., Congedo-Ferrara, T., Kieck, K., Schimmel, T. and Scott, R. (1997a). Cryopreservation of single human spermatozoa. *Hum. Reprod.* **12**, 994–1001.

Cohen, J., Scott, R., Schimmel, T., Levron, J. and Willadsen, S. (1997b). Birth of infant after transfer of anucleate donor oocyte cytoplasm into recipient eggs. *Lancet* **350**, 186–7.

Cooke, S. Tyler, J. and Driscoll, G. (2003). Meiotic spindle location and identification and its effect on embryonic cleavage plane and early development. *Hum. Reprod.*, in press.

Coskun, S., Tbakhi, A., Jaroudi, K., Uzumcu, M., Merdad, T. and Al-Hussein, K. (2002). Flow cytometric ploidy analysis of testicular biopsies from sperm-negative wet preparations. *Hum. Reprod.* **17**, 977–83.

Coticchio, G. and Fleming, S. (1998). Inhibition of phosphoinositide metabolism or chelation of intracellular calcium blocks FSH-induced but not spontaneous meiotic resumption in mouse oocytes. *Dev. Biol.* **203**, 201–9.

Crabbe, E., Verheyen, G., Tournaye, H. and Van Steirteghem, A. (1997). The use of enzymatic procedures to recover testicular germ cells. *Hum. Reprod.* **12**, 1682–7.

Crabbe, E., Verheyen, G., Silber, S., *et al.* (1998). Enzymatic digestion of testicular tissue may rescue the intracytoplasmic sperm injection cycle in some patients with non-obstructive azoospermia. *Hum. Reprod.* **13**, 2791–6.

Cremades, N., Sousa, M., Bernabeu, R. and Barros, A. (2001). Developmental potential of elongating and elongated spermatids obtained after in-vitro maturation of isolated round spermatids. *Hum. Reprod.* **16**, 1938–44.

De Vos, A., Nagy, Z., Van de Velde, H., Joris, H., Bocken, G. and Van Steirteghem, A. (1997). Percoll gradient centrifugation can be omitted in sperm preparation for intracytoplasmic sperm injection. *Hum. Reprod.* **12**, 1980–84.

Doetschman, T., Eistetter, H., Katz, M., Schmidt, W. and Kamler, R. (1985). The in vitro development of blastocyst-derived embryonic stem cell lines: formation of visceral yolk sac, blood islands and myocardium. *J. Embryol. Exp. Morphol.* **87**, 27–45.

Dozortsev, D., De Sutter, P. and Dhont, M. (1994). Behaviour of spermatozoa in human oocytes displaying no or one pronucleus after intracytoplasmic sperm injection. *Hum. Reprod.* **9**, 2139–44.

Dumoulin, J., Bras, M., Coonen, E., Dreesen, J., Geraedts, J. and Evers, J. (1998). Effect of Ca^{2+}/Mg^{2+}-free medium on the biopsy procedure for preimplantation genetic diagnosis and further development of human embryos. *Hum. Reprod.* **13**, 2880–83.

Dumoulin, J., Coonen, E., Bras, M., *et al.* (2001). Embryo development and chromosomal anomalies after ICSI: effect of the injection procedure. *Hum. Reprod.* **16**, 306–12.

Ebner, T., Moser, M., Yaman, C., Feichtinger, O., Hartl, J. and Tews, G. (1999). Elective transfer of embryos selected on the basis of first polar body morphology is associated with increased rates of implantation and pregnancy. *Fertil. Steril.* **72**, 599–603.

Edwards, R. (1965). Maturation in vitro of mouse, sheep, cow, pig, rhesus monkey and human ovarian oocytes. *Nature* **208**, 349–51.

Eichenlaub-Ritter, U., Shen, Y. and Tinneberg, H. (2002). Manipulation of the oocyte: possible damage to the spindle apparatus. *Reprod. Biomed. Online* **5**, 117–24.

Fishel, S., Green, S., Bishop, M., *et al.* (1995a). Pregnancy after intracytoplasmic injection of spermatid. *Lancet* **345**, 1641–2.

Fishel, S., Lisi, F., Rinaldi, L., *et al.* (1995b). Intracytoplasmic sperm injection (ICSI) versus high insemination concentration (HIC) for human conception in vitro. *Reprod. Fertil. Dev.* **7**, 169–75.

Fleming, S., Green, S., Hall, J. and Fishel, S. (1994). Sperm function and its manipulation for microassisted fertilization. In *Bailliere's Clinical Obstetrics and Gynaecology: Micromanipulation Techniques*, ed. S. Fishel, Vol. 8(1), pp. 43–64. London: Bailliere Tindall.

Fleming, S., Meniru, G., Hall, J. and Fishel, S. (1997). Semen analysis and sperm preparation. In *A Handbook of Intrauterine Insemination*, ed. G.I. Meniru, P.R. Brinsden and I.L. Craft, pp. 129–45. Cambridge: Cambridge University Press.

Galli-Taliadoros, L., Sedgwick, J., Wood, S. and Koerner, H. (1995). Gene knockout technology: a methodological overview for the interested novice. *J. Immunol. Methods* **181**, 1–15.

Gianaroli, L., Magli, M., Ferraretti, A., *et al.* (1996a). Reducing the time of sperm–oocyte interaction in human in-vitro fertilization improves the implantation rate. *Hum. Reprod.* **11**, 166–71.

Gianaroli, L., Fiorentino, A., Magli, M., Ferraretti, A. and Montanaro, N. (1996b). Prolonged sperm–oocyte exposure and high sperm concentration affect human embryo viability and pregnancy rate. *Hum. Reprod.* **11**, 2507–11.

Gimenez, E. and Montoliu, L. (2001). A simple polymerase chain reaction assay for genotyping the retinal degeneration mutation ($Pdeb^{rdl}$) in FVB/N-derived transgenic mice. *Lab. Animals* **35**, 153–6.

Goelz, M., Mahler, J., Harry, J., *et al.* (1998). Neuropathologic findings associated with seizures in FVB mice. *Lab. Anim. Sci.* **48**, 34–7.

Gordon, J. (1993). Production of transgenic mice. In *Methods in Enzymology: Guide to Techniques in Mouse Development*, ed. P. Wassarman and M.L. DePamphilis, pp. 747–81. London: Academic Press.

Gordon, J. and Talansky, B. (1986). Assisted fertilization by zona drilling: a mouse model for correction of oligozoospermia. *J. Exp. Zool.* **239**, 347–54.

Gordon, J., Scangos, G., Plotkin, D., Barbosa, J. and Ruddle, F. (1980). Genetic transformation of mouse embryos by microinjection of purified DNA. *Proc. Natl. Acad. Sci. USA* **77**, 7380–84.

Gordon, J., Grunfeld, J., Garrisi, G., Talansky, B., Richards, C. and Laufer, N. (1988). Fertilization of human oocytes by sperm from infertile males after zona pellucida drilling. *Fertil. Steril.* **50**, 68–73.

Hall, J. and Fleming, S. (2001). Short duration HIC-IVF is beneficial to IVF outcome. Presented at 17th World Congress on Fertility and Sterility in Melbourne, Australia, 25–30 November 2001.

Hall, J., Fishel, S., Green, S., *et al.* (1995a). Intracytoplasmic sperm injection versus high insemination concentration in-vitro fertilization in cases of very severe teratozoospermia. *Hum. Reprod.* **10**, 493–6.

Hall, J., Fishel, S., Timson, J., Dowell, K. and Klentzeris, L. (1995b). Human sperm morphology evaluation pre- and post-Percoll gradient centrifugation. *Hum. Reprod.* **10**, 342–6.

Hamberger, L., Sjogren, A., Lundin, K., *et al.* (1995). Microfertilization techniques – the Swedish experience. *Reprod. Fertil. Dev.* **7**, 263–8.

Handyside, A., Kontogianni, E., Hardy, K. and Winston, R. (1990) Pregnancies from biopsied human preimplantation embryos sexed by Y-specific DNA amplification. *Nature* **344**, 378–379.

Hardarson, T., Lundin, K. and Hamberger, L. (2000). The position of the metaphase II spindle cannot be predicted by the location of the first polar body in the human oocyte. *Hum. Reprod.* **15**, 1372–6.

Harvey, A., Speksnider, G., Baugh, L., Morris, J. and Ivarie, R. (2002). Expression of exogenous protein in the egg white of transgenic chickens. *Nat. Biotechnol.* **20**, 396–9.

Haskell, R. and Bowen, R. (1995). Efficient production of transgenic cattle by retroviral infection of early embryos. *Mol. Reprod. Dev.* **40**, 386–90.

Hawes, S., Sapienza, C. and Latham, K. (2002). Ooplasmic donation in humans: the potential for epigenic modifications. *Hum. Reprod.* **17**, 850–52.

Hogan, B., Beddington, R., Constantini, F. and Lacy, E. (1994). *Manipulating the Mouse Embryo*, 2nd edn. Cold Spring Harbor, NY: Cold Spring Harbor Laboratory Press.

Hooper, M., Hardy, K., Handyside, A., Hunter, S. and Monk, M. (1987). HPRT-deficient (Lesch-Nyhan) mouse embryos derived from germline colonization by cultured cells. *Nature* **326**, 292–5.

Hsu, M., Mayer, J., Aronshon, M., *et al.* (1999). Embryo implantation in in-vitro fertilization and intracytoplasmic sperm injection: impact of cleavage status, morphology grade, and number of embryos transferred. *Fertil. Steril.* **72**, 679–85.

Jacobs, M., Stolwijk, A. and Wetzels, A. (2001). The effect of insemination/injection time on the results of IVF and ICSI. *Hum. Reprod.* **16**, 1708–13.

Jaenish, R. (1988). Transgenic animals. *Science* **240**, 1468–74.

Jeyendran, R., Van der Ven, H., Perez-Pelaez, M., Crabo, B. and Zaneveld, L. (1984). Development of an assay to assess the functional integrity of the human sperm membrane and its relationship to other semen characteristics. *J. Reprod. Fertil.* **70**, 219–28.

Johnson, L., Neaves, W., Barnard, J., Keillor, G., Brown, S. and Yanagimachi, R. (1999). A comparative morphological study of human germ cells in vitro or in situ within seminiferous tubules. *Biol. Reprod.* **61**, 927–34.

Johnson, L., Staub, C., Neaves, W. and Yanagimachi, R. (2001). Live human germ cells in the context of their spermatogenic stages. *Hum. Reprod.* **16**, 1575–82.

Jurisicova, A., Varmuza, S. and Casper, R. (1996). Programmed cell death and human embryo fragmentation. *Mol. Hum. Reprod.* **2**, 93–8.

Koentgen, F., Suss, G., Stewart, C., Steinmetz, M. and Bluthmann, H. (1993). Targeted disruption of the MHC class II A^a gene in C57BL/6 mice. *Int. Immunol.* **5**, 957–64.

Koerner, H., Cook, M., Riminton, D., *et al.* (1997). Distinct roles for lymphotoxin-α and tumour necrosis factor in organogenesis and spatial organization of lymphoid tissue. *Eur. J. Immunol.* **27**, 2600–09.

Kruger, T., Ackerman, S., Simmons, K., Swanson, R., Brugo, S. and Acosta, A. (1987). A quick, reliable staining technique for human sperm morphology. *Arch. Androl.* **18**, 275–7.

Kuczynski, W., Dhont, M., Grygoruk, C., Pietrewicz, P., Redzko, S. and Szamatowicz, M. (2002). Rescue ICSI of unfertilized oocytes after IVF. *Hum. Reprod.* **17**, 2423–7.

Lacham-Kaplan, O., Daniels, R. and Trounson, A. (2001). Fertilization of mouse oocytes using somatic cells as male germ cells. *Reprod. Biomed. Online* **2**, 203–9.

Lanzendorf, S., Maloney, M., Veeck, L., Slusser, J., Hodgen, G. and Rosenwaks, Z. (1988). A preclinical evaluation of pronuclear formation by microinjection of human spermatozoa into human oocytes. *Fertil. Steril.* **49**, 835–42.

Larson, K., Brannian, J., Timm, B., Jost, L. and Evenson, D. (1999). Density gradient centrifugation and glass wool filtration of semen remove spermatozoa with damaged chromatin structure. *Hum. Reprod.* **14**, 2015–19.

Latham, K. and Solter, D. (1993). Transplantation of nuclei to oocytes and embryos. In *Methods in Enzymology: Guide to Techniques in Mouse Development*, ed. P.M. Wassarman and M.L. DePamphilis, pp. 719–44. London: Academic Press.

Laws-King, A., Trounson, A., Sathananthan, H. and Kola, I. (1987). Fertilization of human oocytes by micro-injection of a single spermatozoon under the zona pellucida. *Fertil. Steril.* **48**, 637–42.

Ledermann, B. and Burki, K. (1991). Establishment of a germ-line competent C57BL/6 embryonic stem cell line. *Exp. Cell Res.* **197**, 254–8.

Lemckert, F., Sedgwick, J. and Koerner, H. (1997). Gene targeting in C57BL/6 ES cells. Successful germ line transmission using recipient BALB/c blastocysts developmentally matured in vitro. *Nucleic Acids Res.* **25**, 917–8.

Li, E., Bestor, T. and Jaenisch, R. (1992). Targeted mutation of the DNA methyltransferase gene results in embryonic lethality. *Cell* **69**, 915–26.

Lipitz, S., Rabinovici, J., Goldenberg, M., Bider, D., Dor, J. and Mashiach, S. (1994). Complete failure of fertilization in couples with mechanical infertility: implications for subsequent in vitro fertilization cycles. *Fertil. Steril.* **61**, 863–6.

Lundin, K., Sjogren, A., Nilsson, L. and Hamberger, L. (1994). Fertilization and pregnancy after ICSI of acrosomeless spermatozoa. *Fertil. Steril.* **62**, 1266–7.

Lundin, K., Sjogren, A. and Hamberger, L. (1996). Reinsemination of one-day-old oocytes by use of intracytoplasmic sperm injection. *Fertil. Steril.* **66**, 118–21.

Mahajan, N., Fishel, S., Green, S., Fleming, S. and Thornton, S. (1994). The effect of various concentrations of pentoxifylline on survival and motility of spermatozoa. *Hum. Reprod.* **9**, (Suppl. 3), 6.

Mahler, J., Stokes, W., Mann, P., Takaoka, M. and Maronpot, R. (1996). Spontaneous lesions in aging FVB/N mice. *Toxicol. Pathol.* **24**, 710–16.

Mantoudis, E., Podsiadly, B., Gorgy, A., Venkat, G. and Craft, I. (2002). A comparison between quarter, partial and total laser assisted hatching in selected infertility patients. *Hum. Reprod.* **16**, 2182–6.

Mays-Hoopes, L., Bolen, J., Riggs, A. and Singer-Sam, J. (1995). Preparation of spermatogonia, spermatocytes, and round spermatids for analysis of gene expression using fluorescence-activated cell sorting. *Biol. Reprod.* **53**, 1003–11.

Meisler, M. (1992). Insertional mutation of 'classical' and novel genes in transgenic mice. *Trends Genet.* **8**, 341–4.

Mizuarai, S., Ono, K., Yamaguchi, K., Nishijima, K., Kamihira, M. and Iijima, S. (2001). Production of transgenic quails with high frequency of germ-line transmission using VSV-G pseudotyped retroviral vector. *Biochem. Biophys. Res. Com.* **286**, 456–63.

Montag, M., Rink, K., Delacretaz, G. and van der Ven, H. (2000). Laser-induced immobilization and plasma membrane permeabilization in human spermatozoa. *Hum. Reprod.* **15**, 846–52.

Moohan, J., Winston, R. and Lindsay, K. (1993). Variability of human sperm response to immediate and prolonged exposure to pentoxifylline. *Hum. Reprod.* **8**, 1696–700.

Moomjy, M., Colombero, L., Veeck, L., Rosenwaks, Z. and Palermo, G. (1999). Sperm integrity is critical for normal mitotic division and early embryonic development. *Mol. Hum. Reprod.* **5**, 836–44.

Mortimer, D. (1994). *Practical Laboratory Andrology.* New York: Oxford University Press.

Nagy, A., Rossant, J., Nagy, R., Abramow-Newerly, W. and Roder, J. (1993a). Derivation of completely cell culture-derived mice from early-passage embryonic stem cells. *Proc. Natl. Acad. Sci. USA* **90**, 8424–8.

Nagy, Z., Joris, H., Liu, J., Staessen, C., Devroey, P. and Van Steirteghem, A. (1993b). Intracytoplasmic single sperm injection of 1 day-old unfertilized human oocytes. *Hum. Reprod.* **8**, 2180–84.

Nagy, Z., Liu, J., Joris, H., (1995a). The results of intracytoplasmic sperm injection are not related to any of the three basic sperm parameters. *Hum. Reprod.* **10**, 1123–9.

Nagy, Z., Liu, J., Joris, H., *et al.* (1995b). The influence of the site of sperm deposition and mode of oolemma breakage at intracytoplasmic sperm injection on fertilization and embryo development rates. *Hum. Reprod.* **10**, 3171–7.

Nagy, Z., Liu, J., Cecile, J., Silber, S., Devroey, P. and Van Steirteghem, A. (1995c). Using ejaculated, fresh, and frozen-thawed epididymal and testicular spermatozoa gives rise to comparable results after intracytoplasmic sperm injection. *Fertil. Steril.* **63**, 808–15.

Nagy, Z., Verheyen, G., Tournaye, H., Devroey, P. and Van Steirteghem, A. (1997). An improved treatment procedure for testicular biopsy specimens offers more efficient sperm recovery: case series. *Fertil. Steril.* **68**, 376–9.

Nakagawa, K., Yamano, S., Nakasaka, H., Hinokio, K., Yoshizawa, M. and Aono, T. (2001). A combination of calcium ionophore and puromycin effectively produces human parthenogenones with one haploid pronucleus. *Zygote* **9**, 83–8.

Ng, S., Bongso, A., Ratnam, S., *et al.* (1988). Pregnancy after transfer of sperm under zona. *Lancet* **2**, 790.

Ng, S., Bongso, A. and Ratnam, S. (1991). Microinjection of human oocytes: a technique for severe oligoasthenoteratozoospermia. *Fertil. Steril.* **56**, 1117–23.

O'Brien, D. (1993). Isolation, separation, and short-term culture of spermatogenic cells. In *Methods in Toxicology*, ed. R. Chapin and J. Heindel, Vol. 3A, pp. 246–64. New York: Academic Press.

Ord, T., Marello, E., Patrizio, P., Balmaceda, J., Silber, S. and Asch, R. (1992). The role of the laboratory in the handling of epididymal sperm for assisted reproductive technologies. *Fertil. Steril.* **57**, 1103–6.

Palermo, G., Joris, H., Devroey, P. and Van Steirteghem, A. (1992). Pregnancies after intracytoplasmic injection of single spermatozoon into an oocyte. *Lancet* **340**, 17–18.

Palermo, G., Takeuchi, T. and Rosenwaks, Z. (2002). Technical approaches to correction of oocyte aneuploidy. *Hum. Reprod.* **17**, 2165–73.

Parinaud, J., Vieitez, G., Milhet, P. and Richoilley, G. (1998). Use of a plant enzyme preparation (Coronase) instead of hyaluronidase for cumulus cell removal before intracytoplasmic sperm injection. *Hum. Reprod.* **13**, 1933–5.

Payne, D., Flaherty, S., Jeffrey, R., Warnes, G. and Matthews, C. (1994). Successful treatment of severe male factor infertility in 100 consecutive cycles using intracytoplasmic sperm injection. *Hum. Reprod.* **9**, 2051–7.

Petters, R. and Sommer, J. (2000). Transgenic animals as models for human disease. *Transgenic Res.* **9**, 347–51.

Prather, R., Tao, T. and Machaty, Z. (1999). Development of the techniques for nuclear transfer in pigs. *Theriogenology* **51**, 487–98.

Rawlins, R., Binor, Z., Radwanska, E. and Dmowski, W. (1988). Microsurgical enucleation of tripronuclear human zygotes. *Fertil. Steril.* **50**, 266–72.

Robertson, E. (1987). Embryo-derived stem cell lines. In *Teratocarcinomas and Embryonic Stem Cells: A Practical Approach*, ed. E.J. Robertson, p. 71. Oxford: IRL Press.

Robertson, E., Bradley, A., Kuehn, M. and Evans, M. (1986). Germ-line transmission of genes introduced into cultured pluripotential cells by retroviral vector. *Nature* **323**, 445–8.

Ron-El, R., Strassburger, D., Friedler, S., *et al.* (1997). Extended sperm preparation: an alternative to testicular sperm extraction in non-obstructive azoospermia. *Hum. Reprod.* **12**, 1222–6.

Ron-El, R., Strassburger, D., Friedler, S., Komarovski, D., Bern, O. and Raziel, A. (1998). Repetitive ejaculation before intracytoplasmic sperm injection in patients with absolute immotile spermatozoa. *Hum. Reprod.* **13**, 630–33.

Rosenbusch, B., Schneider, M., Glaser, B. and Brucker, C. (2002). Cytogenetic analysis of giant oocytes and zygotes to assess their relevance for the development of digynic triploidy. *Hum. Reprod.* **17**, 2388–93.

Russell, J., Knezevich, K., Fabian, K. and Dickson, J. (1997). Unstimulated immature oocyte retrieval: early versus midfollicular endometrial priming. *Fertil. Steril.* **67**, 616–20.

Salzbrunn, A., Benson, D., Holstein, A. and Schulze, W. (1996). A new concept for the extraction of testicular spermatozoa as a tool for assisted fertilization (ICSI). *Hum. Reprod.* **11**, 752–5.

Sambrook, J., Fritsch, E. and Maniatis, T. (1989). *Molecular Cloning: A Laboratory Manual*, 2nd edn. Cold Spring Harbor, NY: Cold Spring Harbor Laboratory Press.

Sathananthan, A., Ng, S., Trounson, A., Bongso, A., Laws-King, A. and Ratnam, S. (1989). Human micro-insemination by injection of single or multiple sperm: ultrastructure. *Hum. Reprod.* **4**, 574–83.

Schnieke, R., Harbers, K. and Jaenisch, R. (1983). Embryonic lethal mutation in mice induced by retrovirus insertion into the 19 (I) collagen gene. *Nature* **304**, 315–20.

Shepherd, W., Millette, F. and DeWolf, C. (1981). Enrichment of primary pachytene spermatocytes from the human testes. *Gamete Res.* **4**, 487–98.

Silber, S., Nagy, Z., Liu, J., Godoy, H., Devroey, P. and Van Steirteghem, A. (1994). Conventional in-vitro fertilization versus intracytoplasmic sperm injection for patients requiring microsurgical sperm aspiration. *Hum. Reprod.* **9**, 1705–9.

Silber, S., Van Steirteghem, A. and Devroey, P. (1995). Sertoli cell only revisited. *Hum. Reprod.* **10**, 1031–2.

Silva, C., Kommineni, K., Oldenbourg, R. and Keeje, D. (1999). The first polar body does not predict accurately the location of the metaphase II meiotic spindle in mammalian oocytes. *Fertil. Steril.* **71**, 719–21.

Sjogren, A., Lundin, K. and Hamberger, L. (1995). Intracytoplasmic sperm injection of 1 day old oocytes after fertilization failure. *Hum. Reprod.* **10**, 974.

Smith, A., Heath, J., Donaldson, D., *et al.* (1988). Inhibition of pluripotential embryonic stem cell differentiation by purified polypeptides. *Nature* **336**, 688–90.

Sofikitis, N., Mantzavinos, T., Loutradis, D., Yamamoto, Y., Tarlatzis, V. and Miyagawa, I. (1998). Ooplasmic injections of secondary spermatocytes for non-obstructive azoospermia. *Lancet* **351**, 1177–8.

Sousa, M., Mendoza, C., Barros, A. and Tesarik, J. (1996). Calcium responses of human oocytes after intracytoplasmic injection of leukocytes, spermatocytes and round spermatids. *Mol. Hum. Reprod.* **2**, 853–7.

Stoddart, N. and Fleming, S. (2000). Orientation of the first polar body of the oocyte at 6 or 12 o'clock during ICSI does not affect clinical outcome. *Hum. Reprod.* **15**, 1580–5.

Sultan, K., Munné, S., Palermo, G., Alikani, M. and Cohen, J. (1995). Chromosomal status of uni-pronuclear human zygotes following in-vitro fertilization and intracytoplasmic sperm injection. *Hum. Reprod.* **10**, 132–6.

Svalander, P., Jakobsson, A.-H., Forsberg, A.-S., Bengtsson, A.-C. and Wikland, M. (1996). The outcome of intracytoplasmic sperm injection is unrelated to 'strict criteria' sperm morphology. *Hum. Reprod.* **11**, 1019–22.

Taketo, M., Schroeder, A., Mobraaten, L., *et al.* (1991). FVB/N: an inbred mouse strain preferable for transgenic analyses. *Proc. Natl. Acad. Sci. USA* **88**, 2065–9.

Tesarik, J. and Kopecny, V. (1989). Developmental control of the human male pronucleus by ooplasmic factors. *Hum. Reprod.* **4**, 962–8.

Tesarik, J. and Mendoza, C. (1996). Spermatid injection into human oocytes. I. Laboratory techniques and special features of zygote development. *Hum. Reprod.* **11**, 772–9.

Tesarik, J., Sousa, M. and Testart, J. (1994). Human oocyte activation after intracytoplasmic sperm injection. *Hum. Reprod.* **9**, 511–8.

Tesarik, J., Mendoza, C. and Testart, J. (1995). Viable embryos from injection of round spermatids into oocytes. *N. Engl. J. Med.* **333**, 525.

Tesarik, J., Greco, E., Rienzi, L., *et al.* (1998). Differentiation of spermatogenic cells during in-vitro culture of testicular biopsy samples from patients with obstructive azoospermia: effect of recombinant follicle stimulating hormone. *Hum. Reprod.* **13**, 2772–81.

Tesarik, J., Bahceci, M., Ozcan, C., Greco, E. and Mendoza, C. (1999). Restoration of fertility by in-vitro spermatogenesis. *Lancet* **353**, 555–6.

Tesarik, J., Nagy, Z., Sousa, M., Mendoza, C. and Abdelmassih, R. (2001). Fertilizable oocytes reconstructed from patient's somatic cell nuclei and donor ooplasts. *Reprod. Biomed. Online* **2**, 160–4.

Thomas, K. and Capecchi, M. (1987). Site-directed mutagenesis by gene targeting in mouse embryo-derived stem cells. *Cell* **51**, 503–12.

Trounson, A., Wood, C. and Kausche, A. (1994). In vitro maturation and the fertilization and developmental competence of oocytes recovered from untreated polycystic ovarian patients. *Fertil. Steril.* **62**, 353–62.

Trounson, A., Bongso, A., Szell, A. and Barnes, F. (1996). Maturation of human and bovine primary oocytes in vitro for fertilization and embryo production. *Singapore J. Obstet. Gynecol.* **27**, 78–84.

Tsai, M., Takeuchi, T., Bedford, J., Reis, M., Rosenwaks, Z. and Palermo, G. (2000). Alternative sources of gametes: reality or science fiction? *Hum. Reprod.* **15**, 988–98.

Tsirigotis, M., Redgment, C. and Craft, I. (1994). Late intracytoplasmic sperm injection (ICSI) in in-vitro fertilization (IVF) cycles. *Hum. Reprod.* **9**, 1359.

Urman, B., Alatas, C., Aksoy, S., *et al.* (2002). Transfer at the blastocyst stage of embryos derived from testicular round spermatid injection. *Hum. Reprod.* **17**, 741–3.

Vanderzwalmen, P., Bertin, G. and Geerts, L. (1991). Spermatozoa morphology and IVF pregnancy rate: a comparison between percoll gradient centrifugation and swim-up procedures. *Hum. Reprod.* **6**, 581–8.

Vanderzwalmen, P., Zech, H., Birkenfeld, A., *et al.* (1997). Intracytoplasmic injection of spermatids retrieved from testicular tissue: influence of testicular pathology, type of selected spermatids and oocyte activation. *Hum. Reprod.* **12**, 1203–13.

Verheyen, G., De Croo, I., Tournaye, H., Pletincx, I., Devroey, P. and Van Steirteghem, A. (1995). Comparison of four mechanical methods to retrieve spermatozoa from testicular tissue. *Hum. Reprod.* **10**, 2956–9.

Verheyen, G., Joris, H., Crits, K., Nagy, Z., Tournaye, H. and Van Steirteghem, A. (1997). Comparison of different hypo-osmotic swelling solutions to select viable immotile spermatozoa for potential use in intracytoplasmic sperm injection. *Hum. Reprod. Update* **3**, 195–203.

Wang, W., Meng, L., Hackett, R., Odenbourg, R. and Keefe, D. (2001a). The spindle observation and its relationship with fertilization after intracytoplasmic sperm injection in living human oocytes. *Fertil. Steril.* **75**, 348–53.

Wang, W., Meng, L., Hackett, R. and Keefe, D. (2001b). Developmental ability of human oocytes with or without birefringent spindles imaged by Polscope before insemination. *Hum. Reprod.* **16**, 1464–8.

Wang, W., Meng, L., Hackett, R., Odenbourg, R. and Keefe, D. (2001c). Limited recovery of meiotic spindles in living human oocytes after cooling-rewarming observed using polarized light microscopy. *Hum. Reprod.* **16**, 2374–8.

Wang, W., Meng, L., Hackett, R., Odenbourg, R. and Keefe, D. (2001d). Rigorous thermal control during intracytoplasmic sperm injection stabilizes the meiotic spindle and improves fertilization and pregnancy rates. *Fertil. Steril.* **77**, 1274–7.

Wheeler, M. and Walters, E. (2001). Transgenic technology and applications in swine. *Theriogenology* **56**, 1345–69.

Williams, R., Hilton, D., Pease, S., *et al.* (1988). Myeloid leukaemia inhibitory factor maintains the developmental potential of embryonic stem cells. *Nature* **336**, 684–7.

Wilmut, I., Beaujean, N., de Sousa, P., *et al.* (2002). Somatic cell nuclear transfer. *Nature* **419**, 583–6.

Wolf, E., Zakhartchenko, V. and Brem, G. (1998). Nuclear transfer in mammals: recent developments and future perspectives. *J. Biotechnol.* **65**, 99–110.

Wood, S., Allen, N., Rossant, J., Auerbach, A. and Nagy, A. (1993). Non-injection methods for the production of embryonic stem cell-embryo chimaeras. *Nature* **365**, 87–9.

World Health Organization (1999). *WHO Laboratory Manual for the Examination of Human Semen and Sperm–Cervical Mucus Interaction*. Cambridge: Cambridge University Press.

Yamanaka, K., Sofikitis, N., Miyagawa, I., *et al.* (1997). Ooplasmic round spermatid nuclear injection procedures as an experimental treatment for nonobstructive azoospermia. *J. Assist. Reprod. Genet.* **14**, 55–62.

Yazawa, H., Yanagida, K., Katayose, H., Hayashi, S. and Sato, A. (2000). Comparison of oocyte activation and Ca^{2+} oscillation-inducing abilities of round/elongated spermatids of mouse, hamster, rat, rabbit and human assessed by mouse oocyte activation assay. *Hum. Reprod.* **15**, 2582–90.

Yovich, J., Edirisinghe, W., Cummins, J. and Yovich, J. (1990). Influence of pentoxifylline in severe male factor infertility. *Fertil. Steril.* **53**, 715–22.

Zech, H., Vanderzwalmen, P., Prapas, Y., Lejeune, B., Duba, E. and Schoysman, R. (2000). Congenital malformations after intracytoplasmic injection of spermatids. *Hum. Reprod.* **15**, 969–71.

Zhang, J., Wang, C., Krey, L., *et al.* (1999). In vitro maturation of human preovulatory oocytes reconstructed by germinal vesicle transfer. *Fertil. Steril.* **71**, 726–31.

Index

Numbers in italics refer to *tables* and *figures*. Roman numerals indicate glossary pages.

For EU product safety concerns, contact us at Calle de José Abascal, 56–1°,
28003 Madrid, Spain or eugpsr@cambridge.org.

www.ingramcontent.com/pod-product-compliance
Ingram Content Group UK Ltd.
Pitfield, Milton Keynes, MK11 3LW, UK
UKHW051009240426
470322UK00018B/586